Endurance Sports Medicine

Timothy L. Miller

Editor

Endurance Sports Medicine

A Clinical Guide

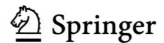 Springer

Editor
Timothy L. Miller
Department of Orthopaedic Surgery
Ohio State University Wexner Medical Center
Gahanna, OH, USA

ISBN 978-3-319-81414-8   ISBN 978-3-319-32982-6   (eBook)
DOI 10.1007/978-3-319-32982-6

Printed on acid-free paper

This Springer imprint is published by Springer Nature
The registered company is Springer International Publishing AG Switzerland

To my family, in particular my wife Nicole and our children Gavin, Ashton, Avery, and Sydney and my parents Tom and Kathleen, for always believing in me and showing patience and understanding when I take on "yet another project."
To the many endurance athletes who have had their seasons and careers cut short due to overuse injuries, know that your hard work and efforts have not gone in vain and, in fact, were the inspiration for this book.

Preface

Endurance Sports Medicine has been in many ways a labor of love for the authors and the editor. It is the culmination of many years of experience with injuries and conditions as athletes, as researchers, and as sports medicine care providers. This textbook compiles the many concepts, experiences, and techniques required to approach and treat the complexities of conditions that affect endurance sports participants. I truly appreciate the contributions of the authors—many of whom are considered pioneers and leaders in the field of sports medicine—who have provided their invaluable insights and pearls. As a developing field of sports medicine, endurance medicine continues to expand its understanding of overuse injuries as athletes continue to push the limits of running, cycling, swimming, wheelchair, skiing, rowing, cross-fit sports, adventure and obstacle course racing, and many other demanding activities. Traditional strategies for treating overuse conditions such as simply stopping the causative activity or sport are no longer considered an acceptable option for many competitive athletes. Alternative training methods including a holistic approach to the evaluation, treatment, and prevention of activity-related conditions are now the standard of care as is evidenced throughout the 21 chapters of this book. This textbook details strategies for not only treating and preventing injuries and conditions but also for optimizing an athlete's performance. Though it is too early to determine whether we can obviate the need to have athletes completely abstain from their sport of choice in response to an injury or condition, we can decrease the time lost from training and competition and allow for a more safe and predictable return to full activity. It is my hope that this textbook will be a valuable guide for sports medicine physicians, orthopedists, athletic trainers, physical therapists, coaches, officials, and athletes in understanding the needs of the determined individuals who participate in endurance sports.

Gahanna, OH, USA   Timothy L. Miller, MD

Contents

Contributors

Geoffrey D. Abrams, MD Department of Orthopedic Surgery, Stanford University, Redwood City, CA, USA

Scott Annett, MD Steadman Hawkins Clinic of the Carolinas, Heritage Internal Medicine and Pediatrics, Greenville Health System, Simpsonville, SC, USA

Chad A. Asplund, MD, MPH, FACSM Health and Kinesiology Director, Athletic Medicine Georgia Southern University Statesboro, GA, USA

Aaron L. Baggish, MD, FACC, FACSM Cardiovascular Performance Program, Division of Cardiology, Massachusetts General Hospital, Boston, MA, USA

Tarryn Bolognani, ATC Vermont Orthopaedic Clinic, Rutland Regional Medical Center, Rutland, VT, USA

Matthew S. Briggs, PT, DPT, PhD, SCS, AT OSU Sports Medicine and Sports Medicine Research Institute, The Ohio State University Wexner Medical Center, Columbus, OH, USA

Darrin Bright, MD, DO Department of Family Medicine/Sports Medicine, OhioHealth, Columbus, OH, USA

Ben Bring, DO Department of Family Medicine, OhioHealth, Columbus, OH, USA

Jacob Michael Bright, DO Family Medicine Residency Program, Eisenhower Army Medical Center, Fort Gordon, GA, USA

Sean Bryan, MD, FAAFP Family Medicine, Greenville Health System, Greenville, SC, USA

Jackie Buell, PhD, RD, CSSD, ATC Department of Medical Dietetics, Ohio State University, Columbus, OH, USA

Alexander Butler, BS Georgetown University School of Medicine, Washington, DC, USA

Jennifer E. Carter, PhD Sports Medicine, Ohio State University Sports Medicine Center and Athletic Department, Columbus, OH, USA

Kyle Cassas, MD Steadman Hawkins Clinic of the Carolinas, Greenville Health System, Greenville, SC, USA

Polly de Mille, BA, BSN, MA Sports Rehabilitation and Performance, Hospital for Special Surgery, New York, NY, USA

Joseph Ferguson, MD Department of Orthopedic Surgery, Medstar Georgetown University Hospital, Washington, DC, USA

Jennifer A. Michaud Finch, DO Cardiovascular Performance Program, Division of Cardiology, Massachusetts General Hospital, Boston, MA, USA

Amanda Gallow, DPT, SCS Sports Rehabilitation Clinic, UW Health at The American Center, Madison, WI, USA

Matthew Gammons, MD Vermont Orthopaedic Clinic, Rutland Regional Medical Center, Rutland, VT, USA

Brian D. Giordano, MD Orthopaedics and Rehabilitation, University of Rochester Strong Memorial, Rochester, NY, USA

Stephen Graef, PhD Sports Medicine, Ohio State University Sports Medicine Center and Athletic Department, Columbus, OH, USA

Joshua D. Harris, MD Houston Methodist Orthopedics and Sports Medicine, Houston, TX, USA

Clinton Hartz, MD Division of Sports Medicine, Department of Family Medicine, Ohio State University, Columbus, OH, USA

Bryan Heiderscheit, PT, PhD Departments of Orthopedics and Rehabilitation and Biomedical Engineering, UW Runners' Clinic, Badger Athletic Performance Research, University of Wisconsin-Madison, Madison, WI, USA

Matt Howland, ATC Vermont Orthopaedic Clinic, Rutland Regional Medical Center, Rutland, VT, USA

Tyler R. Johnston, MD Department of Orthopedic Surgery, Stanford University, Redwood City, CA, USA

Christopher Kempe, MD Division of Pulmonary, Critical Care, and Sleep Medicine, Ohio State University Medical Center, Columbus, OH, USA

Julia Kim, PhD Medicine, Hospital for Special Surgery, New York, NY, USA

Abigail Lang, MD Division of Sports Medicine, Department of Family Medicine, Ohio State University, Columbus, OH, USA

Kelsey Logan, MD, MPH Sports Medicine, Cincinnati Children's Hospital Medical Center, Cincinnati, OH, USA

Jason Machowsky, RD, CSSD, RCEP Sports Rehabilitation and Performance, Hospital for Special Surgery, New York, NY, USA

Aaron Mares, MD Department of Orthopaedic Surgery, University of Pittsburgh Medical Center, Pittsburgh, PA, USA

Timothy L. Miller, MD Department of Orthopaedic Surgery, Ohio State University Wexner Medical Center, Gahanna, OH, USA

Volker Musahl, MD Department of Orthopaedic Surgery, University of Pittsburgh Medical Center, Pittsburgh, PA, USA

Travis Obermire, PT, DPT, SCS, OCS Sports Rehabilitation Clinic, UW Health at The American Center, Madison, WI, USA

Jonathan P. Parsons, MD, MSc Division of Pulmonary, Critical Care, and Sleep Medicine, Ohio State University Medical Center, Columbus, OH, USA

Davis Heart/Lung Research Institute, Columbus, OH, USA

Joshua Pintar, PT, SCS Department of Sports Medicine, The Ohio State University, Columbus, OH, USA

Clinical Outcomes Research Coordinator (CORC) Program, Sports Medicine Research Institute, The Ohio State University, Columbus, OH, USA

Scott Rodeo MD Sports Medicine and Shoulder Service, Department of Orthopedic Surgery, Hospital for Special Surgery, New York, NY, USA

Mike Silverman, PT, MSPT Sports Rehab, Hospital for Special Surgery, New York, NY, USA

Brett Toresdahl, MD Primary Care Sports Medicine Service, Department of Medicine, Hospital for Special Surgery, New York, NY, USA

Gregory Walker, MD Sports Medicine, Cincinnati Children's Hospital Medical Center, Cincinnati, OH, USA

Bryant Walrod, MD Family Medicine, Ohio State University, Columbus, OH, USA

Katherine Wayman, PT, DPT, SCS Department of Sports Medicine, The Ohio State University, Columbus, OH, USA

Clinical Outcomes Research Coordinator (CORC) Program, Sports Medicine Research Institute, The Ohio State University, Columbus, OH, USA

Benjamin M. Weisenthal, MD Orthopedics, Vanderbilt University Medical Center, Nashville, TN, USA

Robin West, MD Sports Medicine, Inova Health System, Falls Church, VA, USA

Jason P. Zlotnicki, MD Department of Orthopaedic Surgery, University of Pittsburgh Medical Center, Pittsburgh, PA, USA

Part I
Medical Conditions

Cardiovascular Evaluation and Treatment of the Endurance Athlete

Jennifer A. Michaud Finch and Aaron L. Baggish

Introduction

Endurance athletes have been the focus of scientific investigation for more than a century. Early investigators, including the Swedish clinician Henschen [1] and Darling [2] of Harvard University, demonstrated increased cardiac dimensions in Nordic skiers and in university rowers, respectively. In the early 1900s, White [3], regarded by some as the father of contemporary cardiology, studied radial contours among Boston Marathon competitors and was the first to report marked resting sinus bradycardia in long-distance runners [4].

Since the work done by these pioneering investigators, advances in our understanding of cardiac adaptations to endurance exercise have largely paralleled advances in diagnostic technology. The development and subsequent widespread availability of chest radiography in the 1950s facilitated studies that demonstrated global cardiac enlargement in trained athletes thereby confirming the earlier physical examination findings of Darling and Henschen by showing global cardiac enlargement in trained athletes [5–7]. In the present era, the electrocardiogram (ECG) and contemporary

noninvasive imaging modalities including echocardiography, cardiac computed tomography, and cardiac magnetic resonance imaging have more comprehensively characterize the electrical, structural, and functional cardiac adaptations that accompany long-term endurance training [8–11].

The last 25 years have seen tremendous increase in endurance sport participation among men and women of all ages as evidenced by the fact that there was a record-setting number of running event finishers, nearly 20 million in the United States, in 2013 [12]. At no time in the past has it been more critical for care providers to possess the fundamental skills required for the care of the active endurance athlete. Effective care of this population requires an understanding of the cardiovascular demands of exercise, a familiarity with training-related cardiovascular adaptations, and a structured approach to the athlete with symptoms suggestive of cardiovascular disease. This chapter is written to provide the clinician with a basic foundation of knowledge in these principal areas of patient care with emphasis on the endurance athlete.

Overview of Normal Physiological Adaptations to Endurance Training

Differentiating adaptive physiology from occult pathology is the most important task for the clinician tasked with caring for endurance athletes.

J.A.M. Finch • A.L. Baggish (✉)
Cardiovascular Performance Program, Division of Cardiology, Massachusetts General Hospital, Yawkey Suite 5B, 55 Fruit St., Boston, MA 02114, USA
e-mail: abaggish@partners.org

© Springer International Publishing Switzerland 2016
T.L. Miller (ed.), *Endurance Sports Medicine*, DOI 10.1007/978-3-319-32982-6_1

As detailed below, sustained endurance training lasting for weeks to years often leads to numerous changes in cardiac structure and function. At times, these changes may be challenging to differentiate from those that occur in the disease processes that place athletes at risk for sudden cardiac death. The process of differentiating adaption from disease necessarily begins with an understanding of what cardiac changes are expected in a healthy endurance athlete and what physiology stimulates these adaptations.

All forms of exercise require an increase in skeletal muscle work. There is a direct relationship between exercise intensity (external work) and the body's demand for oxygen. The oxygen demand during exercise is met by increasing pulmonary oxygen uptake (VO_2). In addition, the cardiovascular system is responsible for transporting oxygen-rich blood from the lungs to the skeletal muscles, a process quantified as cardiac output (in liters per minute). Exercise-induced cardiac remodeling enhances the cardiovascular system's ability to meet the demands of exercising skeletal muscle. The Fick equation (cardiac output $= VO_2 \times$ arterial venous $O_2 \Delta$) can be used to quantify the relationship between cardiac output and VO_2. As suggested by this equation, there is a direct and inviolate relationship between VO_2 and cardiac output in the healthy human.

Cardiac output (CO), the product of stroke volume and heart rate, may increase five- to six-fold during maximal exercise effort. Coordinated autonomic nervous system function, characterized by rapid and sustained parasympathetic withdrawal coupled with sympathetic activation, is required for this process to occur. Heart rate among healthy athletes may range from fewer than 40 beats per minute at rest to greater than 200 beats per minute in a young, maximally exercising athlete. Heart rate increase is responsible for the majority of cardiac output augmentation during exercise. Peak heart rate is determined by age, gender, and genetics and cannot be increased by exercise training. Stroke volume is defined as the quantity of blood ejected from the heart during each contraction. In contrast to heart rate, stroke volume both at rest and during exercise may increase significantly with prolonged exercise training. Cardiac chamber enlargement and

the accompanying ability to generate a large stroke volume are direct results of endurance exercise training and are the cardiovascular hallmarks of the endurance-trained athlete. Stroke volume increases during exercise as a result of increases in ventricular end-diastolic volume and, to a lesser degree, sympathetically mediated reduction in end-systolic volume.

Hemodynamic perturbations that occur during exercise constitute the primary stimulus for exercise-induced cardiac remodeling (EICR). Specifically, changes in cardiac output and peripheral vascular resistance vary widely across sporting disciplines. Although there is considerable overlap and clinically oriented physiology-based sport classification scheme has been developed [13], exercise activity can be classified into two forms with defining hemodynamic differences. Isometric exercise, commonly referred to as strength training, is characterized by short but intense bouts of increased peripheral vascular resistance and normal or only slightly elevated cardiac output. This increase in peripheral vascular resistance causes transient but potentially marked systolic hypertension and left ventricular "pressure" challenge. Strength training physiology is dominant during activities such as weight lifting, track-and-field throwing events, and American-style football. In contrast, isotonic exercise (i.e., endurance exercise) involves sustained elevations in CO, with normal or reduced peripheral vascular resistance. Such activity represents a primary volume challenge for the heart that affects all four chambers. This form of exercise underlies activities such as long-distance running, cycling, rowing, and swimming. It must be emphasized that endurance sports all involve high isotonic stress but that specific disciplines vary considerably as a function of the amount of concomitant isometric stress.

Left Ventricular Adaptations to Endurance Exercise

Enlargement of the left ventricle (LV) is common among endurance-trained athletes. This represents physiologic, eccentric LV hypertrophy (LVH) or eccentric LV remodeling as dictated by endurance discipline [14]. Eccentric LVH is characterized by an increase in LV chamber size accompanied by proportionate increase in LV wall thickness and is common among endurance sports that involve high levels of isometric physiology. Rowing is an example of a sport that has been shown to promote eccentric LVH due to the inherent physiologic combination of sustained high cardiac output and pulsatile surges in systolic blood pressure that occur during the drive phase of each oar stroke [15]. In contrast, long-distance running is an endurance sport discipline characterized by marked and sustained increases in cardiac output coupled with stable and only modestly elevated arterial blood pressure. This physiologic milieu promotes eccentric LV dilation during which LV chamber size may increase and most often do so proportionally more than accompanying adaptive LV wall thickening.

Early cross-sectional data from large heterogeneous cohorts of European athletes demonstrated high prevalence of left ventricular cavity enlargement and increased wall thickness [16, 17]. Markedly dilated LV chambers (defined as >60 mm) were associated with increased body mass and were most common among those participating in endurance sports (cross-country skiing, cycling, etc.). In clinical practice, 55–58 mm is commonly used to define the upper limits of normal for LV end-diastolic dimensions. Thus, approximately 40 % of trained athletes in the above study had LV dimensions that exceeded normal reference points. Within this exclusively white cohort, a small but significant percentage of athletes (1.7 %) had LV wall thicknesses of 13 mm or greater, and all of these individuals had concomitant LV cavity dilation. Sharma and colleagues [18] also reported a low incidence (0.4 %) of LV wall thickness greater than 12 mm in 720 elite junior athletes and confirmed that increased LV wall thickness is associated with increased chamber size in young athletes. More recently, in a study of nearly 500 collegiate athletes, not a single healthy university athlete had LV wall thickness of greater than 14 mm [19]. In summary, LV wall thickness in excess of 13 mm is a rare finding in healthy athletes, although it can be seen in a small number of healthy, highly trained individuals. This finding is more common in athletes with relatively large body size and those of Afro-Caribbean descent [20]. Thickening of the LV, without associated LV chamber dilation, occurs infrequently in trained endurance athletes and should warrant further workup.

Systolic or contractile function of the dilated LV in athletes has also been an area of active investigation. Studies of resting LV systolic function in endurance athletes consistently demonstrate that LV ejection fraction is generally normal in this population [21]. However, a study of 147 cyclists participating in the Tour de France found that 11 % had an LV ejection fraction of 52 % or less [22]. This finding supports our clinical experience in which we often find that healthy endurance athletes demonstrate mildly reduced LV ejection fraction at rest. Exercise testing can be a very useful adjunct to confirm LV augmentation and to document greater than normal exercise capacity in the hearts of trained athletes [23]. Recent advances in functional myocardial imaging, including tissue Doppler and speckle tracking echocardiography, have also suggested that endurance exercise training may lead to changes in regional LV systolic function that are not detected by assessment of a global index, such as LV ejection fraction [24]. Furthermore, changes in LV apical rotation and twist have been identified in a longitudinal study of rowers participating in endurance exercise training [25]. At present, the role of these newer imaging techniques in the clinical assessment of endurance athletes remains uncertain.

LV diastolic function has also been studied in endurance athletes. Endurance exercise training leads to enhanced early diastolic LV filling as assessed by E-wave velocity and mitral annular/LV tissue velocities [26–28]. In an elegant study utilizing invasive hemodynamic measurements, Levine et al. described improved LV chamber compliance in athletes as lesser increases in pulmonary artery capillary wedge pressure for a given increase in end-diastolic volumes [29, 30]. These changes in LV diastolic function are attributable to a combination of enhanced intrinsic myocardial relaxation and training-induced increases in LV preload. Speckle tracking echocardiography has provided further insight into diastolic function, with enhanced peak early diastolic untwisting rate observed in rowers after 90 days of endurance exercise training [25]. This ability of the LV to relax briskly during early diastole is an essential mechanism of stroke volume preservation during exercise at high heart rates.

Right Ventricular Adaptations to Endurance Exercise

Endurance exercise requires both the LV and the right ventricle (RV) to accept and eject large volumes of blood simultaneously. It is therefore not surprising that both the RV and LV remodel during chronic endurance sport participation. Cardiac imaging studies using both echocardiography and magnetic resonance imaging document a high prevalence of right ventricular dilation among endurance-trained athletes [26, 31, 32]. Similar to the left ventricle, resting RV systolic function may be mildly reduced among trained endurance athletes and likely reflects the substantial contractile reserve afforded by physiologic RV dilation [33]. Due to the increased volume load during endurance training, RV volume, mass, and stroke volume have all been observed to increase in endurance athletes, largely based on measurements using cardiac MRI [30].

RV function may also be affected by endurance exercise. In similar fashion to that observed in the LV, it is common to see trained endurance athletes with low-normal to slightly depressed resting RV systolic function. When encountered clinically, the use of exercise testing coupled with noninvasive imaging may be useful to document normal or enhanced contractile reserve [34]. To what degree RV diastolic function is impacted by endurance exercise training and whether this is of clinical or physiologic relevance remain unknown.

Atrial Adaptation to Endurance Exercise

In addition to remodeling of the left and right ventricle, numerous studies have shown that atrial enlargement is frequent among endurance-trained athletes [30]. In an early sentinel report,

Pellicia et al. [35] presented a large data set of atrial measurements in athletes ($n = 1777$) and demonstrated that left atrial enlargement (>40 mm in an anterior/posterior transthoracic echocardiographic view) was present in approximately 20 %. Of note, among athletes with left atrial dilation, few athletes had clinical evidence of supraventricular arrhythmias. In general, atrial enlargement is proportional to the enlargement of the ventricles and is affected by the type of training undertaken [11, 23, 36, 37]. Meta-analysis examining left atrial (LA) size in athletes found that both pooled mean LA diameter and LA volume index were greater than sedentary control subjects. In addition, the LA dilation tracked closely with physiological sporting discipline, with endurance athletes demonstrating the largest differences [38]. Cumulative lifetime exercise training hours have subsequently been shown to be an important determinant of left atrial size [39]. The clinical implications of this finding, particularly with respect to the development of atrial fibrillation, warrant further study.

Endurance training appears to have similar effects on the right atrium (RA) as evidenced by data derived from youthful elite athletes [40], with veteran marathon runners [41], despite the existence of right atrial geometric alterations in endurance athletes; no differences in the right atrial function have yet to be demonstrated [42].

Variability of Exercise-Induced Cardiac Remodeling

The magnitude of exercise-induced cardiac remodeling varies considerably across individual athletes. Obvious explanatory factors including sport type, prior exercise exposure, and training intensity/duration do not explain all of this variability. Additional factors including sex, ethnicity, and genetics are contributory [19, 43, 44]. This appears to be true even when cardiac dimensions are corrected for the typically smaller female body size. Definitive explanation for the sex-specific magnitude of exercise-induced remodeling remains elusive. Race is also an important determinant of remodeling, with black athletes tending to have thicker LV walls than white athletes. A group of white and black athletes have been using echocardiographic imaging and found that nearly 20 % of the black athletes were found to have LV wall thickness of at least 12 mm as compared with 4 % of white athletes. Importantly, 3 % of black athletes in this cohort were found to have wall thickness of greater than 15 mm [45]. Similarly, ethnic-/race-related differences were studied in a group of 440 black and white female athletes using echocardiography. Black female athletes demonstrated significantly greater LV wall thickness and mass compared with the white woman [20].

These numerous adaptations in cardiac structure and function documented above are not exclusive to elite-level athletes. A recent study of middle-aged men who engaged in marathon training also identified biventricular dilation, enhanced left ventricular diastolic function, and favorable changes in non-myocardial determinants of cardiovascular risk after an 18-week recreational running program [46]. The observed structural remodeling in this setting was of sufficient magnitude such that post-training cardiac parameters commonly fell outside the established clinical ranges of normal.

Clinical Implications of Remodeling

Complex cardiovascular demands and adaptations imposed by endurance exercise pose distinct challenges. The overlap between normal, adaptive physiology and pathology and the proper distinction between the two are crucial in the athlete population, where several important causes of athletic sudden cardiac death can be difficult to differentiate from adaptation. The long-term clinical sequela of endurance exercise and the significance of adaptive physiology are still a topic of debate. Although the concept of prolonged endurance exercise participation leading to overuse pathology and premature cardiovascular mortality has been described, there is no definitive evidence to confirm its validity [34, 47–50].

There is a growing body of literature that describes an association between long-term endurance exercise and increased risk of atrial fibrillation [51]. Although routine physical exercise may favorably impact many key determinants of cardiovascular disease (e.g., lipid profiles, blood pressure, and body mass), atrial fibrillation is the exception and has been recognized as a problem for the masters athlete (a group defined as competitors >40 years of age). Numerous underlying mechanisms, including those shared with the general, more sedentary population (e.g., undiagnosed hypertension, excessive alcohol consumption, sleep apnea), and some factors more specific to the aging competitive athlete, including resting vagotonia, chronic inflammation, and left atrial dilation, have been proposed. Greater prevalence of atrial fibrillation among endurance athletes [52] provides an important stimulus for research aimed at better understanding the mechanisms and consequences of endurance exercise. Atrial fibrillation in the endurance athlete will be addressed later in the chapter.

Although cardiac remodeling in response to long-term endurance exercise is often regarded as beneficial, it has been suggested that very extreme exercise bouts could promote permanent structural or functional cardiac changes [34, 48, 53–56]. The RV has been the focus of this debate. We previously reported physiologic RV dilation with focal deterioration of interventricular septal function after a period of intense exercise training [57]. The RV dilation observed may compromise septal function by the way its fibers insert into the LV. Recently, La Gerche and colleagues [48] also demonstrated a relationship between intense endurance exercise and acute reduction in RV function that increased with race duration and correlated with increases in biomarkers of myocardial injury. All immediate postrace right ventricular geometry measurements were increased. According to the Frank–Starling mechanism, the increased volume, area, and dimensions should augment cardiac deformation if contractility is preserved. Therefore, the immediate postrace reductions in the RV may represent a true impairment in RV contractility with acute exercise bouts. In addition, cardiac magnetic resonance imaging with delayed gadolinium enhancement

(DGE) has been used to further characterize RV remodeling.

Septal fibrosis in the locations of RV fiber insertion has been documented in athletes with a longer history of competitive sport, suggesting that repetitive ultra-endurance exercise may lead to more extensive RV change and possible myocardial fibrosis [47, 48]. The cardiac impact of long-term endurance exercise on the RV and the recovery processes may be insufficient to compensate for the extent of injury [34, 48, 58]. This repetitive fatigue may stimulate remodeling and may lead in some to a fibrotic pathologic phenotype. Although the absence of DGE in athletes with modest training histories has been noted, DGE has been reported in 12–50 % of extensively trained veteran athletes [48, 59, 60]. However, the patches of DGE are very small and are focused around the septum and RV insertion points, a region that may indicate local mechanical stresses rather than extensive fibrosis. The relationship between the presence of DGE and long-term outcomes has yet to be defined, and further study is needed.

There has been speculation about whether noninvasive surrogates of cardiac injury may identify athletes at greater risk. Increases in cardiac troponin and beta-type natriuretic peptide after endurance sporting events reflect myocardial injury and have been reported [61]. Significant increases in serological markers, potentially indicating myocardial damage, during and/or directly after a marathon run have been reported [56, 62, 63]. However, the elevated cardiac biomarkers regressed to normal values within a period of 24–48 h and, therefore, may be the result of transient and reversible alterations of the cardiac myocytes without negative clinical consequences [64, 65]. Hanssen et al. [49] combined measurements of cardiac biomarkers with cardiac magnetic resonance, including DGE, demonstrating an absence of detectable myocardial necrosis despite a transient increase in cardiac biomarkers. Further experimental studies are warranted to determine the clinical consequences of these increased cardiac biomarkers.

Electrical Remodeling

In addition to structural and functional myocardial remodeling, electrical remodeling occurs in response to endurance sport training. These adaptations manifest as distinct changes on the 12-lead electrocardiogram (ECG) and are thus important for clinicians to be capable of differentiating ECG patterns which result from training and from those suggestive of the disease which may increase the risk of sudden death during sport participation [30]. The 12-lead ECG provides rapid and relatively inexpensive information about cardiac electrical conduction and myocardial structure. Therefore, the ECG is the initial test of choice in the athletic patient with symptoms suggestive of heart disease and plays an important, though still controversial, role in the pre-participation screening of asymptomatic athletes. Because of the heightened vagal tone that accompanies physical conditioning, trained athletes commonly demonstrate benign arrhythmias and conduction alterations, including sinus bradyarrhythmia, junctional rhythm, first-degree atrioventricular block, and type I second-degree atrioventricular block (i.e., Wenckebach phenomenon) [66].

Clinical criteria for differentiating adaptive/training-related ECG patterns from those suggestive of true pathologic heart disease have undergone considerable evolution over the past two decades. In 1998, Corrado et al. presented the results of a 27-year screening initiative (1979–1996) designed to protect young competitive athletes from sudden cardiac death. This landmark paper represented the first publication in which a comprehensive set of 12-lead ECG criteria was proposed for use in asymptomatic athletes [67]. The European Society of Cardiology (ESC) followed in 2005 with the first consensus document presenting quantitative ECG criteria for use in athletes [68]. Although the use of the 2005 ESC criteria was shown to significantly increase the likelihood of detecting underlying cardiomyopathy in athletes, its use was associated with a prohibitive rate of false-positive testing [8]. Specifically, utilizing transthoracic echocardiography as the gold standard for the presence or absence of structural and valvular heart disease, 12-lead ECG-inclusive screening using the 2005 ESC criteria was associated with a false-positive rate of 16.9 %. The majority of false-positive testing included several common ECG patterns (isolated precordial and limb lead QRS voltage, isolated left atrial enlargement, and incomplete right bundle branch block) and were found almost exclusively among athletes who were found by echocardiography to have evidence of physiologic cardiac remodeling.

The ESC updated their criteria in 2010 [69]. In this update, the writing group divided ECG patterns into two specific groups. "Group 1" was a list of patterns designated as "common and training related" that should not prompt further evaluation for underlying pathology. Key components of the "Group 1" list included sinus bradycardia, first-degree AV block, incomplete right bundle branch block, "early repolarization," and isolated QRS voltage criteria for left ventricular hypertrophy. In parallel, a second group of ECG patterns was designated as those that are "uncommon and training unrelated" among athletes. "Group 2" included many well-established markers of occult structural and electrical diseases including T-wave inversions, ST segment depression, pathologic Q waves, conduction abnormalities including complete bundle branch and left bundle fascicular blocks, gender-specific abnormalities of QT interval duration, and preexcitation.

Most recently, the "Seattle Criteria" [70] and subsequent "revised criteria" [71] have been developed. In sum, these criteria continue to improve the specificity of ECG interpretation in athletes by assigning a benign nature to several common ECG patterns including equivocal QTc intervals, T-wave inversions isolated to leads V1 and V2, and either isolated right axis deviation or right ventricular hypertrophy voltage criteria [72, 73].

Evaluation of the Symptomatic Endurance Athlete

Although participation in sport and regular exercise promotes good health, athletes are not immune to cardiovascular symptoms and disease.

Sudden death of an athlete is a tragic event. These deaths often assume a high public profile because of the youth of the victims and the generally held perception that trained athletes constitute the healthiest segment of society. Sudden death during sport is most commonly caused by occult cardiovascular disease [74], and many of the key cardiovascular diseases responsible for sudden death first manifest as symptoms during exercise. The cardiovascular causes of sudden death in athletes have been well documented, and pathology is often age related [66, 74–77]. In the United States, among people <35 years old, genetic heart diseases predominate, with hypertrophic cardiomyopathy being the most common, accounting for at least one-third of the mortality in autopsy-based athlete study populations [74, 75, 77]. Congenital coronary anomalies (usually those of wrong sinus origin) are second in frequency, occurring in 15–20 % of cases. For older athletes (>35 years of age), atherosclerotic coronary artery disease is the predominant cause of sudden death [74]. Symptoms can first manifest during exercise when there are increased cardiovascular demands. Symptoms may be suggestive of underlying pathology and have long-term prognostic implications. The possibility of coronary or other life-threatening cardiac diseases in "physically fit" endurance athletes who have specific cardiac symptoms must be considered. Symptoms sufficiently severe to interfere with an athlete's performance should be exhaustively investigated, and a cardiac cause must be presumed until disproven. The following sections address the most common cardiovascular issues encountered in the clinical care of the endurance athlete.

Chest Pain

Chest pain is a common complaint seen in athletes across the entire age spectrum, and the underlying etiologies of chest pain are both myriad and referable to many organ systems [78] (Table 1.1). The term "chest pain" encompasses vague sensations that carry a low likelihood of cardiac etiology to typical angina that is commonly

Table 1.1 Common cardiac and noncardiac causes of chest pain among endurance athletes

Common cardiac causes	Typical presenting symptoms
Obstructive CAD	Chest pressure or heaviness; pain radiates to the neck, jaw, shoulder, and/or left arm
Coronary vasospasm	Chest pressure or heaviness; pain radiates to the neck, jaw, shoulder, and/or left arm
Aortic or coronary artery dissection	"Tearing" pain, sudden and excruciating pain in the anterior chest radiating to the back or scapula
Anomalous coronary artery	Exertional chest discomfort at high levels of exertion. Exertional shortness of breath often mislabeled as "asthma." Can manifest as syncope or cardiac arrest without premonitory symptoms
Valvular disease	Exertional chest discomfort at high levels of exertion. Exertional shortness of breath often mislabeled as "asthma." Can manifest as syncope or cardiac arrest without premonitory symptoms
Myo- or pericarditis	Often manifests within days to weeks of a clear noncardiac viral infection. Symptoms variable. Positional chest pain that is most severe when lying supine and relieved at least in part by sitting forward; dyspnea and exercise intolerance
Tachyarrhythmias	Palpitations may be associated with chest pressure or heaviness, shortness of breath, and syncope
Noncardiac causes	
Respiratory	Pulmonary embolism
	Pneumonia/pleurisy
	Pneumothorax
Gastrointestinal	Gastroesophageal reflux disease
	Peptic ulcer disease
	Cholecystitis
	Pancreatitis
Musculoskeletal	Costochondritis
	Trauma
	Strain
Other	Anxiety, depression
	Anemia
	Thyrotoxicosis
	Herpes zoster

associated with pathologic underlying cardiovascular disease.

Athletic patients presenting with chest pain most often experience their symptoms during physical exertion. In patients less than 35 years of age, congenital valvular heart disease; genetic cardiomyopathies, such as hypertrophic cardiomyopathy (HCM); and coronary anomalies/malformations are the leading causes of cardiac chest pain. In contrast, among patients over 35 years of age, obstructive coronary artery disease due to atherosclerosis is the most common cause of exertional chest pain [75, 76]. Chest pain can be divided into two categories: chest pain resulting from myocardial ischemia and chest pain from other causes. Myocardial ischemia results from an imbalance between myocardial oxygen demand and coronary blood flow. The most common causes of ischemic chest pain in athletes include atherosclerotic coronary artery disease (typically in older patients), anomalous coronary arteries (typically in younger patients), and genetic cardiomyopathies, most often HCM. Ischemic chest pain can also be caused by less frequent entities including coronary vasospasm, coronary artery dissection, and valvular heart disease, including aortic stenosis (both congenital and acquired), severe anemia, and thyrotoxicosis. Congenital coronary artery anomalies originating from the contralateral sinus of Valsalva and following a course between the aorta and pulmonary artery are a common cause of exertional chest pain and exercise-related sudden death in athletes younger than 35 years and the literature pertaining to the general population has relevance. Two studies examining atypical chest pain leading to hospital admission found that the causes fell into five categories: musculoskeletal, cardiac, gastrointestinal, respiratory, and miscellaneous. Musculoskeletal causes were the most common (27%) [79], and in our experience, this finding also applies to athletes with chest pain. A careful physical examination of the chest wall can be relied on to differentiate musculoskeletal chest pain from other causes.

There are several important cardiac conditions that can cause chest pain without myocardial ischemia. The most common are pericarditis, myocarditis, and aortic dissection. Pericarditis and myocarditis are inflammatory diseases of the heart lining and muscle, respectively, which are most often caused by infectious agents (most commonly viruses). Both conditions often follow clinically appreciable infectious syndromes and are typically characterized by positional chest discomfort, fatigue, and in some cases palpitations. Aortic dissection, acute tearing of the aortic wall, is a surgical emergency that classically presents with "tearing" chest or back pain, often localized to the mid-scapular region. Among athletes, aortic dissection most commonly occurs in individuals with underlying aortopathy and is usually precipitated by intense isometric actions (i.e., lifting heavy weight) or direct blunt chest wall trauma. Pre-participation screening, whether confined to standard medical history and physical examination or inclusive of a resting or exercise 12-lead ECG, has limited capacity to identify coronary artery anomalies. Therefore, anomalous coronary lesions should be suspected in the athlete who presents with chest discomfort during or immediately after exertion, even if the athlete has been previously screened with a pre-participation exam. When this diagnosis is suspected, direct, noninvasive imaging of the coronary anatomy is required. Transthoracic echocardiographic imaging is capable of accurately defining coronary anatomy in 90% of athletes [80]. Given the absence of radiation exposure and the widespread accessibility of this technique, this is the initial

diagnostic imaging test in this setting. If transthoracic echocardiography does not yield definitive images of the coronary origins and proximal course, magnetic resonance imaging [79, 81, 82] or computed tomography [83] should be considered, based on institutional preferences and insurance reimbursement patterns.

Syncope

Syncope, transient loss of consciousness followed by complete and spontaneous return to baseline mental status, is common among athletes. In a large series of young Italian athletes, approximately 6% experienced some form of syncope during their athletic careers [84]. Etiologies of syncope in the endurance athlete range from the benign neurally mediated collapse to life-threatening pathologic conditions, including structural heart disease and primary arrhythmias.

Most syncopes in athletes are attributable to neurally mediated mechanisms involving predominant and often excessive vagal tone related to chronic exercise training. Syncope frequently occurs in athletes outside of sports participation. Typical triggers include anxiety, sudden postural changes, and painful stimuli. While often recurrent, non-exertional, neurally mediated syncope in the athlete is usually a benign condition. A closely related and common fainting syndrome is "post-exertional" syncope, often informally referred to as exercise-associated collapse. Post-exertional syncope occurs following abrupt cessation of exercise, most commonly moderate- to high-intensity endurance exercise, and is caused by a rapid reduction in central venous return. This reduction in venous return, caused by both the cessation of skeletal muscle contraction and altered sympathetic/parasympathetic balance, causes transient cerebral hypoperfusion. The affected athlete typically reports prodromic feelings of warmth, light-headedness, or diaphoresis, which begin within seconds of exercise termination and rapidly culminate in a loss of consciousness lasting from several seconds to a minute. Athletes predisposed to this condition should be

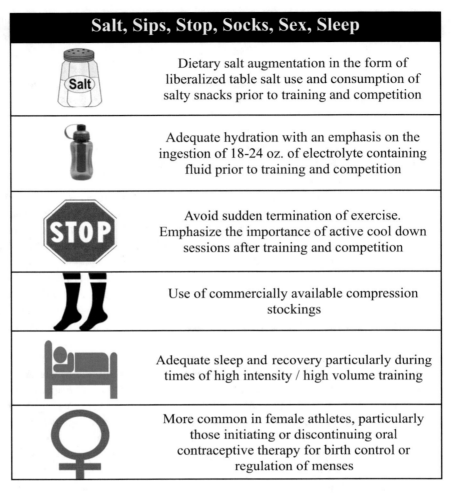

Fig. 1.1 Conservative steps for the clinical management of neurally mediated syncope among endurance athletes

counseled as this problem has a high rate or recurrence in the absence of avoidance-based therapy. In our practice, we employ the "6-S" algorithm (salt, sips, stop, socks, sex, sleep) as shown in Fig. 1.1.

Syncope that occurs during intense exercise, either with or without prodromal symptoms, should raise suspicion for underlying cardiac disease. Traumatic injury secondary to syncope should further increase the index of suspicion for underlying disease. Current American College of Cardiology/American Heart Association (ACC/AHA) guidelines recommend that the approach to the athlete with exertional syncope begin with a meticulous history, physical examina-

tion, resting 12-lead electrocardiogram, and echocardiogram [85]. The medical history should characterize potential triggers, the timing and duration of the event, and the risks associated with future episodes of loss of consciousness. Physical examination should be directed toward signs, most often pathologic murmurs, of occult heart muscle and valve diseases. The resting 12-lead ECG should be inspected for abnormalities of conduction (QT prolongation, preexcitation, pathologic right bundle branch block with early precordial ST elevations suggestive of Brugada syndrome) and findings suggestive of structural heart disease (left bundle branch block, LVH with repolarization abnormalities, diffuse

T-wave inversion). Transthoracic echocardiography is recommended to exclude structural and valvular heart disease in individuals with syncope, especially if any abnormality is detected during medical history, physical examination, or ECG interpretation.

The comprehensive assessment of true exertional syncope often extends far beyond these basic measures and must be tailored to exclude underlying structural and electrical heart disease. We recommend such evaluations be conducted under the supervision of a cardiovascular specialist with expertise in the care of athletic patients. Provocative and customized exercise testing is often high yield and should be designed to approximate the exercise conditions in which the syncope occurred. Careful attention should be given to the exercise ECG for the detection of explanatory arrhythmias. When lab-based exercise testing is inconclusive, ambulatory rhythm monitoring may be necessary. There are numerous ambulatory rhythm monitoring devices available, and the choice should be dictated by the frequency and duration of syncope on an individual patient basis. The use of tilt-table testing in athletes, due to high rates of false-positive testing, is of limited value. In very select cases, most often in the setting of a documented arrhythmia syndrome, invasive electrophysiologic study (EPS) may be both diagnostic and potentially therapeutic [86].

Management of the athlete with syncope is dictated by cause. Individuals with significant structural or valvular heart disease should be managed with appropriate sport restriction, medication, EPS with or without ablation, implantable defibrillator placement, or surgery on the basis of specific pathology [83]. Neurally mediated post-exertional syncope can often be avoided by mandating an active cooldown period after exertion and by paying attention to hydration and supplemental salt intake. In athletes with recurrent neurally mediated syncope despite these first-line treatments, postural training or pharmacologic therapy may be reasonable; however, these should be prescribed only after careful consideration of rules delineating banned substances in athletes.

Palpitations

Palpitations are a frequent complaint in athletes. The heightened vagal tone that accompanies routine exercise training commonly results in marked sinus bradycardia, and the relatively lengthy time period between sinus beats may facilitate an increase in ectopic atrial and ventricular beats. Slow resting heart rate coupled with the keen body awareness that is typical among athletic patients often leads to sensing of these spontaneous depolarizations. In the majority of cases, resting palpitations that are suppressed with exercise, particularly among athletes with no findings during medical history, physical examination, and 12-lead ECG, are a benign phenomenon that requires no further evaluation [87].

The athlete presenting either with palpitations that are exacerbated by exercise or with other findings suggestive of occult cardiac disease requires a comprehensive evaluation by a cardiovascular specialist with expertise in the care of athletic patients. A broad differential diagnosis must be considered. Noninvasive cardiac imaging, customized exercise testing designed to stimulate the demands of training and competition, and ambulatory rhythm monitoring play a key role in the evaluation. The choice of a specific ambulatory rhythm monitoring device is crucial and requires individualized decision making. For symptoms that predictably recur within a 24-h period, simple Holter monitoring may be adequate. If the athlete experiences less frequent, more intermittent symptoms, they are best evaluated with a continuous loop recorder or event (patient-triggered) monitor. For those with very infrequent or elusive symptoms (>1 month between symptoms), an implantable loop recorder may be required.

Palpitations due to benign atrial and/or ventricular ectopy that occur at rest are suppressed by exercise, are not accompanied by primary structural or electrical diseases, and are best managed conservatively. Often counseling geared toward patient reassurance and avoidance of potential triggers including alcohol, caffeine, and stimulants are sufficient. Among athletic patients with palpitations caused by pathology, disease-specific therapies designed to reduce the burden of arrhythmia (i.e., pharmacologic suppression, intracardiac ablation) and to reduce the risk of sudden cardiac death (i.e., sports restriction, implantable defibrillator placement) are often indicated.

Atrial Arrhythmias

Atrial fibrillation (AF) is the most common arrhythmia in the general population [88]. A rapidly growing body of literature suggests that long-standing participation in endurance exercise may increase the prevalence of atrial fibrillation in athletes [89]. Mechanistic underpinning of this observation remains unknown but is likely multifactorial with contributions from age, years of training, structural remodeling (atrial stretch), scarring, atrial inflammation, changes in the autonomic nervous system (increased vagal tone), hypovolemia, genetic predisposition, and illicit drug use.

A meta-analysis of six studies that involved 655 athletes engaging in diverse sporting disciplines reported a fivefold risk of AF [90]. A recent large study of 52,000 long-distance cross-country skiers demonstrated that atrial fibrillation was the most common arrhythmia (1.3 %) and was related to the number of races competed and faster finishing times, surrogates of endurance training volume and duration, respectively [91]. This has been supported by others who documented lone atrial fibrillation with endurance athletes (mean age 44 years) who report a lifetime practice of sport exceeding 1500 h [92–94].

In an effort to identify as potential modulators and triggers of arrhythmias, Wilhelm studied a cohort of 70 randomly selected athletes entering a ten-mile running race and demonstrated an increase in left atrial volume and P-wave prolongation as evidence of altered atrial substrate and increased vagal tone and atrial ectopy, respectively [39]. The alterations seen in the atria with chronic endurance training may also adversely affect the sinoatrial and atrioventricular nodes.

Treatment and prognostication of endurance athletes with atrial fibrillation is difficult due to the paucity of large-scale prospective, randomized clinical trials and guidelines focusing directly on this population. In the absence of such resources, current guidelines for the management of atrial fibrillation in the general population must be considered when caring for endurance athletes. Therapeutic options for athletes with AF must be individualized and may include strategies including restriction of endurance exercise dose, rhythm maintenance pharmacotherapy, and intracardiac ablation. We routinely assess the risk–benefit balance of anticoagulation pharmacotherapy for all athletes with AF and develop an individualized strategy that emerges from a shared decision-making strategy.

Long-Term Effect of Chronic Endurance Training

Regular exercise is highly effective for prevention and treatment of many chronic diseases and improves cardiovascular (CV) health and longevity. The American Heart Association recommends at least 30 min of moderate-intensity aerobic activity at least 5 days per week for a total of 150 min for overall cardiovascular health. Moderate-intensity exercise is considered to be any activity causing a raised heart rate and increased breathing but being able to speak comfortably and includes a brisk walk at 4 mph or cycling at 10–12 mph. The intensity of physical exercise is usually expressed in terms of energy expenditure or metabolic equivalents (METs). One MET represents an individual's energy expenditure while sitting quietly for 1 min (equivalent to about 1.2 kcal/min for a person weighing 72 kg). Moderate-intensity exercise is equivalent to 3–6 METs, whereas athletes typically perform in excess of 15 METs [95]. The "dose" of exercise consists of a number of factors, including intensity (how hard), duration (how long), and frequency (how often).

People who exercise regularly have markedly lower rates of disability and a mean life expectancy that is 7 years longer than that of their physically inactive contemporaries [96–98]. It is clear that mild to moderate exercise is better from a health outcomes perspective than no exercise; it remains unknown and actively debated whether an upper limit of exercise dose exists above which adverse effects outweigh benefits [50]. Preliminary data suggests that there may be a U-shaped relationship between exercise dose and adverse cardiovascular events [99, 100]. Among 1000 joggers prospectively studied, those who ran for 30–45 min, three times a week, had a lower mortality than sedentary non-joggers, while more strenuous joggers had a mortality rate that was not statistically different from this study's sedentary group. Similarly, a 15-year observational study of 52,000 adults found that runners had a 19 % lower risk of all-cause mortality compared with non-runners, with U-shaped mortality curves for distance, speed, and frequency. Running distances of about 1–20 miles per week, speeds of 6–7 miles per hour, and frequencies of 2–5 days per week were associated with lower all-cause mortality, whereas higher mileage, faster paces, and more frequent runs were not associated with better survival [101]. In our opinion, these data generate important hypotheses that will require further work to confirm or refute.

Sudden Death During Endurance Competition

Sudden cardiac death (SCD) during endurance sporting events is a rare phenomenon. Collectively, this topic has been most thoroughly examined in the context of marathon running as summarized in Table 1.2. The largest database documenting sudden death during marathon run-

ning was comprised by the RACER study group. Kim et al. [62] investigated the incidence and outcome of cardiac arrests during marathon and half-marathon races in the United States during the decade spanning from 2000 to 2010. In the 10.9 million runners examined, 59 cases of cardiac arrest occurred in association with either marathon or half-marathon races. Men were significantly more likely to experience cardiac arrest and SCD than women. The event rates were significantly correlated with the age of the runners and significantly more frequent in "full" marathon runs (42.195 km) than in "half"-marathon runs. Notably, more than half the cases of sudden cardiac death occurred in the final mile.

The RACER authors calculated that the incidence rates of cardiac arrest and sudden death during long-distance running races were 1 per 184,000 and 1 per 259,000 participants, respectively. Thus, event rates among marathon and half-marathon runners are relatively low, as compared with other athletic populations, including collegiate athletes (1 death per 43,770 participants per year) [102], triathlon participants (1 death per 52,630 participants) [103], and previously healthy middle-aged joggers (1 death per 7620 participants) [104], suggesting that the risk associated with long-distance running events is no higher and may be lower when compared with other vigorous physical activities. These rates compare favorably with those presented by other investigators.

Conclusion

In summary, since the days of Henschen and Darling, understanding of sport-specific changes in cardiac structure and exercise-induced cardiac remodeling has advanced significantly. In order to define the natural history of endurance-induced cardiac remodeling, longer-duration longitudinal study is required. Examination of prolonged exposures to exercise training will be necessary to determine normative values across the age and training spectrums of athletic patients.

Table 1.2 Major reports

Studies	Race	# of runners	Deaths N (rate)	Cardiac arrest N (rate)	Mean age (years)	Male (%)	Etiology
RACE Paris registry (2006–2012) [105]	Marathon, half-marathon, 20 K	511,880	2 (0.4/100,000)	9 (1.8/100,000)	42.8	100	Eight MI, three arrhythmias, one ARVD, five heat stroke
RACER (2000–2010) [62]	Marathon, half-marathon	10,900,000	42 (0.4/100,000)	59 (0.5/100,000)	42	86	14 HCM +/− other, one heat stroke, one ARVC, two hyponatremias, seven presumed dysrhythmias, seven MI, three unknown
Webner (1976–2009) [106]	Marathon	1,710,052	10 (1/171,005)	30 (1/57,002)	49.7	93	Seven CAD, one ACA, one unknown, one no autopsy
Redelmeier and Greenwald (1975–2004) [107]	Marathon	3,292,268	26 (0.8/100,000)	N/A	41	81	21 CAD, four electrolyte abnormalities, two ACA, one heat stroke
Maron and Roberts (1976–1994) [108]	Marathon	215,413	4 (0.5/100,000)	0.9/100,000	39	75	Three CAD, one ACA
Maron and Roberts (1995–2004) [109]	Marathon	220,606	1 (0.45/100,000)	3 (1.4/100,000)	47	100	Three CAD, one mitochondrial myopathy

HCM hypertrophic cardiomyopathy, *ARVC* arrhythmogenic right ventricular cardiomyopathy, *CAD* coronary artery disease, *ACA* anomalous coronary artery, *MI* myocardial infarction

This information, coupled with the impact of detraining, will help to more clearly distinguish the boundary between physiology and pathology in athletic patients.

References

1. Henschen S. Skidlauf und skidwettlauf:eine medizinische sportsudie. Mitt Med Klin Upsala. 1899: 2.
2. Darling E. The effects of training: as study of Harvard University crews. Boston Med Surg J. 1899;161:229–33.
3. White P. The pulse after a marathon race. JAMA. 1918;71:1047–8.
4. White P. Bradycardia in athletes, especially long distance runners. JAMA. 1942;120:642.
5. Roskamm H, et al. Relations between heart size and physical efficiency in male and female athletes in comparison with normal male and female subjects. Arch Kreislaufforsch. 1961;35:67–102.
6. Reindell H, et al. The heart and blood circulation in athletes. Med Welt. 1960;31:1557–63.
7. Bulychev VV, et al. Roentgenological and instrumental examination of the heart in athletes. Klin Med. 1965;43:108–14.
8. Baggish AL, et al. Cardiovascular screening in college athletes with and without electrocardiography: across-sectional study. Ann Intern Med. 2010;152:269–75.
9. Magalski A, et al. Cardiovascular screening with electrocardiography and echocardiography in collegiate athletes. Am J Med. 2011;124:511–8.
10. Weiner R, et al. Performance of the 2010 European Society of Cardiology criteria for ECG interpretation in athletes. Heart. 2011;97:1573–7.
11. Baggish A, Wood M. Athlete's heart and cardiovascular care of the athlete scientific and clinical update. Circulation. 2011;123:2723–35.
12. Running USA. 2015 state of the sport. 2015. U.S. Race Trends, http://www.runningusa.org/2015-state-of-sport-us-trends?returnTo=annual-reports
13. Maron B, et al. Eligibility and disqualification recommendations for competitive athletes with cardiovascular abnormalities. Circulation. 2015;66:2343–450.
14. Wasfy M, et al. Endurance exercise-induced cardiac remodeling: not all sports are created equal. J Am Soc Echocardiogr. 2015;28(12):1434–40.
15. Clifford PS, et al. Arterial blood pressure response to rowing. Med Sci Sports Exerc. 1994;6(26):715–9.
16. Pelliccia A, et al. Physiologic left ventricular cavity dilation in elite athletes. Ann Intern Med. 1999;130:23–31.
17. Pelliccia A, et al. The upper limit of physiologic cardiac hypertrophy in highly trained elite athletes. N Eng J Med. 1991;324:295–301.
18. Sharma S, et al. Physiologic limits of left ventricular hypertrophy in elite junior athletes: relevance to differential diagnosis of athlete's heart and hypertrophic cardiomyopathy. J Am Coll Cardiol. 2002;40:1431–6.
19. Weiner R, et al. The feasibility, diagnostic yield, and learning curve of portable echocardiography of out-of-hospital cardiovascular disease screening. J Am Soc Echocardiogr. 2012;25:568–75.
20. Rawlins J, et al. Ethnic differences in physiological cardiac adaptation to intense physical exercise in highly trained female athletes. Circulation. 2010;121:1078–85.
21. Douglas PS, et al. Left ventricular structure and function by echocardiography in ultraendurance athletes. Am J Cardiol. 1986;58:805–9.
22. Abergel E, et al. Serial left ventricular adaptations in world-class professional cyclist: implications for disease screening and follow up. J Am Coll Cardiol. 2004;44:144–9.
23. Weiner R, Baggish AL. Cardiovascular adaptation and remodeling to rigorous athletic training. Clin Sports Med. 2015;34:405–18.
24. Baggish AL, et al. The impact of endurance exercise training on left ventricular systolic mechanics. Am J Physiol Heart Circ Physiol. 2008;296:H1109–16.
25. Weiner RB, et al. The impact of endurance training on left ventricular torsion. JACC Cardiovasc Imaging. 2010;3:1001–3.
26. Baggish AL, et al. Differences in cardiac parameters among elite and subelite rowers. Med Sci Sports Exerc. 2010;42:1215–20.
27. D'Andrea A, et al. Left ventricular myocardial velocities and deformation indexes in top-level athletes. J Am Soc Echocardiogr. 2010;23:1281–8.
28. Caso P, et al. Pulsed doppler tissue imaging in endurance athletes: relation between left ventricular preload and myocardial regional diastolic function. Am J Cardiol. 2000;85:1131–6.
29. Levine BD, et al. Left ventricular pressure-volume and Frank-Startling relations in endurance athletes. Implications for orthostatic tolerance and exercise performance. Circulation. 1991;84:1016–23.
30. Prior D, La Gerche A. The athlete's heart. Heart. 2012;98:947–55.
31. Oxborough D, et al. The right ventricle of the endurance athlete: the relationship between morphology and deformation. J Am Soc Echocardiogr. 2012;25:263–71.
32. D'Andrea A, et al. Range of right heart measurements in top-level athletes: the training impact. Int J Cardiol. 2013;164:48–57.
33. La Gershe A, et al. Exercise strain rate imaging demonstrates normal right ventricular contractile reserve and clarifies ambiguous resting measures in endurance athletes. J Am Soc Echocardiogr. 2012;25:253–62.
34. D'Andrea A, et al. Right Heart Structural and Functional Remodeling in Athletes. Echocardiography. 2015;23:11-S22.

35. Pellicia A, et al. Prevalence and clinical significance of left atrial remodeling in competitive athletes. J Am Coll Cardiol. 2005;46:690–6.
36. D'Andrea A, et al. Left atrial volume index in highly trained athletes. Am Heart J. 2010;159:1155–61.
37. Weiner RB, Baggish AL. Exercise-induced cardiac remodeling. Prog Cardiovasc Dis. 2012;54:380–6.
38. Iskandar A, et al. Left atrium size in elite athletes. J Am Coll Cardiol Img. 2015;8:753–62.
39. Wilhelm M, et al. Atrial remodeling, autonomic tone, and lifetime training hours in nonelite athletes. Am J Cardiol. 2011;108:580–5.
40. Grunig E, et al. Reference values for and determinants of right atrial area in healthy adults by 2-dimensional echocardiography. Circ Cardiovasc Imaging. 2013;6:117–24.
41. Wilhelm M, et al. Long-term cardiac remodeling and arrhythmias in nonelite marathon runners. Am J Cardiol. 2012;110:129–35.
42. Pagourelias E, et al. Right atrial and ventricular adaptations to training in male Caucasian athletes: an echocardiographic study. J Am Soc Echocardiogr. 2013;26:1344–52.
43. Pellicia A, et al. The genetics of left ventricular remodeling in competitive athletes. J Cardiovasc Med. 2006;7:267–70.
44. Pelliccia A, et al. Athlete's heart in women. Echocardiographic characterization of female athletes. JAMA. 1996;376:211–5.
45. Basavarajaiah S, et al. Ethnic differences in left ventricular remodeling in highly-trained athletes relevance to differentiating physiologic left ventricular hypertrophy from hypertrophic cardiomyopathy. J Am Coll Cardiol. 2008;51:2256–62.
46. Zelinski J, et al. Myocardial adaptations to recreational marathon training among middle-aged men. Circ Cardiovasc Imaging. 2015;8.
47. La Gerche A, et al. Can intense endurance exercise cause myocardial damage and fibrosis? Curr Sports Med Rep. 2013;12(2):63–9.
48. La Gerche A, et al. Exercise-induced right ventricular dysfunction and structural remodelling in endurance athletes. Eur Heart J. 2012;33:998–1006.
49. Hanssen H, et al. Magnetic resonance imaging of myocardial injury and ventricular torsion after marathon running. Clin Sci. 2011;120:143–52.
50. O'Keefe JH, et al. Potential adverse cardiovascular effects from excessive endurance exercise. Mayo Clin Proc. 2012;87(6):587–95.
51. Sorokin AV, et al. Atrial fibrillation in endurance-trained athletes. Br J Sports Med. 2011;45:185–8.
52. Link M. Arrhythmias and sport practice. Heart. 2010;96:398–405.
53. La Gerche A, et al. Biochemical and functional abnormalities of left and right ventricular function after ultra-endurance exercise. Heart. 2008;94:860–6.
54. Mousavi N, et al. Relation of biomarkers and cardiac magnetic resonance imaging after marathon running. Am J Cardiol. 2009;103:1467–72.
55. Neilan TG, et al. Myocardial injury and ventricular dysfunction related to training levels among nonelite participants in the Boston marathon. Circulation. 2006;114:2325–33.
56. Neilan TG, et al. Persistent and reversible cardiac dysfunction among amateur marathon runners. Eur Heart J. 2006;27:1079–84.
57. Baggish AL, et al. The impact of endurance exercise training on left ventricular systolic mechanisms. Am J Physiol. 2008;395:H1109–16.
58. Heidbuchel H, et al. Ventricular arrhythmias associated with long-term endurance sports: what is the evidence? Br J Sports Med. 2012;46 Suppl 1:i44–50.
59. Möhlenkamp S, et al. Running: the risk of coronary events: prevalence and prognostic relevance of coronary atherosclerosis in marathon runners. Eur Heart J. 2008;29:1903–10.
60. Wilson M, et al. Diverse patterns of myocardial fibrosis in lifelong, veteran endurance athletes. J Appl Physiol. 1985;110:1622–6.
61. Heidbuchel H, et al. Can intensive exercise harm the heart? Circulation. 2014;130:992–1002.
62. Kim JH, et al. Race Associated Cardiac Arrest Event Registry (RACER) Study Group. Cardiac arrest during long-distance running races. N Engl J Med. 2012;366:130–40.
63. Whyte G, et al. Treat the patient not the blood test: the implications of an increase in cardiac troponin after prolonged endurance exercise. Br J Sports Med. 2007;41:613–5.
64. Scharhag J, et al. Reproducibility and clinical significance of exercise-induced increase in cardiac troponins and N-terminal pro brain natriuretic peptide (NT-proBNP) in endurance athletes. Eur J Cardiovasc Prev Rehabil. 2006;13:388–97.
65. Wilson M, et al. Biological markers of cardiac damage are not related to measure of cardiac systolic and diastolic function using cardiovascular magnetic resonance and echocardiography after acute bout of prolonged endurance exercise. Br J Sports Med. 2011;45:780–4.
66. Maron BJ, Pelliccia AM. The heart of trained athletes cardiac remodeling and the risks of sports, including sudden death. Circulation. 2006;114:1633–44.
67. Corrado D, et al. Screening for hypertrophic cardiomyopathy in young athletes. N Engl J Med. 1998;336(6):364–9.
68. Corrado D, et al. Cardiovascular pre-participation screening of young competitive athletes for prevention of sudden death: proposal for a common European protocol. Eur Heart J. 2005;26(5):516–24.
69. Corrado D, et al. Recommendations for interpretation of 12-lead electrocardiogram in the athlete. Eur Heart J. 2010;31:243–59.
70. Drezner JA, et al. Abnormal electrocardiographic findings in athletes: recognising changes suggestive

of primary electrical disease. Br J Sports Med. 2013;47(3):153–67.

71. Sharma S, et al. Comparison of ECG criteria for the detection of cardiac abnormalities in elite black and white athletes. Circulation. 2014;129(16):1637–49.

72. Wasfy MM, et al. ECG findings in competitive rowers: normative data and the prevalence of abnormalities using contemporary screening recommendations. Br J Sports Med. doi:10.1136/bjsports-2014-093919, Published Online First 9/8/14.

73. Brosnan M, et al. Modest agreement in ECG interpretation limits the application of ECG screening in young athletes. Heart Rhythm. 2015;12:130–6.

74. Maron BJ, et al. Sudden death in young competitive athletes: clinical, demographic and pathologic profiles. JAMA. 1996;276:199–204.

75. Maron BJ. Sudden death in young athletes. N Engl J Med. 2003;349:1064–75.

76. Maron BJ, et al. Prevalence of sudden cardiac death during competitive sports activities in Minnesota high school athletes. J Am Coll Cardiol. 1998;32:1881–4.

77. Maron BJ, et al. Sudden deaths in young competitive athletes: analysis of 1866 deaths in the United States, 1980–2006. Circulation. 2009;119:1085–92.

78. Pellicia A. CHest pain in athletes. Clin Sports Med. 2003:37–50.

79. Spalding L, et al. Cause and outcome of atypical chest pain in patients admitted to hospital. J R Soc Med. 2003;96(3):122–5.

80. Pelliccia A, et al. Prospective echocardiographic screening for coronary artery anomalies in 1,360 elite competitive athletes. Am J Cardiol. 1993;72:978–9.

81. McConnell MV, et al. Identification of anomalous coronary arteries and their anatomic course by magnetic resonance coronary angiography. Circulation. 1995;92:3158–62.

82. Pelliccia A. Chest pain in athletes. Clin Sports Med. 2003;22:37–50.

83. Pelliccia A, et al. European Society of Cardiology consensus document: recommendations for competitive sports participation in athletes with cardiovascular disease. Eur Heart J. 2005;26:1422–45.

84. Colivicchi F, et al. Epidemiology and prognostic implications of syncope in young competitive athletes. Eur Heart J. 2004;25(19):1749–53.

85. Strickberger SA, et al. AHA/ACCF scientific statement on the evaluation of syncope. Circulation. 2006;113:316–27.

86. Colivicchi F, et al. Exercise-related syncope in young competitive athletes without evidence of structural heart disease. Clinical presentation ad long-term outcome. Eur Heart J. 2002;23(14):1125–30.

87. Lawless C. Palpitations in athletes. Sports Med. 2008;38(8):687–702.

88. Wehrens HT, et al. Chronic exercise: a contributing factor to atrial fibrillation? Am J Cardiol. 2013; 62:78–80.

89. Turagam MK, et al. Atrial fibrillation in athletes. Am J Cardiol. 2012;109:296–302.

90. Abdulla J, et al. Is the risk of atrial fibrillation higher in athletes than in the general population? A systematic review and meta-review. Europace. 2009;11:1156–9.

91. Andersen K, et al. Risk of arrhythmias in 52755 long-distance cross-country skiers: a cohort study. Eur Heart J. 2013;34:3624–31.

92. Elosua R, et al. Sport practice and the risk of lone atrial fibrillation: a case-controlled study. Int J Cardiol. 2006;108:332–7.

93. Drca N, et al. Atrial fibrillation is associated with different levels of physical activity levels at different ages in men. Heart. 2014;100:1037–42.

94. Mont L, et al. Long-lasting sport practice and lone atrial fibrillation. Eur Heart J. 2002;23:477–82.

95. Levine B. Exercise dose. J Appl Physiol. 2014;116: 736–45.

96. Chakravarty EF, et al. Reduced disability and mortality among aging runners: a 21-year longitudinal study. Arch Intern Med. 2008;168(15):1638–46.

97. Wen CP, et al. Minimum amount of physical activity for reduced mortality and extended life expectancy: a prospective cohort study. Lancet. 2011;378(9798): 1244–53.

98. O'Keefe JH, et al. Exercise and life expectancy. Lancet. 2012;379(9818):800–1.

99. Sharma S, et al. The U-shaped relationship between exercise and cardiac morbidity. Trends Cardiovasc Med. 2015; doi:10.1016/j.tcm.2015.06.005.

100. Schnohr P. Dose of jogging and long-term mortality. J Am Coll Cardiol. 2015;65:411–9.

101. Lee J, et al. Running and all-cause mortality risk: is more better? Med Sci Sports Exerc. 2012;44(6):990–4.

102. Harmon KG, et al. Incidence of sudden cardiac death in National Collegiate Athletic Association athletes. Circulation. 2011;123:1594–600.

103. Harris KM, et al. Sudden death during the triathlon. JAMA. 2010;303:1255–7.

104. Thompson PD, et al. Incidence of death during jogging in Rhode Island from 1975 through 1980. JAMA. 1982;247:2535–8.

105. Gerardin B, et al. Registry on acute cardiovascular events during endurance running races: the prospective RACE Paris registry. Eur Heart J. 2015; doi:10.1093/eurheartj/ehv675.

106. Webner D, et al. Sudden cardiac arrest and death in United States marathons. Med Sci Sports Exerc. 2012; doi:10.1249/MMS.0b013e318 258b59a.

107. Redelmeier DA, Greenwald JA. Competing risks of mortality with marathons: retrospective analysis. BMJ. 2007.

108. Maron B, Poliac L, et al. Risk for sudden cardiac death associated with marathon running. JACC. 1996;28(2):428–31.

109. Roberts WO, Maron BJ. Evidence for decreasing occurrence of sudden cardiac death associated with the marathon. JACC. 2005;46(7):1373–7.

Exercise-Induced Bronchoconstriction and Vocal Cord Dysfunction

Christopher Kempe and Jonathan P. Parsons

Exercise-induced bronchoconstriction (EIB) describes acute, transient airway narrowing that occurs in association with exercise. EIB is characterized by symptoms of cough, wheezing, or chest tightness during or after exercise. Exercise is one of the most common triggers of bronchospasm in patients with underlying asthma, and approximately 80 % of individuals with chronic asthma have experienced exercise-induced respiratory symptoms [1]. However, EIB also occurs in up to 10 % of people who are not known to be atopic or asthmatic [2]. These patients do not have the typical features of chronic asthma (i.e., frequent daytime symptoms, nocturnal symptoms, impaired lung function), and exercise may be the only stimulus that causes respiratory symptoms.

EIB occurs quite commonly in athletes, and prevalence rates of bronchospasm related to exercise in athletes range from 11 to 50 % [3]. Holzer and colleagues [4] found 50 % of a cohort of 50 elite summer athletes had EIB. Wilber and associates

[5] found that 18–26 % of Olympic winter sport athletes and 50 % of cross-country skiers had EIB. The US Olympic Committee reported an 11.2 % prevalence of EIB in all athletes who competed in the 1984 Summer Olympics [6].

Despite numerous studies that investigate the prevalence of EIB in athletes, few studies have investigated the prevalence of EIB in cohorts of athletes without known history of asthma or EIB. Mannix and associates [7] found that 41 of 212 subjects (19 %) in an urban fitness center, none of whom had a previous diagnosis of asthma, had EIB. Rupp and colleagues [8] evaluated 230 middle and high school student athletes and, after excluding those with known EIB, found that 29 % had EIB. These studies suggest that EIB occurs commonly in subjects who are not known to have asthma and likely is underdiagnosed clinically.

The prevalence of EIB may be further underestimated because patients with asthma and EIB have been shown to be poor perceivers of symptoms of bronchospasm [9, 10]. Specifically, athletes often suffer from lack of awareness of symptoms suggestive of EIB [11, 12]. Health-care providers and coaches also may not consider EIB as a possible explanation for respiratory symptoms occurring during exercise. Athletes are generally fit and healthy, and the presence of a significant medical problem often is not considered. The athlete is often considered to be "out of shape," and vague symptoms of chest discomfort, breathlessness, and fatigue are not interpreted as a manifestation of EIB. Athletes themselves are often not aware that

C. Kempe
Division of Pulmonary, Critical Care, and Sleep Medicine, Ohio State University Medical Center, Columbus, OH 43210, USA

J.P. Parsons (✉)
Division of Pulmonary, Critical Care, and Sleep Medicine, Ohio State University Medical Center, Columbus, OH 43210, USA

Davis Heart/Lung Research Institute,
473 W., 12th Avenue, Columbus, OH 43210, USA
e-mail: jonathan.parsons@osumc.edu

© Springer International Publishing Switzerland 2016
T.L. Miller (ed.), *Endurance Sports Medicine*, DOI 10.1007/978-3-319-32982-6_2

they may have a physical problem. Furthermore, if they do recognize they have a medical problem, they often do not want to admit to health personnel that a problem exists because of fear of social stigma or losing playing time.

Athletes that compete in high-ventilation or endurance sports may be more likely to experience symptoms of EIB than those who participate in low-ventilation sports [13]; however, EIB can occur in any setting. EIB is prevalent in endurance sports in which ventilation is increased for long periods of time during training and competition such as cross-country skiing, swimming, and long-distance running [13]. EIB also occurs commonly in winter sport athletes [5]. In addition, environmental triggers may predispose certain populations of athletes to an increased risk for development of EIB. Chlorine compounds in swimming pools [14] and chemicals related to ice-resurfacing machinery in ice rinks [15], such as carbon monoxide and nitrogen dioxide, may put exposed athletic populations at additional risk. These environmental factors may act as triggers and exacerbate bronchospasm in athletes who are predisposed to EIB. Thus, it is important for athletes, coaches, and athletic trainers supervising athletes in these sports to be aware of these important environmental issues.

The clinical manifestations of EIB are extremely variable and can range from mild impairment of performance to severe bronchospasm and respiratory failure. Common symptoms include coughing, wheezing, chest tightness, and dyspnea. More subtle evidence of EIB includes fatigue, symptoms that occur in specific environments (e.g., ice rinks or swimming pools), poor performance for conditioning level, and avoidance of activity (Table 2.1).

Table 2.1 Common symptoms of EIB

Symptoms of EIB
Dyspnea on exertion
Chest tightness
Wheezing
Fatigue
Poor performance for conditioning level
Avoidance of activity
Symptoms in specific environments (e.g., ice rinks, swimming pools)

Generally, exercise at a workload representing at least 80 % of the maximal predicted oxygen consumption for 5–8 min is required to generate bronchospasm in most athletes [16]. Typically, athletes experience transient bronchodilation initially during exercise, and symptoms of EIB begin later or shortly after exercise. Symptoms often peak 5–10 min after exercise ceases and can remain significant for 30 min or longer if no bronchodilator therapy is provided [17]. However, some athletes spontaneously recover to baseline airflow within 60 min, even in the absence of intervention with bronchodilator therapy [17]. Unfortunately, it is currently impossible to predict which athletes will recover without treatment. Athletes who experience symptoms for extended periods often perform at suboptimal levels for significant portions of their competitive or recreational activities.

The presence of EIB can be challenging to recognize clinically because symptoms are often nonspecific. Complete history and physical examination should be performed on each athlete with respiratory complaints associated with exercise. However, despite the value of a comprehensive history of the athlete with exertional dyspnea, the diagnosis of EIB based on self-reported symptoms alone has been shown to be inaccurate. Hallstrand and colleagues [18] found that screening history identified subjects with symptoms or a previous diagnosis suggestive of EIB in 40 % of the participants, but only 13 % of these persons actually had EIB after objective testing. Similarly, Rundell and associates [12] demonstrated that only 61 % EIB-positive athletes reported symptoms of EIB, whereas 45 % of athletes with normal objective testing reported symptoms. The poor predictive value of the history and physical examination in the evaluation of EIB strongly suggests that clinicians should perform objective diagnostic testing when there is a suspicion of EIB.

Other medical problems that can mimic EIB and that need to be considered in the initial evaluation of exertional dyspnea include vocal cord dysfunction, gastroesophageal reflux disease, and allergic rhinitis. Cardiac pathology such as arrhythmia, cardiomyopathy, and cardiac shunts are rarer,

Table 2.2 Mimics of EIB

Mimics of EIB
Vocal cord dysfunction
Gastroesophageal reflux disease
Allergic rhinitis
Cardiac disease

but need to be considered as well (Table 2.2). A comprehensive history and examination is recommended to help rule out these other disorders, and specific testing such as echocardiography may be required. A history of specific symptoms in particular environments or during specific activities should be elicited. Timing of symptom onset in relation to exercise and recovery is also helpful. A thorough family and occupational history should be obtained because a family history of asthma increases the risk for other family members developing asthma [19].

Objective testing should begin with spirometry before and after inhaled bronchodilator therapy, which will help identify athletes who have asthma. However, many people who experience EIB have normal baseline lung function [20]. In these patients, spirometry alone is not adequate to diagnose EIB. Significant numbers of false-negative results may occur if adequate exercise and environmental stress are not provided in the evaluation for EIB. In patients being evaluated for EIB who have a normal physical examination and normal spirometry, bronchoprovocation testing is recommended [21]. A positive bronchoprovocation test indicates the need for treatment of EIB. Specific tests have varying positive values, but in general, a change (usually $\geq 10\%$ decrease in forced expiratory volume in 1 s [FEV_1]) between pretest and posttest values is suggestive of EIB [22]. In a patient with persistent exercise-related symptoms and negative physical examination, spirometry, and bronchoprovocation testing, we recommend reconsidering alternative diagnoses.

Not all bronchoprovocation techniques are equally valuable or accurate in assessing EIB in athletes. The International Olympic Committee recommends eucapnic voluntary hyperventilation (EVH) challenge to document EIB in Olympians

[23]. EVH involves hyperventilation of a gas mixture of 5 % CO_2 and 21 % O_2 at a target ventilation rate of 85 % of the patient's maximal voluntary ventilation in 1 min (MVV). The MVV is usually calculated as 35 times the baseline FEV_1. The patient continues to hyperventilate for 6 min, and assessment of FEV_1 occurs at specified intervals up to 20 min after the test. This challenge test has been shown to have a high specificity [24] for EIB. EVH has also been shown to be more sensitive for detecting EIB than methacholine [4] or field- or lab-based exercise testing [24].

Field-exercise challenge tests that involve the athlete performing the sport in which he or she is normally involved and assessing FEV_1 after exercise have been shown to be less sensitive than EVH [25] and allow for little standardization of a protocol. Pharmacologic challenge tests, such as the methacholine challenge test, have been shown to have a lower sensitivity than EVH for detection of EIB in athletes [4] and are also not recommended for first-line evaluation of EIB.

Pharmacologic therapy for EIB has been studied extensively. The most common therapeutic recommendation to minimize or prevent symptoms of EIB is the prophylactic use of short-acting bronchodilators (selective β-adrenergic receptor agonists) such as albuterol shortly before exercise [21]. Treatment with two puffs of a short-acting β-agonist shortly before exercise (15 min) will provide peak bronchodilation in 15–60 min and protection from EIB for at least 3 h in most patients.

Long-acting bronchodilators work in a similar manner pharmacologically as short-acting bronchodilators; however, the bronchoprotection afforded by long-acting β-agonists has been shown to last up to 12 h, whereas that of short-acting agents is no longer significant by 4 h [26]. However, long-acting bronchodilators are not recommended as monotherapy in EIB given increased risk of adverse outcomes [21].

Inhaled corticosteroids are first-line therapy in terms of controller medications for patients who have chronic asthma and also experience EIB [27]. Airway inflammation is also often present in athletes who have EIB but do not have chronic asthma [14, 28]; therefore, inhaled corticosteroids are an effective medicine for treatment in this population as well.

Leukotriene modifiers have also been shown to be effective in treating EIB [29]. Leff and colleagues [30] evaluated the ability of montelukast, a leukotriene receptor antagonist, to protect asthmatic patients against EIB. Montelukast therapy offered significantly greater protection against EIB than placebo therapy and was also associated with a significant improvement in the maximal decrease in FEV_1 after exercise. In addition, tolerance to the medication and rebound worsening of lung function after discontinuation of treatment were not seen. Leukotriene modifiers are an effective second-line agent for treatment of EIB.

Mast cell stabilizers have been studied extensively for the prophylaxis of EIB. These medications prevent mast cell degranulation and subsequent histamine release. In a meta-analysis of the prevention of EIB in asthmatic patients, nedocromil sodium was found to improve FEV_1 by an average of 16 % and to shorten the duration of EIB symptoms to less than 10 min [31]. Although these agents are effective, they are often used as a second-line treatment because of their cost, lack of availability in the United States, and their decreased duration of action and efficacy compared with β_2-agonists.

Many athletes find that a period of precompetition warm-up reduces the symptoms of EIB that occur during their competitive activity. It has been shown by investigators that this refractory period does occur in some athletes with asthma and that athletes can be refractory to an exercise task performed within 2 h of an exercise warm-up [32, 33]. However, the refractory period has not been consistently proven across different athletic populations [34].

Other nonpharmacologic strategies can be employed to help reduce the frequency and severity of symptoms of EIB. Wearing a face mask warms and humidifies inspired air when outdoor conditions are cold and dry and is especially valuable to elite and recreational athletes who exercise in the winter [35]. In addition, people with knowledge of triggers (e.g., freshly cut grass) should attempt to avoid them if possible.

Dietary modifications (low-sodium diet, supplementation with vitamin C, lycopene, or fish oil) have all been studied with mixed results [21].

Vocal Cord Dysfunction

Vocal cord dysfunction (VCD) is an abnormal physiologic response to physical and emotional stimuli that culminates in an inappropriate adduction of the vocal cords during inspiration [36]. This leads to clinical manifestations including wheezing, stridor, and dyspnea [36]. Early in the history of this disease, it was believed to be entirely psychogenic in nature. Reports of the disease suggested that it was a conversion disorder, factitious disorder, or variant of Munchausen [36]. More recent research has also revealed, however, that many nonpsychiatric triggers exist as well including exercise [37]. The overall prevalence of this disorder in athletes is unknown; however, in one of the largest cohorts of 370 athletes, the estimated prevalence was roughly 5.1 % [38]. VCD commonly mimics and coexists with asthma and can be difficult to diagnose. Diagnosis typically requires direct visualization of the vocal cords during video laryngoscopy. Treatment typically entails controlling comorbid conditions exacerbating VCD and formal laryngeal control therapy under the care of experienced speech therapists.

Although the prevalence of VCD is unknown, it is estimated that between 11 and 59 % of the general population have VCD [39, 40]. Studies have shown that typically, patients are young females from 20 to 40 years old [41]. These patients tend to have type A personality traits, strong drive for personal achievement, and other psychological stressors. Despite being more common in females, VCD has been diagnosed in males as well and in all age groups [40, 41].

The most common presenting symptoms and physical exam findings are listed in Table 2.3. VCD is often misinterpreted as underlying asthma as it frequently presents as dyspnea, wheezing, chest tightness, and cough provoked by exercise. Exercise-induced voice changes, throat tightness, and frank stridor also can be

Table 2.3 Symptoms of VCD

Symptoms of VCD
Wheezing
Dyspnea
Stridor (predominantly inspiratory but can be expiratory)
Chest pain/tightness (more common in EIB)
Neck or throat tightness (more common in VCD)
Cough
Hoarseness
Failure to respond to standard therapy for bronchospasm (inhaled beta-agonists, corticosteroids)

Table 2.4 Common comorbid conditions associated with VCD

Common comorbid conditions associated with VCD[a]
Asthma, most common—28–74%
Gastroesophageal reflux disease—17–56%
Allergic rhinitis—43%
Psychiatric disease—17%

[a]Estimates of prevalence of comorbid conditions were drawn from two of the larger cohort studies evaluating patients with VCD [40, 44]

signs of vocal cord dysfunction. The presentation in athletes is similar to that of nonathletes, in that wheezing and inspiratory stridor are the most common symptoms. For athletes, however, typically the symptoms of VCD manifest during and interfere with exercise and aerobic performance. Symptoms typically are self-reported in this cohort of patients, and VCD is commonly misdiagnosed as EIB.

In contrast to exercise-induced bronchoconstriction (EIB), symptoms can be very abrupt in onset and resolution. It may only require a very brief amount of activity to trigger an episode of vocal cord dysfunction, whereas it often takes 15–20 min of exercise to trigger an episode of EIB.

The pathogenesis or etiology of VCD appears to be multifaceted. Review of the current literature suggests that there are many inciting factors that can lead to VCD. However, it should be noted that none of these proposed mechanisms have been prospectively proven in the literature. The most common comorbid conditions associated with VCD are listed below in Table 2.2.

It has been suggested that for patients with psychologically mediated VCD, there is a dysregulation of the central respiratory mechanism that is triggered by anxiety or panic [42].

One study demonstrated that nearly half of all patients diagnosed with VCD also have concomitant asthma [43]. This substantial overlap may be a result of the fact that gastroesophageal reflux disease and rhinitis are frequent comorbid conditions in patients with asthma, and these conditions can also confound or exacerbate underlying vocal cord dysfunction (Table 2.4).

Another common mechanism that has been proposed involves irritation of the larynx which results in laryngeal hyperactivity. This laryngeal hyperactivity can be a consequence of acid exposure in patients with gastroesophageal reflux disease (GERD) or secretions from the nasal cavity in patients with sinus disease or rhinitis. It is believed that the acid or nasal secretions result in irritation of the larynx, which in turns alters the closure reflex of the glottis. This has also been seen in response to noxious olfactory stimuli in patients with chronic rhinosinusitis [45]. This abnormal glottic closure can happen at rest, but may be more likely to occur when the upper airway is irritated by large volumes of air passing through it during vigorous exercise.

Multiple difficulties arise when attempting to diagnose VCD. One of the most common barriers to diagnosis is that VCD often masquerades as asthma. It has been shown that VCD alone may cause wheezing; however, a significant proportion of patients diagnosed with VCD also have concomitant asthma. Unfortunately, no formal standard algorithm exists between centers to allow for uniform diagnosis, adding to the clinical challenge represented by VCD [43].

The initial step in evaluation begins with symptom recognition. Given the strong personal drive and committed nature of athletes, some patients may not identify that they have symptoms. Instead, they may blame training setbacks on themselves or other external reasons and fail to recognize that the exercise limitations may indeed be secondary to an underlying issue such as VCD or EIB. Once symptom recognition occurs, then the initial step would involve a history and physical exam A. After determining that the patients' symptoms are suggestive of possible EIB or VCD, the next step in management is pulmonary function testing. Pulmonary function testing includes spirometry with a flow volume loop, lung volumes, and a diffusion capacity. The lung volumes and diffusion capacity will allow the clinician to rule out any occult pulmonary parenchymal or pulmonary vascular process that could contribute to dyspnea on exertion. Spirometry will help to identify obstructive lung disease, such as asthma, but does not completely rule it out if testing is normal.

In the evaluation of VCD, the flow volume loop will sometimes be the first clue that the patient may have VCD. Figure 2.1 illustrates an example of a normal flow volume loop, and Fig. 2.2 shows a flow volume loop from a patient with VCD. At first glance, the VCD loop appears normal, but on closer inspection, the inspiratory limb is flattened, suggesting a limitation to inspired airflow. This has been referred to as the "sail sign," or "up arrow," as the shape of the flow volume loop appears to point upward. This pattern suggests a variable extrathoracic obstruction. While such a pattern is not diagnostic of VCD, VCD is the most common disease to cause this pattern on the flow volume loop.

If pulmonary function testing is normal, bronchoprovocation testing should occur next as

outlined earlier in this chapter. If bronchoprovocation testing is nondiagnostic for EIB or if clinical suspicion for vocal cord dysfunction still remains, direct visualization during video laryngoscopy should be performed at this point.

To confirm the diagnosis of suspected VCD, direct visualization during video laryngoscopy is used. This also serves to rule out other causes of variable extrathoracic obstruction, such as structural lesions. Diagnostic criteria for VCD on videolaryngostroboscopy (VLS) include the following [41, 43]:

1. Adduction of the vocal cords during inspiration (or both inspiration and expiration)
2. >50 % closure of the cords
3. Diamond-shaped "chink" (narrow opening at the base of cords) in the posterior one-third of the vocal cords, not always present

Generally speaking, otolaryngologists perform the VLS exam, usually in the office, as an outpatient procedure. The VLS exam also allows for the physician to evaluate the presence of exacerbating or contributing factors such as

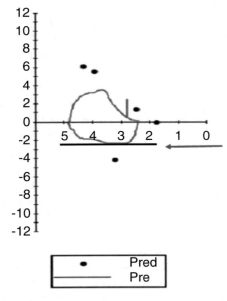

Fig. 2.2 Flow volume loop suggestive of VCD. *Red arrow* points to the *black line* below the expiratory limb of the loop. The flattening of the expiratory limb suggests a variable extrathoracic obstruction

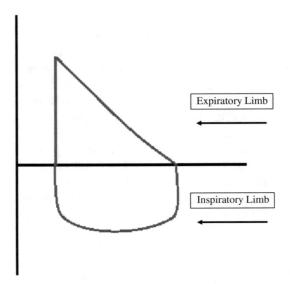

Fig. 2.1 Normal flow volume loop

reflux disease, vocal cord polyps, or chronic sinusitis. In patients with suspected exercise-induced VCD, the VLS exam should occur after a period of exercise in an attempt to induce an episode of VCD. This will help to reduce the false-negative rate of VLS in exercise-induced VCD if simply performed at rest.

The treatment for VCD has two main components. The first important step in treating VCD is identifying and treating any comorbid conditions that may exacerbate or cause VCD. This includes ruling out concomitant exercise-induced bronchospasm or exercise-induced asthma with bronchoprovocation testing. Also treating existing gastroesophageal reflux, allergic rhinitis and chronic rhinosinusitis will also improve VCD. For athletes in particular, overall hydration status may also improve VCD [46].

The second component, of treatment for VCD is laryngeal control therapy (LCT) [46, 47]. Speech therapists are responsible for administering LCT. This involves an overarching theme of retraining the respiratory muscles to focus more on abdominal breathing and less on tight/constricted pharyngeal breathing. Some of the techniques used to aid in retraining include biofeedback, direct visualization, and practice exercises.

During biofeedback, the patient is allowed to view their vocal cords (transmitted to a display screen via video laryngoscopy), while speech therapy teaches them to relax their pharyngeal and laryngeal muscles while taking deep breaths. Typically, the patient inhales through the nose and exhales through pursed lips. They are told to focus on expanding their abdomen during inspiration, and then relaxing their abdomen, neck, and shoulders during expiration. The purpose behind biofeedback is that the patient is able to see when they perform the maneuver correctly and create internal feedback loop to perfect the technique. The breathing exercises include diaphragmatic breathing, "sniffing" respirations, and tightening/relaxation exercises of the abdominal muscles.

Direct visualization can refer to the above biofeedback technique, but it can also refer to self-monitoring in a mirror during breathing exercises. This allows the patient to visualize their neck and abdominal musculature during the exercises and monitor for correct technique.

After the patient is taught LCT, the patient is taught to practice these exercises 3–5 times per day at home. They are also encouraged to use these exercises during activity, at the first sign of dyspnea or throat tightness, signaling onset of VCD.

The overall prognosis for VCD is excellent. The majority of patients respond to the interventions listed above. In a study evaluating the success of therapy in athletes, it was shown that 69 % of patients had improvement in symptoms [47]. It should be noted that recurrence of symptoms is common and patients should be warned about such recurrences before they occur to mitigate their psychological consequences. However, by continuing the LCT exercises even when asymptomatic, recurrences will be less frequent and more easily controlled [48].

References

1. Parsons JP, Craig TJ, Stoloff SW, Hayden ML, Ostrom NK, Eid NS, et al. Impact of exercise-related respiratory symptoms in adults with asthma: exercise-Induced Bronchospasm Landmark National Survey. Allergy Asthma Proc. 2011;32(6):431–7.
2. Gotshall RW. Exercise-induced bronchoconstriction. Drugs. 2002;62(12):1725–39.
3. Rundell KW, Jenkinson DM. Exercise-induced bronchospasm in the elite athlete. Sports Med. 2002;32(9):583–600.
4. Holzer K, Anderson SD, Douglass J. Exercise in elite summer athletes: challenges for diagnosis. J Allergy Clin Immunol. 2002;110(3):374–80.
5. Wilber RL, Rundell KW, Szmedra L, Jenkinson DM, Im J, Drake SD. Incidence of exercise-induced bronchospasm in Olympic winter sport athletes. Med Sci Sports Exerc. 2000;32(4):732–7.
6. Voy RO. The U.S. Olympic Committee experience with exercise-induced bronchospasm, 1984. Med Sci Sports Exerc. 1986;18(3):328–30.
7. Mannix ET, Roberts M, Fagin DP, Reid B, Farber MO. The prevalence of airways hyperresponsiveness in members of an exercise training facility. J Asthma. 2003;40(4):349–55.
8. Rupp NT, Guill MF, Brudno DS. Unrecognized exercise-induced bronchospasm in adolescent athletes. Am J Dis Child. 1992;146(8):941–4.
9. Barnes PJ. Poorly perceived asthma. Thorax. 1992; 47(6):408–9.

10. Barnes PJ. Blunted perception and death from asthma. N Engl J Med. 1994;330(19):1383–4.

11. Parsons JP, Kaeding C, Phillips G, Jarjoura D, Wadley G, Mastronarde JG. Prevalence of exercise-induced bronchospasm in a cohort of varsity college athletes. Med Sci Sports Exerc. 2007;39(9):1487–92.

12. Rundell KW, Im J, Mayers LB, Wilber RL, Szmedra L, Schmitz HR. Self-reported symptoms and exercise-induced asthma in the elite athlete. Med Sci Sports Exerc. 2001;33(2):208–13.

13. Holzer K, Brukner P. Screening of athletes for exercise-induced bronchoconstriction. Clin J Sport Med. 2004;14:134–8.

14. Helenius IJ, Rytila P, Metso T, Haahtela T, Venge P, Tikkanen HO. Respiratory symptoms, bronchial responsiveness, and cellular characteristics of induced sputum in elite swimmers. Allergy. 1998;53(4):346–52.

15. Rundell KW. High levels of airborne ultrafine and fine particulate matter in indoor ice arenas. Inhal Toxicol. 2003;15(3):237–50.

16. Parsons JP, Mastronarde JG. Exercise-induced bronchoconstriction in athletes. Chest. 2005;128(6):3966–74.

17. Brudno DS, Wagner JM, Rupp NT. Length of postexercise assessment in the determination of exercise-induced bronchospasm. Ann Allergy. 1994;73(3):227–31.

18. Hallstrand TS, Curtis JR, Koepsell TD, Martin DP, Schoene RB, Sullivan SD, et al. Effectiveness of screening examinations to detect unrecognized exercise-induced bronchoconstriction. J Pediatr. 2002;141(3):343–9.

19. London SJ, James Gauderman W, Avol E, Rappaport EB, Peters JM. Family history and the risk of early-onset persistent, early-onset transient, and late-onset asthma. Epidemiology. 2001;12(5):577–83.

20. Rundell KW, Wilber RL, Szmedra L, Jenkinson DM, Mayers LB, Im J. Exercise-induced asthma screening of elite athletes: field versus laboratory exercise challenge. Med Sci Sports Exerc. 2000;32(2):309–16.

21. Parsons JP, Hallstrand TS, Mastronarde JG, Kaminsky DA, Rundell KW, Hull JH, et al. An official American Thoracic Society clinical practice guideline: exercise-induced bronchoconstriction. Am J Respir Crit Care Med. 2013;187(9):1016–27.

22. Crapo RO, Casaburi R, Coates AL, Enright PL, Hankinson JL, Irvin CG, et al. Guidelines for methacholine and exercise challenge testing-1999. This official statement of the American Thoracic Society was adopted by the ATS Board of Directors, July 1999. Am J Respir Crit Care Med. 2000;161(1):309–29.

23. IOC Medical Commission. Beta2 adrenoceptor agonists and the Olympic Games in Beijing. 2008. http://multimedia.olympic.org/pdf/en_report_1302.pdf.

24. Eliasson AH, Phillips YY, Rajagopal KR, Howard RS. Sensitivity and specificity of bronchial provocation testing. An evaluation of four techniques in exercise-induced bronchospasm. Chest. 1992;102(2):347–55.

25. Mannix ET, Manfredi F, Farber MO. A comparison of two challenge tests for identifying exercise-induced bronchospasm in figure skaters. Chest. 1999;115(3):649–53.

26. Bronsky EA, Yegen U, Yeh CM, Larsen LV, Della Cioppa G. Formoterol provides long-lasting protection against exercise-induced bronchospasm. Ann Allergy Asthma Immunol. 2002;89(4):407–12.

27. Expert Panel Report 3 (EPR-3): guidelines for the Diagnosis and Management of Asthma-Summary Report 2007. J Allergy Clin Immunol. 2007;120 Suppl 5:S94–138.

28. Parsons JP, Baran CP, Phillips G, Jarjoura D, Kaeding C, Bringardner B, et al. Airway inflammation in exercise-induced bronchospasm occurring in athletes without asthma. J Asthma. 2008;45(5):363–7.

29. Philip G, Villaran C, Pearlman DS, Loeys T, Dass SB, Reiss TF. Protection against exercise-induced bronchoconstriction two hours after a single oral dose of montelukast. J Asthma. 2007;44(3):213–7.

30. Leff JA, Busse WW, Pearlman D, Bronsky EA, Kemp J, Hendeles L, et al. Montelukast, a leukotriene-receptor antagonist, for the treatment of mild asthma and exercise-induced bronchoconstriction. N Engl J Med. 1998;339(3):147–52.

31. Kelly KD, Spooner CH, Rowe BH. Nedocromil sodium versus cromoglycate for the pre-treatment of exercise induced bronchoconstriction in asthma. Cochrane Database Syst Rev. 2000;2, CD002169.

32. Anderson SD, Schoeffel RE. Respiratory heat and water loss during exercise in patients with asthma. Effect of repeated exercise challenge. Eur J Respir Dis. 1982;63(5):472–80.

33. McKenzie DC, McLuckie SL, Stirling DR. The protective effects of continuous and interval exercise in athletes with exercise-induced asthma. Med Sci Sports Exerc. 1994;26(8):951–6.

34. Rundell KW, Spiering BA, Judelson DA, Wilson MH. Bronchoconstriction during cross-country skiing: is there really a refractory period? Med Sci Sports Exerc. 2003;35(1):18–26.

35. Schachter EN, Lach E, Lee M. The protective effect of a cold weather mask on exercised-induced asthma. Ann Allergy. 1981;46(1):12–6.

36. Maschka DA, Bauman NM, McCray Jr PB, Hoffman HT, Karnell MP, Smith RJ. A classification scheme for paradoxical vocal cord motion. Laryngoscope. 1997;107(11 Pt 1):1429–35.

37. Newman KB, Mason 3rd UG, Schmaling KB. Clinical features of vocal cord dysfunction. Am J Respir Crit Care Med. 1995;152(4 Pt 1):1382–6.

38. Rundell KW, Spiering BA. Inspiratory stridor in elite athletes. Chest. 2003;123(2):468–74.

39. Doshi DR, Weinberger MM. Long-term outcome of vocal cord dysfunction. Ann Allergy Asthma Immunol. 2006;96(6):794–9.

40. Morris MJ, Christopher KL. Diagnostic criteria for the classification of vocal cord dysfunction. Chest. 2010;138(5):1213–23.

41. Wilson JJ, Wilson EM. Practical management: vocal cord dysfunction in athletes. Clin J Sport Med. 2006;16(4):357–60.

42. Balkissoon R, Kenn K. Asthma: vocal cord dysfunction (VCD) and other dysfunctional breathing disorders. Semin Respir Crit Care Med. 2012; 33(6):595–605.

43. Forrest LA, Husein T, Husein O. Paradoxical vocal cord motion: classification and treatment. Laryngoscope. 2012;122(4):844–53.

44. Parsons JP, Benninger C, Hawley MP, Philips G, Forrest LA, Mastronarde JG. Vocal cord dysfunction: beyond severe asthma. Respir Med. 2010;104(4):504–9.

45. Bucca C, Rolla G, Scappaticci E, Chiampo F, Bugiani M, Magnano M, et al. Extrathoracic and intrathoracic airway responsiveness in sinusitis. J Allergy Clin Immunol. 1995;95(1 Pt 1):52–9.

46. Newsham KR, Klaben BK, Miller VJ, Saunders JE. Paradoxical vocal-cord dysfunction: management in athletes. J Athl Train. 2002;37(3):325–8.

47. Marcinow AM, Thompson J, Chiang T, Forrest LA, deSilva BW. Paradoxical vocal fold motion disorder in the elite athlete: experience at a large division I university. Laryngoscope. 2014;124(6):1425–30.

48. Matrka L. Paradoxic vocal fold movement disorder. Otolaryngol Clin North Am. 2014;47(1):135–46.

Evaluation and Treatment of Heat- and Altitude-Related Illness

3

Matthew Gammons, Tarry Bolognani,
and Matt Howland

Heat-related illnesses are common worldwide, accounting for more than 600 deaths annually [1]. A heat-related illness can be defined as a pathophysiologic process that occurs to the body from exposure to elevated environmental temperatures [2]. Sporting activities, particularly endurance events, performed in the heat may increase the risk of heat-related illness, and in this setting, the condition is defined as exertional heat illness (EHI) [3]. EHI may present with symptoms ranging from mild to severe and can potentially become fatal due to an elevate core body temperature [1, 3, 4]. The body maintains a temperature of 37 °C during homeostasis, when the bodily systems are balanced. When body temperature increases at a faster rate than the body is able to remove heat, an individual begins to suffer from a heat-related illness. As the core temperature increases, cells can no longer function properly; cellular proteins start to denature, metabolic functions stop, and the body beings to shut down.

The body regulates temperature through a process called thermoregulation. Thermoregulation allows for heat to be transported from the skin to the environment through four mechanisms [5]. These four mechanisms include conduction, convection, radiation, and evaporation. Conduction is the transfer of heat from a cooler object to a warmer object through direct contact [6]. Convection is the transfer of heat via air circulation or water molecules across the body surface [6]. Radiation is the transfer of heat energy via electromagnetic radiation or infrared rays [5]. Evaporation is the most common heat transfer mechanism; it refers to the transfer of heat between objects that requires energy to change phases. The body releases sweat through the skin as a liquid, which then evaporates off the skin as a vapor when attempting to decrease core body temperature [5]. When an individual is exercising in a hot environment, the body attempts to regulate its own temperature, mainly through evaporation. This is why sweating occurs; the hypothalamus detects elevation in core body temperature and triggers sweating to occur, allowing for heat to dissipate [5]. Heat illnesses occur when the body can no longer cool itself through heat transfer, and body core temperature becomes elevated due impeding physiological functions.

Endurance athletes often participate in hot and humid environments for prolonged periods, and this makes them susceptible to exertional heat illness. Although endurance athletes are physically fit and well conditioned, this alone is not protective of heat illness, and heat can be one of the biggest dangers to endurance athletes [7].

M. Gammons (✉) T. Bolognani • M. Howland
Vermont Orthopaedic Clinic, Rutland Regional
Medical Center, 158 Chapel Ridge Place, Rutland,
VT 05701, USA
e-mail: mgammons@rrmc.org

© Springer International Publishing Switzerland 2016
T.L. Miller (ed.), *Endurance Sports Medicine*, DOI 10.1007/978-3-319-32982-6_3

While some acclimatization is possible, it often takes several weeks to begin adjusting to hot and humid conditions. Early recognition of the symptoms of heat illness is crucial. If symptoms escalate before body cooling occurs, a mild heat illness can turn into heat stroke which is considered a medical emergency [4].

Heat illness classifications progress from mild to severe; the most severe can be life-threatening [3, 4, 8] (Fig. 3.1). The mildest forms of heat illness include heat rash (prickly heat or miliaria rubra), heat edema, and heat syncope. The important distinguishing feature of these three types of heat illness is that the core body temperature is not significantly elevated. Heat rash occurs as pinpoint-popular erythematous or patches of small red bumps appearing, commonly underneath clothing [8]. When there is profuse sweating, the sweat ducts on the skin become saturated and clog, resulting in the leakage of eccrine sweat into the epidermis of the skin creating the rash [8]. Heat edema is described by soft tissue swelling usually occurring in the lower extremities. Vasodilation occurs as the body tries to release heat and can lead to pooling of fluid in the interstitial spaces. Heat syncope refers to a heat illness categorized by a person's blood pressure falling while in a standing position [3, 8, 9]. It causes an individual to become extremely light-headed and dizzy and to lose postural control due to venous pooling in the lower extremities. It commonly occurs after stopping exercise. An individual suffering from heat syncope is usually able to recover their mental status quickly after being placed in a supine position allowing blood to flow back to the central nervous systems (CNS) [3, 8, 9]. Knowledge of these mild heat illnesses, understanding of the symptoms, and proper treatment can help to keep heat illnesses under control.

Moderate heat-related illnesses include heat cramps and heat exhaustion. Heat cramps are common after excessive heat exposure causing muscle spasms and cramps. Heat cramps have been thought to occur due to profuse sweating and prolonged exercise with lack of proper hydration being a contributing factor. The term exercise-associated muscle cramps (EAMC) better fits this condition since exertional cramping can occur in the presence of lower environmental and near-normal core temperatures [8, 9]. Therefore, the exact mechanism of cramping is not completely understood, may have a centrally mediated component, and is likely multifactorial [10]. Heat exhaustion has several contributing factors but is defined as inability to exercise effectively in the heat [9]. Heat exhaustion is typically characterized by an elevated body temperature between 37 and 40 °C as well as fatigue and dizziness [8, 9]. Other symptoms may include nausea, vomiting, fainting, and cold clammy skin. If an individual is experiencing these symptoms, it is critical to evaluate an individual's core temperature and neurological status. Cooling the body down is imperative, helping alleviate the risk of heat exhaustion developing into heat stroke. If moderate heat illnesses are not diagnosed and treated promptly, they can develop into more serious heat illnesses and potentially become fatal.

Heat injury, also commonly known as heat stroke, is the most severe heat illness. If unrecognized, heat exhaustion can progress into heat stroke and become a serious problem [8, 9]. Heat injury is categorized by an elevated core body temperature of 40 °C or more, coinciding with dysfunction of the central nervous system. The body temperature rises to a critical level that causes cellular and systematic functions to occur [1, 2, 9]. Symptoms of heat injury usually include irritability, change in mental status, hot skin, and confusion. During the acute phase, the body responds to heat stress by releasing interleukins, cytokines, and proteins as an inflammatory response [1]. The release of these proteins alters blood flow, causes injury to tissues, and impairs the body's ability to maintain thermoregulation. Based on pathological differences, heat stroke can be divided into two categories: exertional heat injury (EHI) and classical heat injury (CHI) [2]. EHI occurs due to strenuous activities or occupations that expose individuals to heat during exertion [2, 9]. These activities can include marathons, long-distance cycling, obstacle course races, etc., and occupations include firefighters, military personnel, and individuals who are constantly working in hot environments. Environmental factors cause an increase in internal

HEAT ILLNESS CLASSIFICATION	SYMPTOMS	BODY TEMPERATURE
Heat edema	Swelling in the lower extremities	Normal - 37°C
Heat rash	Skin eruptions over clothed areas	Normal - 37°C
Heat syncope	Dizziness, body weakness Loss of postural control	Normal - 37°C
Heat cramps	Painful muscle contractions (calf, quadriceps) Muscle firmness	Normal - 37°C
Heat exhaustion	Dizziness, fatigue, fainting, nausea, vomiting, headache Flushed skin, profuse sweating, cold clammy skin	Slightly elevated-37°C - 40°C
Heat stroke/injury	Hot skin, possible perspiration, confusion, irritability, coma Multi-organ failure	Elevated > 40°C

Fig. 3.1 Heat illness classification chart

temperature that the body cannot regulate, leading to heat stroke. CHI occurs when heat cannot be dissipated from the body due to impaired physiological mechanisms [2]. An individual can be predisposed to this impairment if they have metabolic or cardiac conditions where the body cannot regulate its own temperature because of decreased cardiac function. Individuals also at risk for CHI include people who suffer from substance abuse and psychiatric or physical challenges because they are unable to remove themselves from a hot environment. Endurance athletes may be at increased risk as they often push themselves for

long periods in hot environments and may not recognize the symptoms of more serious heat illness. The treatment of the two is the same: reduce heat and cool the body as quickly as possible [8].

A vital measurement to take into consideration if an individual is suspected to be suffering from a heat-related illness is their core body temperature. An increase in body temperature correlates with the severity of heat illness an individual may have. The most accurate way to measure this is through the use of a rectal thermometer [9]. Body temperature can also be measured by oral, axillary, skin sensing, and tympanic membrane methods, but these methods often do not reflect core temperature well and may underestimate the severity [2].

The treatment of heat-related illnesses is indicative of what severity of heat illness an individual has. Individuals showing signs of mild heat illnesses may suffer from mild dehydration. The individual should be removed from a hot environment and given a wet towel to place on the forehead, neck, groin, and axillae area [9, 11]. It is important to replace lost fluids with sodium-containing fluids (sports drinks are good to consume during the recovery of a heat illness especially in endurance athletes who are expending energy and losing fluids for the long periods of time). For moderate heat illnesses such as exercise-associated muscle cramps, athletes should stop activity and rehydrate with high-sodium sports drinks. The athlete should then do light stretching of the muscle along with light massage. If an athlete is suffering from brief fainting and dizziness, and there is no elevated core body temperature, they are most likely experiencing heat syncope. The individual should be moved to a shaded area, placed in a supine position with their legs elevated [9]. The body should also be cooled down with cold cloths. Vital signs should be measured so the heat condition severity does not increase. When dealing with an individual who is potentially suffering from heat exhaustion, with slight cognitive changes, rectal core temperature should be measured if possible [9]. It is important to have prompt recognition of these symptoms and understand how to stabilize the patient in a cool environment [9, 11]. Excessive clothes should be removed; they should be taken to a shaded area and cooled with cold cloths, ice bags, and fans. Once cooling has begun, fluid replacement should take place as well. When dealing with an individual who is suffering from suspected heat exhaustion, vital signs should be measured including blood pressure, heart rate, and body temperature (rectally), and cognitive function should be assessed [9, 11]. If the individual's status remains the same or worsens within 20–30 min after administering treatment, advanced medical care needs to take place to keep the individual's case from advancing to heat stroke [9, 11]. Heat injury is the most severe heat illness and is considered a medical emergency. This condition must be recognized and treatment administered promptly; rapid and aggressive cooling is key in preventing fatality in heat stroke cases [9, 11]. When dealing with an individual suspected to be suffering from exertional heat stroke, rectal temperature should be measured [9, 11]. The body temperature should be lowered as quickly as possible; clothes should be removed, and the body should be submerged into a tub of cold water. Submersion should not be delayed for clothing or equipment removal as this can be done in the water if necessary. Cold water immersion is the most effective and fastest method in lowering body temperature [9, 12]. If full immersion is not possible, then partial immersion, ice and/or cold towels, or cold water dousing should be initiated. This treatment should be on-site; time may be lost, and the condition may worsen when transferring an individual to the hospital. Vital signs should be measured continuously during recovery along with rectal temperature. When the temperature returns to 38.3–38.9 °C, the individual can be removed from the cold water immersion [9]. An individual experiencing exertional heat stroke should see a physician, so their vital signs and fluid replacement can be monitored by a medical professional in a controlled environment.

The best treatment for all types of heat illness is prevention [9, 11]. Exercising in high heat and humidity are major risk factors of developing a heat-related illness. Coaches and athletes must be aware of the risk of exercise-induced heat illness and understand predisposing factors [9, 11]. It is important for athletes, coaches, and medical staff to be aware that heat acclimatization can occur and will take athletes up to several weeks to fully adjust. For traveling athletes, scheduling may not allow this process to occur, so close monitoring and accommodations are important. Some predisposing factors are uncontrollable such as outdoor temperature and the environment; these are known as external factors [8]. These factors may also include excessive clothing or equipment used during training and activity level of the athlete or individual. Clothing worn by athletes participating in the heat should not restrict heat evaporation [7]. Other predisposing factors such as internal factors are controllable as they relate to the athlete [8]. These factors include medical conditions, hydration status, recent illnesses, sleeping habits, sun exposure, and body weight conditions, among others. Dehydration is a major component in developing a heat-related illness. Dehydration occurs when the body experiences inadequate fluid consumption and excessive fluid loss [8]. Athletes especially runners who are recovering from illness should not participate in hot environments [7]. When recovering from illness, an individual is more susceptible to developing heat-induced conditions due to inadequate fluid retention and recovering altered body functions.

Using the wet-bulb globe temperature (WBGT) to assess environmental conditions can help to prevent heat illnesses due to environmental factors [8]. This device is used to measure ambient temperature, radiant heat, and humidity [11]. The calculation of WBGT is as follows [2]:

$$\text{WBGT index} = (\text{DBT} \times 0.1)$$
$$+ (\text{WBT} \times 0.7) + (\text{GT} \times 0.2)$$

DBT = dry-bulb temperature, refers to true ambient air temperature; WBT = wet-bulb temperature is measured by covering a thermometer with a white cloth kept wet by wicking; GT = globe temperature is a measure of radiant heat from the sun. WBGT above 27.8 °C refers to a high-risk environment for developing a heat illness. WBGT between 22.8 and 27.8 °C refers to a high-risk environment, and a WBGT between 18.3 and 22.8 °C refers to a moderate-risk environment. A WBGT of 18.3 °C or below refers to a low-risk environment for developing a heat-related illness [2]. This measuring device can help to determine if the environment endurance athletes are participating is safe. Knowing the heat and humidity measures along with limiting predisposing factors, heat illnesses can be prevented and controlled.

Return to activity for athlete should be guided by the severity of the illness. For mild to moderate illness, return to activity may begin once symptoms have resolved although same day return is not generally recommended [9]. For those athletes who experience heat stroke/injury, the return is less clear. There are no evidence-based guidelines, but most recommend the athlete be asymptomatic, have normal blood work, and then may begin a gradual return to activity. For endurance athletes who will be returning to competition in hot environments, consideration can be given to heat-tolerance testing. This testing however still has limitations and should be used with caution and under supervision of an experienced healthcare provider [9].

With the increase in interest in endurance events worldwide, athletes may be exposed to high altitudes. Athletes who live at lower altitudes need to be aware of the issues of competing and training at altitude as high-altitude illness (HAI) may be performance limiting and even life-threatening. Most endurance events at altitude will be held in the high range (1500–3500 m). At this level, with time to acclimatize, the risk of HAI and performance deficits can be limited. Very high altitude (3500–5500 m) and extreme altitude (>5500 m) require additional acclimatization and the use of adjunct equipment. HAI is used to define a wide category of both cerebral and pulmonary conditions that effect individuals who are unacclimatized and ascend to altitude too quickly. High-altitude headache (HAH), acute mountain sickness (AMS), and high-altitude cerebral edema (HACE) refer to conditions affecting cerebral function. High-altitude pulmonary edema (HAPE) refers to the condition that affects pulmonary function [13].

Anytime an unacclimatized individual ascends to an altitude of above 2500 m, there is a risk to develop some form of HAI. However, both clinical evidence and prior studies have shown that individuals who are considered susceptible for HAI can develop both AMS and HAPE at elevations much lower, as low as 2000 m [14].

The primary risk factors in developing HAI are rate of ascent and altitude achieved, especially sleeping altitude, in unacclimatized individuals. Other factors influencing the onset of HAI include living at low altitude and physical exertion upon reaching altitude. Also a previous history of HAI puts an individual at higher risk for developing symptoms on subsequent visits to altitude. Children and adults under age 50 appear to be equally susceptible to experiencing HAI; however, that risk appears to drop after the age of 50 [13]. While individuals with high fitness levels do show an increased ability to perform exertion at altitude, there is no evidence that it confers a benefit and reduces the risk of developing HAI [15].

Identifying HAI is sometimes difficult as the symptoms of early illness are subtle and very nonspecific. Oftentimes, early stages of HAI can be confused with dehydration, fatigue, hypothermia, flulike illness, and migraine or be mistaken for an alcohol hangover. As there is no specific test for early-stage HAI, subjective reporting of symptoms is used based on the Lake Louise Consensus Criteria (see Table 3.1) [15, 16].

(High-altitude headache (HAH) is usually the first, and most common, symptom that susceptible individuals will experience as they ascend to altitude. Oftentimes, HAH is the only adverse effect that people will complain of when exposed to altitude. HAH is the primary symptom of AMS and is described as being severe, throbbing, and bitemporal [17]. Each year in the United States, millions of people ascend to high altitude. Of these individuals, up to 80 % will report experiencing a high-altitude headache [18]. HAH can be treated by a variety of medications. Over-the-counter NSAID treatment using ibuprofen has been shown to be the standard treatment of HAH and the benchmark that all other treatments are measured [18, 19]. Both aspirin and naproxen have been proven to be effective in treating HAH as well [20, 21]. However, NSAIDs carry the risk of gastrointestinal side effects including nausea, which is a defining feature of AMS. In individuals

with a history of GI bleeding or with allergies or sensitivities to that prior, NSAID use in combination with prior regular exercise in young men may increase the risk of developing HAPE. Additionally, there may be an increased risk of exertional hyponatremia in endurance athletes who use NSAIDs although this risk is not currently understood or quantified [22]. As an alternative to NSAIDs, acetaminophen has been shown to be as effective as ibuprofen in treating HAH and does not have the same risk of side effects as most NSAIDs do not seem to increase the risk of HAPE [17].

AMS is a condition of nonspecific, subjective symptoms that occurs in unacclimatized individuals ascending to altitude of above 2500 m. While the symptoms of AMS can oftentimes be severe and extremely limiting of activity in the onset, typically they will resolve within 24–48 h as the body begins to acclimatize to altitude [23]. The Lake Louise Consensus Group defines AMS as the presence of a headache and the presence of one or more of the following symptoms: nausea, vomiting, anorexia, dizziness, lassitude, fatigue, or insomnia (see Table 3.1) [15, 16, 24]. Physical exam of individuals experiencing AMS is generally unremarkable [25]. Symptoms of AMS generally appear within 6–12 h after arriving at altitude but can develop in as little as 2 h. Likewise, symptoms of AMS may take an upward of 36 h to 4 days before symptoms develop [26–28]. Several studies have shown rates of occurrence of HAI to range from 9 % to as high as 58 %. There has been shown to be a higher occurrence of illness as the level of altitude increases [28].

HACE is a potentially life-threatening condition that is commonly considered to be the end

Table 3.1 Lake Louise Consensus Score for AMS and HACE

Symptom score	Headache	Gastrointestinal symptoms	Fatigue and weakness	Dizziness and light-headedness	Difficulty sleeping
0	None	None	None	None	None
1	Mild	Poor appetite or nausea	Mild	Mild	Did not sleep as well as usual
2	Moderate	Moderate nausea or vomiting	Moderate	Moderate	Woke many times, poor sleep
3	Severe	Severe nausea or vomiting	Severe	Severe	Unable to sleep at all

Lake Louise AMS Score mild AMS (2–4) moderate–severe AMS (5–15)

stage of AMS. While AMS is a completely subjective diagnosis, HACE is very much a clinical diagnosis [13, 15, 24]. Most commonly, HACE develops from AMS over a course of 24–48 h [29]. Although rare, HACE is most common with a rapid ascent to higher than 3000 m. The mean onset of HACE occurred at 4730 m, but occurred at a lower altitude of 3920 m in individuals with concurrent HAPE [30]. In those individuals suffering from HAPE, severe hypoxemia can rapidly transition AMS to HACE [24]. The primary symptoms of HACE are confusion and ataxic gait. Other symptoms may include fatigue, apathy and lassitude, anorexia, and nausea. Physical findings include any of the symptoms that are present with AMS, retinal hemorrhage, papilledema, and neurological deficits [15, 24]. If left untreated, HACE can progress to coma and death.

The exact pathophysiology of AMS and HACE is unclear despite many studies to understand the mechanism behind them. While HACE is considered to be the end stage of AMS, there is uncertainty as to whether AMS and HACE share the same pathophysiology. This in part is due to the relatively low numbers of HACE cases available to research. As such, many conclusions concerning AMS and HACE have come from the similarities of reported symptoms from both sever AMS and beginning HACE [23].

The main component of high-altitude illness from a physiological standpoint is the decrease in barometric pressure as altitude increases combined with the decrease in the partial pressure of oxygen (PO_2). As the inspired PO_2 decreases, so too does the PO_2 in the arterial blood leading to tissue hypoxia [31, 32]. Features of AMS include hypoventilation, impaired gas exchange, increased sympathetic activity, fluid retention and redistribution, and elevated intracranial pressure [13].

Investigators have studied the pathophysiology of AMS and HACE and have developed a model to explain the mechanism behind them. In their proposed model, hypoxemia causes neurohumoral and hemodynamic responses that raise cerebral blood flow, change the permeability of the blood-brain barrier, and lead to cerebral edema [24]. This cerebral edema may be cytotoxic edema, vasogenic edema, or a combination

Table 3.2 Risk categories for acute mountain sickness (From the WMS practice guidelines for the prevention and treatment of acute mountain illness 2014 update) [14]

Risk category	Description
Low	Individual with no prior history of altitude illness and ascending to ≤2800 m
	Individuals taking ≥2 days to arrive at 2500–3000 m with subsequent increases in sleeping elevation <500 m/day and an extra day for acclimatization every 1000 m
Moderate	Individual with prior history of AMS and ascending to 2500–2800 m in 1 day
	No history of AMS and ascending to >3500 m in 1 day
	All individuals ascending >500 m/day (increase in sleeping altitude) above 3000 m but with an extra day of acclimatization every 1000 m
High	Individuals with a history of AMA and ascending to >2800 m in 1 day
	All individuals with a prior history of HACE
	All individuals ascending to 3500 m in 1 day
	All individuals ascending >500 m/day (increase in sleeping altitude) above >3000 m without extra days for acclimatization
	Very rapid ascents

of both. While it does not explain AMS or early HACE, in the late stages of HACE, cytotoxic edema may be present due to the increased cerebral-spinal fluid pressure, decreased perfusion, and focal ischemia. HACE however may present with vasogenic edema, as there has been some evidence of that on MRI [13].

The Wilderness Medical Society (WMS) has developed guidelines for the prevention and treatment of AMS and HACE based on the relative risk of individual susceptibility (Table 3.2). In low-risk individuals, gradual ascent is an effective way to prevent the onset of altitude illness without the need to use prophylactic medications. In planning a gradual ascent, the individual's sleeping altitude is much more important than the maximum altitude attained during the individual's waking hours. Above the 3000 m mark, individuals should not ascend to a new sleeping altitude of more than

500 m per day. At this elevation and following the rate of ascent guidelines, individuals should have a day of rest (no gain in sleeping elevation is attained) every 3–4 days. If individuals need to ascend more than 500 m per day, it is recommended that a rest day be taken either before or after such an ascent [14].

In individuals with a moderate to high risk of developing HAI, medications should be considered in conjunction with a gradual ascent. The preferred medication for the prevention of illness is acetazolamide at 125 mg twice a day for an adult and 2.5 mg/kg/dose every 12 h in children. In adults that are unable to take acetazolamide due to intolerance or adverse reaction, dexamethasone can be substituted as an alternative. In the extremely rare event that rapid ascent of over 3500 m and physical activity are required, the use of both acetazolamide and dexamethasone may be considered. This approach, however, should be reserved only for emergency circumstances that require a very rapid ascent (Table 3.3).

The WMS guidelines to treating HAI begin with a halt in the ascent of altitude. Individuals suffering from mild AMS may remain at their current altitude and treat themselves symptomatically. Over-the-counter NSAIDs and acetaminophen can be used to treat HAH and antiemetics to treat gastrointestinal discomfort. Acetazolamide may also be used to treat mild AMS. Individuals suffering moderate to severe AMS can be more effectively treated with dexamethasone combined with descent to an altitude prior to the onset of symptoms. Once the symptoms of AMS have resolved, the individual may be given acetazolamide and begin ascending again [14].

Individuals developing HACE within populated areas with access to appropriate healthcare facilities should be started on dexamethasone and supplemental oxygen. In remote areas where access to medical treatment is not available, limited descent should be initiated in conjunction with supplemental oxygen and dexamethasone. If descent is not possible, the use of supplemental oxygen and a hyperbaric chamber should be considered. Individuals with HACE should not resume ascent until they are asymptomatic and have stopped the use of dexamethasone [14] (Table 3.4).

HAPE is a life-threatening condition that develops within 2–5 days of arrival to high altitude between 2500 and 3000 m, and it is the most common cause of death in altitude-related illness [33]. HAPE rarely occurs in individuals who

Table 3.3 WMS recommended medications and doses for the prevention of HAI [14]

Medication	Indication for prevention	Dose and route
Acetazolamide	AMS, HACE	Adult—125 mg BID (oral)
		Pediatric—2.5 mg/kg Q12 h (oral)
Dexamethasone	AMS, HACE	2 mg Q6 h (oral) or 4 mg Q12 h (oral)
		Should not be used in pediatrics as prophylaxis
Nifedipine	HAPE	30 mg extended release Q12 h (oral)
Tadalafil	HAPE	10 mg BID (oral)
Sildenafil	HAPE	50 mg Q8 h (oral)
Sameterol[a]	HAPE	125 μg BID (inhaled)

[a]Should not be used as monotherapy but in conjunction with oral medications

Table 3.4 WMS recommended medications for the treatment of HAI [14]

Medication	Indication for treatment	Dose and route
Acetazolamide	AMS, HACE[a]	Adult—250 mg BID (oral)
		Pediatric 2.5 mg/kg Q12 h (oral)
Dexamethasone	AMS, HACE	AMS, adult—4 mg Q6 h (oral, IV, IM)
		HACE, adult—8 mg initially then 4 mg Q6 h (oral, IV, IM)
		Pediatrics—0.15 mg/kg/dose Q6 h (oral, IV, IM)
Nifedipine	HAPE	30 mg extended release Q12 h
Supplemental O₂	HAPE	Via facemask or nasal cannula

[a]Can be used as an adjunct treatment for HACE but dexamethasone remains the primary treatment method

remain at the same altitude for more than 4–5 days likely due to the body acclimating and remodeling to the high-altitude environment. While commonly developed in unacclimatized individuals rapidly ascending in altitude, another form of HAPE, named reentry HAPE, can occur in individuals who reside at high altitude, travel to low altitude, and return to high altitude [34].

According to the Lake Louise Consensus Group, HAPE can be diagnosed in the presence of high altitude and has at least two of the following symptoms: cough, chest tightness, dyspnea at rest, and reduced exercise capacity and the presence of two of the following signs, tachycardia, tachypnea, central cyanosis, or pulmonary crackles. Upon X-ray, there may be evidence of patchy opacities or interstitial edema [35].

The WMS-suggested approach to the prevention of HAPE is to assume a gradual ascent profile. The recommendations put forth in the AMS/HACE prevention also serve as a guideline for HAPE prevention as well. For susceptible individuals with a previous history of HAPE, nifedipine is the recommended medication. Usage of nifedipine should begin a day before ascent begins and should be continued until the individual has remained at a constant altitude for 4 days or until the individual descends. If the ascent profile is faster than the recommended ascent rate, the use of nifedipine should be extended out to 7 days at the individual's target elevation. While there is limited data on the use of acetazolamide in prophylaxis of HAPE, there is clinical experience that supports its use and is a rational choice. Salmeterol may be considered as a supplement to nifedipine in individuals with a prior history of HAPE and are considered high risk [14].

The WMS guidelines for treating HACE begin with ruling out other causes of respiratory illness that may occur at high altitudes. Descent is the first and primary method of treatment in individuals with HAPE. If descent is not possible, then use of supplemental oxygen and a portable hyperbaric chamber should be initiated. Individuals that have access to a healthcare facility may not need to descend further and can be treated at their current elevation. If no healthcare facility is available, nifedipine can be administered as an adjunct to descent, oxygen therapy, and a hyperbaric chamber. The use of nifedipine should only be used as the primary treatment method if none of the other treatment options are available. If nifedipine is not available, phosphodiesterase inhibitor may be used instead, but use of multiple vasodilators is not recommended. In the healthcare setting, CPAP can be administered as an adjunct to oxygen, and nifedipine can be added in individuals that fail to respond with oxygen therapy alone [14].

Individuals may resume ascent to higher altitudes when their symptoms have resolved and they can maintain a stable oxygenation rate at rest and with mild exertion while off of oxygen and vasodilators. Upon resuming ascent, it may be appropriate to use nifedipine or another pulmonary vasodilator upon resuming ascent. In individuals with both HAPE and HACE, dexamethasone should be added into treatment. Nifedipine and vasodilators can be used as treatment in patients with both HACE and HAPE, although the individual should be monitored to ensure that mean arterial pressure is not lowered, increasing the risk of cerebral ischemia [14].

Worldwide, there are over 300 million individuals with sickle-cell trait (SCT). In the United States, up to 10 % of the African-American community is SCT positive compared to only 0.05 % of the white population [36, 37]. In general, individuals with SCT are asymptomatic, and many are unaware that they are SCT positive.

Splenic syndrome is a condition that may occur in an individual with SCT that is exposed to high altitudes. Splenic syndrome occurs primarily in men of non-African-American descent and often at altitudes ranging from 2000 to 3000 feet above the individual's living altitude [38, 40].

Symptoms include left upper quadrant pain, difficulty or painful breathing, nausea, vomiting, and fever. On X-ray, sympathetic effusion in the left lung may be noted as well. Ultrasound or CT scan of the spleen may show evidence of splenic infarction [37].

Treatment of splenic syndrome can be managed conservatively. In individuals suffering splenic syndrome at altitude, descent is recommended.

In conjunction with descent, individual can be managed and supported with hydration, oxygen, and analgesia. Splenectomy is not recommended unless there is evidence of a spleen rupture, abscess, refractory sequestration, or symptomatic splenomegaly. It is recommended that individuals that experience splenic syndrome be followed up and monitored for the formation of an abscess [36].

In planning for endurance events at altitude, athletes and healthcare providers should consider several factors for both safety and performance. Pre-altitude evaluation should look for risk factors such as cardiac or lung disease [39]. A management strategy will often allow athletes with these conditions to still participate. Additionally, a previous history of HAI is an important predictor of recurrence. Education on acclimatization time and strategies should be discussed. Even brief exposures to real or simulated altitude leading up the training or competition can help improve performance and decrease risk in addition to the previously discussed acclimatization strategy recommendations. The use of medication should be done with caution as some athletes may be subject to testing. Some medications may be banned or required a therapeutic use exemption. The effect of these medications on performance has not been well studied.

Athletes with mild illness may return to activity when symptoms have resolved. No evidence-based guidelines exist to guide the return of athletes who have experienced HACE or HAPE. It is generally recommended that athletes be symptom free and be slow return to activity and altitude.

References

1. Lipman GS, Eifling KP, Ellis MA, Gaudio FG, Otten EM, Grissom CK. Wilderness medical society practice guidelines for the prevention and treatment of heat related illness: 2014 update. Wilderness Environ Med. 2014;25:S55–65.
2. Atha W. Heat-related illness. Emerg Med Clin North Am. 2013;31:1097–108.
3. Pryor RR, Bennett BL, O'Connor FG, Young JM, Asplund CA. Medical evaluation for exposure extremes: heat. Clin J Sport Med. 2015;25:437–42.
4. Becker JA, Stewart LK. Heat-related illness. Am Fam Physician. 2011;83:1325–30.
5. Noonan B, Bancroft RW, Dines JS, Bedi A. Heat and cold-induced injuries in athletes: evaluation and management. J Am Acad Orthop Surg. 2012;20:744–54.
6. Nichols AW. Heat-related illness in sports and exercise. Curr Rev Musculoskelet Med. 2014;7:355–65.
7. Bergeron M. Heat stress and thermal strain challenges in running. J Orthop Sports Phys Ther. 2014;44:831–38.
8. Howe AS, Boden BP. Heat-related illness in athletes. Am J Sports Med. 2007;35:1384–95.
9. Casa DJ, Demartini JK, Bergeron MF, Csillan D, Eichner ER, Lopez RM, et al. National athletic trainers' association position statement: exertional heat illnesses. J Athl Train. 2015;50:986–1000.
10. Miller KC, Stone MS, Huxel KC, Edwards JE. Exercise-associated muscle cramps: causes, treatment and prevention. Sports Health. 2010;2:279–83.
11. Miners AL. The diagnosis and emergency care of heat related illness and sunburn in athletes: a retrospective case series. J Can Chiropr Assoc. 2010;54:107–17.
12. Sloan BK, Kraft EM, Clark D, Schmeissing SW, Byrne BC, Rusyniak DE. On-site treatment of exertional heat stroke. Am J Sports Med. 2015;20:1–7.
13. Basnyat B, Murdoch D. High altitude illness. Lancet. 2003;361:1967–74.
14. Luks AM, McIntosh SE, Grissom CK, Auerbach PS, Rodway GW, Schoene RB, et al. Wilderness Medical Society practice guidelines for the prevention and treatment of acute altitude illness: 2014 update. Wilderness Environ Med. 2014;25:s4–14.
15. Derby R, deWeber K. The athlete and high altitude. Curr Sports Med Rep. 2010;0902:79–85.
16. Eide III RP, Asplund CA. Altitude illness: update on prevention and treatment. Curr Sports Med Rep. 2012;11(3):124–30.
17. Harris SN, Wenzel RP, Thomas SH. J Emerg Med. 2003;2404:383–7.
18. Lopez JI, Holdridge A, Mendizabal JE. Altitude headache. Curr Pain Headache Rep. 2013. doi:10.1007/s11916-013-0383-2.
19. Broome JR, Stoneham MD, Beeley JM, Milledge JS, Hughes MB. High altitude headache: treatment with ibuprofen. Aviat Space Environ Med. 1994;65:19–20.
20. Burtscher M, Likar R, Nachbauer W, Philadelphy M. Aspirin for the prophylaxis against headache at high altitudes: randomized, double blind, placebo controlled trial. BMJ. 1998;316:1057–8.
21. Burtscher M, Likar R, Nachbauer W, Philadelphy M. Naproxen for treatment of high altitude headache. 11th International Hypoxia Symposium, Jasper 1999, abstracts. p. 144.
22. Armstrong LE, Casa DJ, Watson G. Exertional hyponatremia. Curr Sports Med Rep. 2006;5:221–2.
23. Imray C, Wright A. Subudhi A, Roach R. Acute mountain sickness: pathophysiology, prevention, and treatment. Prog Cardiovasc Dis. 2010;52:467–84.

24. Hackett PH, Roach RC. High-altitude illness. N Engl J Med. 2001;34502:107–18.
25. DeFranco MJ, Baker CLIII, DaSilva JJ, Piasecki DP, Bach BR. Environmental issues for team physicians. Am J Sports Med. 2008;3611:2226–37.
26. Zafren K. Prevention of high altitude illness. Travel Med Infect Dis. 2014;12:29–39.
27. Honigman B, Theis MK, Koziol-McLain J, Roach R, Yip R, Houston C, et al. Ann Intern Med. 1993; 11808:587–92.
28. Taylor AT. High-altitude illnesses: physiology, risk factors, prevention, and treatment. Rambam Maimonides Med J. 2011; 0201. doi:10.5041/RMMJ.10022.
29. Hackett PH, Roach RC. High altitude cerebral edema. High Alt Med Biol. 2004;0502:136–46.
30. Hultgren H. High altitude medicine. 1st ed. Stanford, CA: Hultgren; 1997.
31. West JB. Early history of high-altitude physiology. Ann N Y Acad Sci. 2015. doi:10.1111/nyas.12719.
32. Luks AM. Physiology in medicine: a physiological approach to prevention and treatment of acute high-altitude illness. J Appl Physiol. 2015;11805. doi:10.1153/japplphysiol.oo955.2014.
33. Bhagi S, Srivastava S, Singh SB. High-altitude pulmonary edema: review. J Occup Health. 2014;56:235–43.
34. Maggiorini M. Prevention and treatment of high-altitude pulmonary edema. Prog Cardiovasc Dis. 2010;52:500–06.
35. Basnyat B. High altitude cerebral and pulmonary edema. Travel Med Infect Dis. 2004;3:199–211.
36. Scordino D, Kirsch T. Splenic infarction at high altitude secondary to sickle cell trait. J Emerg Med. 2013;31:446e1–3.
37. Sheikha A. Splenic syndrome in patients at high altitude with unrecognized sickle cell trait: splenectomy is often unnecessary. Can J Surg. 2005;4805:377–81.
38. Lane P, Githens J. Splenic syndrome at mountain altitudes in sickle cell trait. Its occurrence in nonblack persons. JAMA. 1985;253:2251.
39. Campbell AD, McIntosh SE, Nyberg A, Powell AP, Schoene RB, Hackett P. Risk stratification for athletes and adventurers in high-altitude environments: recommendations for preparticipation evaluation. Clin J Sports Med. 2015;25:404–11.
40. Goldberg NM, Dorman JP, Riley CA, Armbruster EJ. Altitude related splenic infarction in sickle cell trait – case reports of a father and son. West J Med. 1985;14302:670–2.

Pregnancy and the Endurance Athlete

4

Jacob Michael Bright and Chad A. Asplund

Introduction

Exercise is encouraged as part of a healthy lifestyle. Endurance sports are a very popular way for people to exercise with participation growing. Many women who become pregnant wonder if exercise is safe during their pregnancy, especially endurance exercise. Some women will enter pregnancy already with a regular endurance exercise routine, while others will choose pregnancy as an opportunity to modify their lifestyles to become healthier and include exercise into their practice. It has been noted that habits adopted during pregnancy could affect a woman's health across her life-span [1]. Traditional medical advice has been for women to engage in only moderate physical activity during pregnancy; however, with the increase in endurance athletes, who become pregnant, what should be the guidance for these athletes? The purpose of this chapter will be to explore the changes in physiology with pregnancy and with exercise, discuss some concerns of exercise during pregnancy, review existing consensus guidelines, and provide guidance on how to prescribe endurance exercise during pregnancy.

Pregnancy Physiology

There are profound changes in cardiovascular, respiratory, and renal physiology and in the regulation of fluid and electrolytes during pregnancy. These changes occur in early pregnancy before there is an increase in demand, so in the first trimester the increase in cardiac output is greater than the increase in oxygen demand [2]. Cardiac output is the result of stroke volume and heart rate. During pregnancy, maternal cardiac output increases by 30–50 % above the antepartum baseline with approximately half of this increase occurring before 8 weeks estimated gestational age. Studies demonstrate that the heart rate increases early in pregnancy and stays elevated throughout the pregnancy. An expected increase of 10–15 beats per minute is typically observed relative to the preconception resting heart rate. However, the chief component of the calculated cardiac output that increases is the stroke volume [3]. There is also an increase in stroke volume secondary to relaxation of the left ventricle, which may be estrogen dependent [4].

In addition there are pulmonary changes brought about by pregnancy. Changes in the thorax and diaphragm have been documented to

J.M. Bright
Family Medicine Residency Program, Eisenhower Army Medical Center, 300 East Hospital Road, Fort Gordon, GA 30909, USA

C.A. Asplund, MD, MPH (✉)
Associate Professor, Health and Kinesiology Director, Athletic Medicine Georgia Southern University Statesboro, GA, USA
e-mail: chad.asplund@gmail.com

occur quite early in pregnancy, much earlier than could be explained by the mechanical disadvantage of a gravid uterus filling an abdominal cavity [5]. Minute ventilation increases by almost 50 % early during pregnancy and stays elevated until the postpartum period. While there is relative maternal hyperventilation during the first trimester, the primary drive responsible for increased minute ventilation is a nearly 40 % increase in tidal volume (V_T), most of which occurs during the first trimester. The early changes observed in tidal volume as well as diaphragmatic height are most likely in response to increasing progesterone levels, a known stimulant of respiratory drive.

As pregnancy progresses, functional residual capacity declines secondary to elevation of the diaphragm by the growing uterus. During pregnancy, the functional residual capacity (expiratory reserve volume + residual capacity) decreases by approximately 20 %. The inspiratory capacity (inspiratory reserve volume + tidal volume) is mildly increased during pregnancy. As the uterus grows throughout pregnancy, the functional residual capacity steadily declines, primarily to the diaphragm's mechanical disadvantage caused by the uterus. This causes total lung volume to decrease from an average of 4.2 L in a healthy, adult female to 4.0 in the average pregnant female at term without underlying respiratory pathology. During pregnancy, the forced expiratory volume in 1 s (FEV1) remains unchanged as a result of the large airways being unaffected by pregnancy.

During pregnancy, there are changes to the renal and vascular systems that impact blood volume and blood pressure. Blood volume begins to increase so that by term the plasma volume has increased by 50 %. The notable expansion in plasma volume starts in the fourth week of gestation and continues to increase until peaking between 32 and 34 weeks estimated gestational age. For the plasma volume to increase, there must be salt and water retention, which occurs due to upregulation of the renin-angiotensin-aldosterone system. Red blood cell mass also increases in pregnancy, starting between 8 and 10 weeks and steadily rising throughout pregnancy. However, the rise in red blood cell mass does not increase to the same proportion as the expanding plasma volume, resulting in a dilutional ("physiologic") anemia when retained plasma volume peaks as the mother reaches term. Under normal circumstances, this would act as a signal for the increased production of erythropoietin (EPO), but the renal blood flow is dramatically increased during early pregnancy which delays this increase in EPO, which maintains the relative anemia. This volume expansion serves multiple benefits to the fetus and mother. It protects the mother from the hardships and potential morbidities associated with vaginal delivery, mainly postpartum hemorrhage. Also, the expanded plasma volume and increased red blood cell mass contribute to a nutrient-rich environment optimal for fetal growth.

Finally there are musculoskeletal adaptations to pregnancy, the most obvious are the weight gain and shift in the center of gravity, which may alter balance and may predispose to increased falls. The recommended weight gain during maternal gestation for a woman with a normal prepregnancy body mass index is 25–35 pounds; this excess weight imparts distinct alterations in the biomechanical stresses placed on the axial skeleton, pelvis, and large joints of the lower extremity. In biomechanical studies, this weight gain has been associated with the force on the joints of the lower extremity increasing twofold compared to prepregnancy weight [6]. The increased weight associated with pregnancy increases stress on the joints but also creates an increased demand on the cardiovascular system.

Also, the increase in estrogen and relaxin during pregnancy increases ligamentous laxity, which may lead to a higher risk of sprains. Relaxin specifically causes increased laxity in the anterior and posterior longitudinal ligaments of the lumbar spine, which may predispose to paraspinal muscle strain during activities that place that stress low back flexibility. However, relaxation caused by excess relaxin and estrogen in the pelvis impart biomechanical advantages as the mother nears the end of her pregnancy and is preparing for vaginal delivery. There has been documented widening of sacroiliac joints and the pubic symphysis, thus increasing the mobility of each

Table 4.1 Changes in maternal physiology during pregnancy

Cardiovascular:
   Increased HR by 10–15 bpm
   Increased SV
   Increased CO by up to 50 %
   Increased RBC mass

Pulmonary:
   Increased tidal volume (V_T)
   Increased minute ventilation by 50 %
   Decreased functional residual capacity
   Increased work of breathing

Renal/vascular
   Upregulation of RAAS
   Salt retention
   Water retention
   Plasma volume increased by 50 %
   Increased renal blood flow (prevents EPO release)
   Physiologic anemia

Increased progesterone:
   Smooth muscle relaxation
   Increased venous compliance
   Decreased peripheral vascular resistance

Musculoskeletal:
   Weight gain of 25–35 pounds (ideal)
   Ligamentous laxity
   Increased joint stress
   Predisposition to falls (new center of gravity)
   Increased lumbar and (compensatory) cervical lordosis
   Compression of neurovascular structures (median nerve, ulnar nerve)

respective site and increasing the overall rotation of the pelvis. In the latter portions of pregnancy, maternal use of several muscle groups increases in response to the increased anterior tilt of the pelvis that occurs in response to the enlarging uterus. These muscle groups placed at increased stress during the latter portion of pregnancy include maternal hip extensors, hip abductors, and ankle plantar flexors. Subconsciously, maternal resting stance and gait also become wider in an effort to maintain trunk stability. Lastly, the aforementioned fluid retention and drastic increase in plasma volume can have unfortunate consequences for the musculoskeletal system. This excessive circulating volume can cause compression of vulnerable neurovascular structures, such as the median nerve, leading to diagnosis of, or worsening of, previously diagnosed, peripheral neuropathies such as carpal tunnel syndrome.

A brief summary of these physiologic changes can be found in Table 4.1.

Endurance Physiology

Endurance can be defined as the ability to withstand stress over periods of time. Endurance exercise can therefore be termed exercise that takes a long time to complete or may also be defined as sports that are highly aerobic such as running, cycling, and swimming. The main source of energy for endurance sport is the metabolism of carbohydrates (glycogen) and fats in the form of free fatty acids. Energy may also be supplied from the anaerobic metabolism of glycogen to form lactate and from the intramuscular store of high-energy phosphates.

In order to continue to exercise for prolonged durations, oxygen uptake must increase. Some of this occurs simply by increasing cardiac output (increased heart rate and stroke volume). Maintenance of a stable hemoglobin concentration is also vital to ensure that oxygen can be delivered by the red blood cells to the muscles. Finally, enzymatic activation and increase in muscle capillary density complete the adaptations required for endurance sport.

As can be noted from the physiological changes of pregnancy described above, there can be some competing demands on the body when a pregnant female participates in endurance sports.

Physiological Concerns of Exercise During Pregnancy

The proper delivery and exchange of oxygen, nutrients, and waste products at the maternal-fetal interface (placenta) serves as the primary maternal stimulus for health fetal growth. During pregnancy, sustained exercise can cause reductions in oxygen and nutrient delivery to the fetus by as much as 50 %, but regular exercise has been theorized to improve oxygen and substrate delivery at rest.

Maternal Physiologic Concerns

Exercise in early and midpregnancy has been shown to stimulate fetal growth, while the relative amount of exercise in late pregnancy determines fetal growth. It was previously theorized that thermal response to maternal exercise could negatively impact fetal growth and development. However, rectal temperature monitoring is performed in 18 female recreational athletes before, during, and after 20 min of continuous exercise prior to conception and every 6–8 weeks throughout pregnancy. This study showed that decreased peak rectal temperature reached during exercise decreased by 0.3 °C (0.54 °F) at 8 weeks estimated gestational age and decreased by 0.1 °C (0.18 °F) monthly until reaching 37 weeks estimated gestational age. This study showed that the maternal physiologic adaptations to pregnancy helped reduce the thermal response to exercise and thus reduce any exercise-associated thermal stress to the fetus [7].

Another common myth regarding exercise during pregnancy is that the continuation of regular aerobic exercise in the latter portion (third trimester) of pregnancy has negative impact on the duration of pregnancy and the outcomes of labor. Several studies have tested this hypothesis but one study [8] in particular enrolled 131 well-conditioned recreational athletes prior to conception. Each participant's daily exercise regimen was quantified prior to conception, and then they were followed throughout pregnancy. Eighty-seven of these women continued to exercise regularly at or above 50 % of their preconception level of activity, while the remaining 44 women completely discontinued their exercise regimen before the end of the first trimester. The incidence of preterm labor was similar between the two groups (9 % in each group). However, the incidence of cesarean delivery (6 % for exercising patients vs. 30 % for non-exercising patients) and operative (vacuum or forceps-assisted) vaginal delivery (6 % vs. 20 %) was significantly lower in patients who exercised throughout their pregnancy. In those who went on to deliver vaginally, exercising patients had much shorter active labor (264 ± 149 min) compared to their non-exercising counterparts (382 ± 275 min). Finally, clinical evidence of acute fetal stress as defined as meconium-stained amniotic fluid, fetal heart pattern of category II or III strip, and APGAR scores was less frequent in the exercise group (50 % vs. 26 %), although birth weight was reduced (3369 ± 318 g vs. 3776 ± 401 g).

Fetal Physiological Concerns

Regular sustained exercise in pregnancy has been viewed as a cause for concern as it could potentially change the homeostasis of the maternal-fetal unit and may adversely affect the fetus. In addition to concerns regarding exposure to elevated maternal temperatures discussed above, there are several physiologic concerns of exercise with respect to fetal development from exercise during pregnancy.

The fetus is wholly dependent on the mother for normal development. This includes the supply of oxygen and nutrients but also the removal of waste products—therefore, maternal exercise-induced changes may affect the fetus.

The availability and rate of delivery of oxygen and nutrients play an important role in fetal development. The placenta modulates vascular and tissue growth based on nutrient and oxygen availability through growth-regulatory peptides [9]. Exercise influences the functional placental volume secondary to substrate availability. While acute exercise diverts placental blood to the muscles and skin, recurrent exercise may lead to different placental growth similar to that seen by those who have anemia or live at altitude [10]. Increased levels of insulin growth factors lead to increased functional placental mass and may upregulate placental nutrient transporters. Functional placental size may also be altered by the timing of exercise during the course of pregnancy. Those who exercised more in early to midpregnancy and reduced their volume in late pregnancy had a greater level of functional placental tissue compared to those that increased the volume of exercise as pregnancy continued [11].

Fetal heart rate (FHR) and breathing are considered important indices of fetal well-being with a normal FHR between 120 and 160 beats per minute (bpm). Fetal heart rate can be affected by a number of stimuli including hypoxia. Therefore, it may lead to the question, does the decreased uterine blood flow during exercise increase fetal heart rate or decrease delivery of oxygen to the fetus? Several studies have evaluated this and the results are variable. In general in healthy late pregnant females, the heart rate was stable after a step test, after a cycle ergometry test, and after treadmill walking [12]. Running seemed to elevate fetal heart rate, but the studies have had some limitations. Further, there is no consistent data to demonstrate any long-term abnormalities in fetal breathing following exercise [12].

Well-conditioned recreational athletes who continue a program of vigorous exercise into late gestation have on average a 310 g reduction in fetal weight compared to non-exercising controls. However, this reduction in fetal weight was caused entirely by reduction in fat mass—there was no difference in lean mass between the groups [8]. In contrast, those non-exercisers who started an exercise program in pregnancy actually saw an increase of 260 g in fetal weight [13]. Further, two very large population-based cohort studies with over 120,000 total subjects [14, 15] suggest that the independent effect of exercise in pregnancy has only a minimal effect on birth weight. Fetal body fat is primarily laid down during the third trimester, so the timing of exercise may play a role. Women who perform vigorous exercise early in the pregnancy and then back off toward late pregnancy delivered significantly heavier (460 g) than controls, while those that increase the intensity of exercise as pregnancy develops delivered infants with an average birth weight 100 g smaller than those infants delivered by the control group [11].

Another common concern among women is that physical activity during pregnancy will lead to preterm birth. A large epidemiologic study in Europe included over 87,000 women who self-reported their physical exercise during a singleton pregnancy from 1996 to 2002. Hazard ratios for preterm birth according to (1) hours of exercise per week, (2) type of exercise, and (3) metabolic equivalent hours per week were calculated and found a reduced risk of preterm birth among the women who engaged in some kind of exercise during pregnancy (39 % of women; hazard ratio = 0.82, 95 % confidence interval: 0.76, 0.88). However, this study did not find any dose-dependent response to exercise; additionally, the results were not affected by the type of exercise performed [16].

It would seem that exercise may lead to short-term alterations in fetal physiology, but that over the long term, there is a beneficial fetal effect to maternal exercise. Further, women should continue with exercise during the first two trimesters and should consider reducing the volume and intensity of exercise after 28 weeks.

Risks/Benefits of Exercise During Pregnancy

Moderate-intensity aerobic exercise has been shown to be safe during pregnancy, and exercise confers several benefits. Additionally, more recent data suggest that regular exercise during pregnancy is associated with lower birth weight and lower concentrations in serum concentrations of IGF-I and IGF-II levels in cord blood samples. This data suggests that exercise has an influence on endocrine influences on fetal growth regulation. However, there was no observed association between maternal insulin sensitivity and exercise [17]. There are several hypothesized risks of exercising during pregnancy and include fetal anomalies secondary to maternal hyperthermia, as well as possible smaller birth weight for infants born to mothers who participate in vigorous physical exercise into late pregnancy. However, there appears to be no difference in lean body mass in infants born to vigorous exercisers [13]. While several studies discussed in this chapter have published since its release, the most recent *Cochrane Review* declared that regular aerobic exercise in pregnancy could improve or maintain maternal physical fitness, but there was insufficient data to infer risk/benefits to the mother and infant [18]. Although there have no reports of fetal injury or death secondary to contact sports, the risk of blunt abdominal trauma does exist with participation in certain activities or secondary to falling due to balance issues in pregnancy [19]. For these reasons, it is important that a thought-out individualized exercise prescription be crafted for active females who become pregnant.

Physical Activity in Pregnancy

Prior to developing an exercise prescription to the pregnant patient, it is important to gauge the activities she is most interested continuing from her pre-pregnancy exercise habits and routines or what new activities she hopes to begin. Research has demonstrated that nonpregnant females and male patients are more likely to continue an exercise prescription if it involves activities they have an interest in. Thus, it is essential that the physician outlines the patient's desired activity/interest she hopes to pursue or continue during her pregnancy. A number of professional athletes have competed in various sports *during* their pregnancy. Olympic

beach volleyball gold medalist Kerri Walsh, WNBA athlete Candace Parker, and LPGA golf professional Catriona Matthew have all competed during pregnancy. Matthew won the Brazil Cup when she was five months pregnant [20].

Table 4.2 outlines sports in which participation has absolute or relative contraindications during pregnancy; sports generally considered safe during pregnancy are also included. Of note, it is recommended that women never scuba dive during pregnancy as there are no maternal mechanisms to protect the fetus from decompression sickness or gas embolism. The other activities listed in Table 4.2 as absolute contraindications are from expert opinion based on the risk of harm secondary to risk of falls, loss of balance, or other abdominal trauma that could lead to fetal injury or fetal demise or result in situations requiring expedited delivery or immediate care such as premature rupture of membranes (PROM), preterm premature rupture of membranes (PPROM), or placental abruption. For the listed relative contraindications, avid hikers should be counseled that risk of abdominal trauma from falls is the chief concern with this activity. Limited studies have shown that under normal circumstances with appropriate hydration, moderate exercises at altitudes up to 6000–8250 feet (1800–

Table 4.2 Sport/activity participation during pregnancy

Absolute contraindications	Relative contraindications	Activities to encourage
Scuba diving	Basketball	Low-impact aerobics
Mixed martial arts (MMA)	Soccer (field positions)	Traditional yoga
Wrestling	Bicycling	Stationary cycling
Boxing	Bikram (hot) yoga	Swimming
Kickboxing	Distance running below maximal exertion	Walking
(American) football	Volleyball or beach volleyball	Jogging at moderate or low intensity
Ice hockey	Tennis	Golfing
Rugby	Rowing	
Soccer (goalie)	Hiking (in locations where falls may occur)	
Jumping events in track and field (high jump, pole vault, long jump)		
Aquatic diving		
Horseback riding		
Downhill skiing or snowboarding		
Skateboarding or other "extreme" sports		
Gymnastics		

2500 m) do not appear to cause significant maternal or fetal stress. Women who do not live at high altitude but plan on exercising at any altitude above 2500 m should undergo appropriate acclimatization.

Of note, Sports Medicine Australia published guidelines [21] addressing exercise in pregnant women and also participation in non-contact, limited contact, and a third category of unlimited contact and collision sports. The Australian Guidelines define a non-contact sport as one with "virtually no risk of falling or contact with projectile/person" and cite swimming, low-impact aerobics, and stationary cycling as examples. They place no limitations on these activities aside from controlling degree of exertion and only participating under appropriate medical supervision in the absence of any contraindications to exercise. Limited contact sports are defined in the Australian Guidelines as any sport in which contact occurs minimally (legally or illegally), and there is a small risk of falls or contact with a projectile, citing netball and racquet sports as examples. These are described as suitable during the first trimester with ongoing participation into the second trimester being possible under the supervision of an obstetrician and sports medicine physician.

"Unlimited contact" and collision sport participation is much more restrictive in the Australian Guidelines, similar to the expert opinions of American [22, 23] and Canadian societies [19]. The Sports Medicine Australia Guideline [21] defines these as any sport in which contact or collision is frequent and has the potential to be "quite forceful" and places the athlete at high risk for falls, blunt trauma to the abdomen, or contact with projectiles. These cited sports in the Australian Guideline are soccer, softball/baseball, Australian rules football, American football, martial arts, and gymnastics. They also recommend maternal exclusion from any sport, exercise, or activity that carries a high risk of falls or physical trauma. The guideline explicitly states that women should not participate in scuba diving, downhill skiing, ice skating, horseback riding, martial arts, or gymnastics once she knows

Table 4.3 Warning signs to stop exercise

Vaginal bleeding
Shortness of breath before exertion
Headache
Chest pain
Dizziness
Calf swelling, redness, asymmetry, or pain
Uterine contractions
Amniotic fluid leakage (or suspected rupture)
Decreased fetal movement

Adapted from ACOG committee opinion: exercise during pregnancy and the postpartum period

she is pregnant or if she suspects she is pregnant until confirming she is in fact not pregnant.

The Sports Medicine Australia Guideline [21] for participation of the pregnant athlete additionally addresses maternal risk of overheating during exercise and suggests the avoidance of exercise during the hottest or most humid portions of the day; if climate is not suited for this, they recommend exercise in an indoor facility that has central cooling and is well ventilated.

Whatever their chosen sport or activity, it is important that pregnant women be properly counseled regarding what warning signs and symptoms warrant immediate cessation of activity/exercise and seeking immediate medical attention (Table 4.3). These warning signs were introduced by ACOG [23] and have been adopted by virtually every other sports medicine or exercise physiology society in America, Canada, New Zealand, Australia, and Europe; they can be classified as general medical problems and obstetric problems.

Exercise Prescriptions

Prior to prescribing an exercise prescription in pregnancy, it is important to identify any absolute or relative contraindications to exercise during pregnancy. It is important for pregnant women to understand that certain conditions (placenta previa) may only become a contraindication to exercise in the latter stages of pregnancy or may develop later in a previously normal pregnancy (pregnancy-induced hypertension). While it is

Table 4.4 Contraindications to exercise

Absolute contraindications—maternal medical conditions:
Hemodynamically significant heart disease
Restrictive lung disease
Absolute contraindications—obstetric complications:
Known cervical incompetence or having undergone placement of cervical cerclage
Rupture of membranes
Premature labor during current pregnancy
Hypertensive disorders of pregnancy (pregnancy-induced hypertension, preeclampsia, or HELLP syndrome)
Known intrauterine growth restriction of fetus
High-order multiple gestations (≥3 fetuses)
Placenta previa during or after the 26th week of estimated gestational age
Persistent second or third trimester bleeding
Relative contraindications—maternal medical conditions:
Unevaluated maternal cardiac arrhythmia
Chronic bronchitis
Poorly controlled type I diabetes
Extreme morbid obesity
Extreme underweight (prepregnancy BMI < 12)
History of extremely sedentary lifestyle
Poorly controlled chronic hypertension
Orthopedic limitations
Heavy smoker
Poorly controlled seizure disorder
Poorly controlled thyroid disorders
Thyroid disease
Relative contraindications—obstetric medical conditions:
Severe anemia (hemoglobin value of ≤10)
IUGR during current pregnancy

unethical and impractical to have random controlled, double-blind trials comparing the exercise habits of pregnant women with high-risk pregnancies, several conditions have been identified as exclusion criteria for subjects identified in previously conducted research studies. As such, the following conditions are considered absolute contraindications to exercise during pregnancy based on expert opinion outlined in ACOG guidelines [23] and adopted or endorsed by several other medical societies (Table 4.4). It is often helpful to think of these as maternal medical conditions or obstetric complications, although some overlaps may occur.

The guidance and outline of relative contraindications to exercise during pregnancy also rely upon expert opinion with most societies adopting or endorsing ACOG guidelines. Simply put, any condition in which the relative risk of exercise would outweigh the benefits of exercise during pregnancy should be considered a relative contraindication to exercise. Any women with a relative contraindication to exercise identified should only make the decision to participate in physical activity based on the advice and counseling of the physician providing their prenatal care. These relative contraindications predominantly focus on chronic maternal medical conditions, with the exception of anemia (which could be acute or chronic) and current intrauterine growth restriction (IUGR).

Additionally, when helping to develop an exercise prescription during pregnancy, it is important to consider the aforementioned changes in maternal physiology, mainly the increased resting heart rate and as a result blunted heart rate response to exercise. The *Canadian Society for Exercise Physiology* created modified heart rate target zones for women who desire to perform aerobic exercise during pregnancy; this recommendation has been endorsed by other organizations as well [19]. For women without access to heart rate monitoring devices, a simple modification could be the use of the "talk test" to assess maternal exertion—the patient should be able to maintain a conversation during exercise; if not, she should decrease her exercise intensity. This also provides an opportunity for the physician to encourage the patient's spouse, father of the child, or members of her social support circle to exercise with the patient to help improve the health of everyone who will be involved with the support and care of the mother during pregnancy and newborn following discharge from the hospital.

Women who desire to maintain aerobic fitness and/or continue frequent aerobic exercise in pregnancy should be counseled; when studied, pregnant runners report a reduction in total training but very few reported injuries during pregnancy. Of 110 long-distance runners who ran competitively prior to pregnancy, only 31 % ran during their third trimester and overall women reduced their training intensity by one half [24]. Another interesting finding of the same study was that women who ran during breastfeeding were less likely to be diagnosed with postpartum depression, but there was no statistically significant difference in the rate of postpartum depression in women who ran during pregnancy versus those who did not run.

Exercise Prescription During Pregnancy

The Sedentary or Non-exercising Patient

Regular exercise is an essential part of a healthy lifestyle and should be encouraged in all patients, including pregnant patients. Exercise may help prevent the development of conditions that can complicate pregnancy and negatively impact fetal well-being, including excess maternal weight gain, gestational diabetes, and LGA infants. In the 2008 *Physical Activity Guidelines for Americans* [25], the US Department of Health and Human Services (HHS) recommended that women who have not been exercising prior to pregnancy should not begin a vigorous exercise program during pregnancy. The US Department of Health and Human Services 2008 Physical Activity Guideline for Americans and the American College of Obstetricians and Gynecologists (ACOG) committee opinion on exercise during pregnancy [23] both discuss, but do not explicitly define, "vigorous" or "strenuous" exercise in the pregnant patient or immediate postpartum patient. The US Department of HHS defines "vigorous" as either anything greater than 6.0 metabolic equivalents (METs) or 60–84% of the maximum heart rate estimate based on age.

Further, research supports that when compared with regularly or highly active pregnant females, previously sedentary females were able to increase their time to fatigue on a treadmill with intrapartum exercise and when performing moderate exercise did not demonstrate any signs of fetal or maternal morbidity. Those regularly active or highly active (non-sedentary) females were able to perform vigorous exercise without adverse consequences. In all of the groups, postexercise fetal heart rate tracings were reactive (category I) within 20 min and biophysical profiles were reassuring [26]. Walking has been cited in obstetric and sports medicine literature as the most popular activity during pregnancy.

A recent study [27] examined the effect of a walking program of low intensity (30 % of maximum heart rate) versus high intensity (70 % of maximum heart rate) during on a standard treadmill. Normal-weight pregnant women were randomized to low-intensity, high-intensity, or control groups and then underwent standard submaximal treadmill test at 16–20 weeks gestational age (study entry) and tested again at 34–36 weeks gestation to evaluate changes in cardiorespiratory responses. Increased body mass was similar between all groups studied; pre- and post-walking program intervention revealed an unchanged VO2 and VCO2 in the low-intensity group but decreased values in the high-intensity group. This study demonstrated that previously inactive pregnant women could have unchanged (low-intensity group) or decreased (high-intensity group) energy cost/demand from walking in the latter stages of their pregnancy. This demonstrated that aerobic conditioning response was conferred despite similar body mass at time of post-intervention testing in all groups. All participants in this study delivered healthy, viable infants.

The Regular Exercising Patient

Regular exercising patients may continue to exercise at the previous rate and intensity of exercise while pregnant without adverse consequence. A study of highly active and regularly active pregnant females between 28 and 32 weeks gestational age with treadmill exercise evaluated fetal well-being before and after exercise. Fetal well-being was measured with pre- and immediate post-exercise umbilical artery Doppler, fetal heart rate tracing, fetal heart rate, and biophysical profile. There were statistically significant decreases in immediate post-exercise umbilical artery Doppler flow in each group; however, post-exercise fetal heart rate tracings were all reactive and category 1 within 20 min for both groups with normal biophysical profiles [26].

Regular exercising patients should be written a FITT exercise prescription similar to sedentary patients except with greater frequency and duration (time). They should be advised to exercise

3–5 times per week at 65–80 % of maximum heart rate and may perform activities that are not a contraindication to participation in their stage in pregnancy (running/jogging, tennis, cross-country skiing) and/or low-impact exercises that would be prescribed to the sedentary patient.

The Elite Athlete

Females that participate in sport as elite athletes have dedicated many years of training and competition to achieve this level of success. Further, their financial livelihood may depend on their ability to train or compete while pregnant. However, the ACOG reports that quality research on strenuous or vigorous intensity exercise during pregnancy is scarce and such activities require close medical supervision. No professional guidelines or any other available data identify an upper limit of safety with regard to exercise during pregnancy; also, neither guidelines address maximal exercise in high-level athletes.

When high-functioning or elite athletes address exercise with their provider during pre-natal counseling and routine obstetric care, the physician is unable to provide an evidence-based answer to patient inquiry. While expert opinion only offers vague guidance for joint decision making between patient and provider, recent research studies provide some limited insight into the effects of strenuous exercise during the second and third trimester of pregnancy.

Although there is not a wealth of evidence on exercise in elite-level females, a recent study suggests that fetal well-being may be compromised during near-maximal exercise among pregnant elite athletes. Six Olympic-level females, who reported performing 15–20 h per week of strenuous training before they were pregnant, were tested at 60–90 % of maximal oxygen consumption during the second trimester. During the test, mean uterine artery blood flow was reduced during the exercise testing; however, the fetal heart rate stayed within normal limits. But, when the women exercised at greater than 90 % of their VO2 max, the mean uterine artery was decreased to below 50 % of the pre-exercise levels [28].

Further, another study [29] demonstrated that in previous highly active pregnant females, a small subset of highly active women demonstrated transient FHR decelerations and alterations in umbilical and uterine artery Doppler indices immediately after near-maximal exercise. Therefore, it is reasonable to recommend that elite female athletes should not exercise at higher than 90 % of MHR during pregnancy. Because of the lack of evidence and the differences in maximal heart rate per individual athlete, pregnant athletes—particularly elite athletes—may benefit from individualized exercise prescriptions. The key aspect of the exercise prescription in these women is to set boundaries so they do not overexert themselves and reach a level of exertion or maximal heart rate that could compromise fetal well-being (Table 4.5).

Table 4.5 Summary of fetal responses to strenuous maternal exercise

Study	Maternal testing	Measures of fetal well-being	Population studied	Observed results
Salvesen et al. [28]	VO2 maximum testing during peak treadmill test to volitional fatigue	Doppler U/S of uterine and umbilical arteries before, during, and after exercise	6 Olympic-level athletes at 23–29 weeks EGA	Fetal bradycardia at ≥90 % of maternal oxygen consumption by VO2 maximum

Szymanski and Satin [29]	Peak treadmill test to volitional fatigue	Umbilical and uterine artery Doppler U/S, fetal heart rate tracing, and BPP pre- and post-exercise	45 women, varying activity levels
			  15 sedentary
			  15 regular exercisers
			  15 highly active patients at 28–32 weeks EGA
				Transient fetal heart rate deceleration in one-third of highly active women immediately after exercise

Conclusion

Exercise is an important aspect of a healthy, well-balanced lifestyle for all women, including those of childbearing age. Aerobic exercise during pregnancy has the ability to influence maternal and fetal health. The acute physiologic changes during exercise and long-term adaptations from repeated bouts of exercise can have a considerable impact on fetal development and maternal well-being. In the absence of contraindicated obstetric or maternal medical conditions, data demonstrates that aerobic exercise can safely be performed during pregnancy in all women, regardless of their prepregnancy level of activity. It should be noted that certain activities may place the fetus in physical or physiologic danger secondary to risk of blunt abdominal trauma and/or the lack of maternal physiologic safeguards to protect the developing fetus from stress. It is universally recommended that such activities be avoided during pregnancy, which are outlined in Table 4.2. Additionally, there is limited data to suggest that reaching near-maximal levels of exertion in highly active and elite athletes can create physiologic circumstances which can compromise fetal well-being.

Prior to engaging in an exercise program, it is recommended that all pregnant women consult with their obstetric provider to develop an exercise prescription that will promote further maternal and fetal health while mitigating the risk of exercise. Exercise, especially in the first and second trimester, has been associated with lower evidence of fetal distress, shorter duration of labor, and overall improved maternal and fetal well-being. All providers who regularly interact with obstetric patients should encourage patients to participate in a safe form of exercise during their pregnancy. Exercise prescriptions written by these providers can help set up safe boundaries for women to avoid overexertion which could potentially compromise fetal or maternal well-being.

References

1. Artal R, O'Toole M. Guidelines of the American College of Obstetricians and Gynecologists for exercise during pregnancy and the postpartum period. Br J Sports Med. 2003;37(1):6–12.
2. Lumbers ER. Exercise in pregnancy: physiological basis of exercise prescription for the pregnant woman. J Sci Med Sport. 2002;5(1):20–31.
3. Capeless EL, Clapp JF. Cardiovascular changes in early phase of pregnancy. Am J Obstet Gynecol. 1989;161(6):1449–53.
4. Morton MJ, Paul MS, Campos GR, Hart MV, Metcalfe J. Exercise dynamics in late gestation: effects of physical training. Am J Obstet Gynecol. 1985;151(1):91–7.
5. Gilroy RJ, Mangura BT, Lavietes MH. Rib cage and abdominal volume displacements during breathing in pregnancy. Am Rev Respir Dis. 1988;137(3):668–72.
6. Karzel RP, Freedman MJ. Orthopedic injuries in pregnancy. In: Artal R, Wiswell RA, Drinkwater BL, editors. Pregnancy. 2nd ed. Baltimore: Lippincott Williams & Wilkins; 1991.
7. Clapp III JF. The changing thermal response to endurance exercise during pregnancy. Am J Obstet Gynecol. 1991;165(6):1684–9.
8. Clapp III JF. The course of labor after endurance exercise during pregnancy. Am J Obstet Gynecol. 1990;163(6):1799–805.
9. Jeffreys RM, Wtepanchak W, Lopez B, Haris J, Clapp 3rd JF. Uterine blood flow during supine rest and exercise after 28 weeks of gestation. Br J Obstet Gynaecol. 2006;113(11):1239–47.
10. Clapp 3rd JF, Schmidt S, Paranjape A, Lopez B. Maternal insulin-like growth factor-I levels (IGF-I) reflect placental mass and neonatal fat mass. Am J Obstet Gynecol. 2004;190(3):730–6.
11. Clapp III JF, Kim H, Burciu B, Schmidt S, Petry K, Lopez B. Continuing regular exercise during pregnancy: effect of exercise volume on fetoplacental growth. Am J Obstet Gynecol. 2002;186(1):142–7.
12. Gorski J. Exercise during pregnancy: maternal and fetal responses. A brief review. Med Sci Sports Exerc. 1985;17(4):407–16.
13. Clapp III JF, Kim H, Burciu B, Lopez B. Beginning regular exercise in early pregnancy: effect of fetoplacental growth. Am J Obstet Gynecol. 2000;183(6):1484–8.
14. Fleten C, Stigum H, Magnus P, Nystad W. Exercise during pregnancy, maternal prepregnancy body mass index and birth weight. Obstet Gynecol. 2010;115(2):331–7.

15. Juhl M, Olsen J, Andersen PK, Nohr EA, Andersen AM. Physical exercise during pregnancy and fetal growth measures: as study within the Danish National Birth Cohort. Am J Obstet Gynecol. 2012;202(1):63.e1–8.

16. Juhl M, Andersen PK, Olsen J, Madsen M, Jorgensen T, Nohr EA, et al. Physical exercise during pregnancy and the risk of preterm birth: a study within the Danish National Birth Cohort. Am J Epidemiol. 2008; 167(7):859–66.

17. Hopkins SA, Baldi JC, Cutfield WS, McCowan L, Hofman PL. Exercise training in pregnancy reduces offspring size without changes in maternal insulin sensitivity. J Clin Endocrinol Metabol. 2010;95(5):2080–8.

18. Kramer MS, McDonald SW. Aerobic exercise for women during pregnancy. Cochrane Database Syst Rev. 2006;19(3), CD000180.

19. Davies GA, Wolfe LA, Mottola MF, MacKinnon C. Joint SOGC/CSEP clinical practice guidelines: exercise in pregnancy and the postpartum period. Can J Appl Physiol. 2003;28(3):329–41.

20. Lavigne P. Pregnant athletes don't have to sit out. ESPN.com. 2009. http://sports.espn.go.com/espn/otl/news/story?id=4693739. Accessed 1 July 2015.

21. Australia SM. SMA statement the benefits and risk of exercise during pregnancy. J Sci Med Sport. 2002;5(1):11–9.

22. Artal R, Clapp III JF, Vigil DV. ACSM current comment: exercise during pregnancy. https://www.acsm. org/docs/current-comments/exerciseduringpregnancy.pdf?sfvrsn=4. Accessed 1 July 2015.

23. ACOG Committee Obstetric Practice. ACOG Committee opinion, number 267, January 2002: exercise during pregnancy and the postpartum period. Obstet Gynecol. 2002;99(1):171–3.

24. Tenforde AS, Toth KE, Langen E, Freddericson M, Sainani KL. Running habits of competitive runners during pregnancy and breastfeeding. Sports Health. 2015;7(2):172–6.

25. Haskell WL, Nelson ME. 20080 U.S. Department of Health and Human Services Physical Activity Guidelines Advisory Committee Report. http://health.gov/paguidelines/pdf/paguide.pdf. Accessed 1 July 2015.

26. Syzmanski LM, Satin AJ. Exercise during pregnancy: fetal responses to current public health guidelines. Obstet Gynecol. 2012;119(3):603–10.

27. Ruchat SM, Davenoport MH, Giroux I, Hillier M, Batada A, Sopper MM, et al. Walking program of low or vigorous intensity during pregnancy confers an aerobic benefit. Int J Sports Med. 2012;33(8):661–6.

28. Salvesen KA, Hem E, Sundgot-Borgen J. Fetal well-being may be compromised during strenuous exercise among pregnant elite athletes. Br J Sports Med. 2012;46(4):279–83.

29. Szymanski LM, Satin AJ. Strenuous exercise during pregnancy: is there a limit? Am J Obstet Gynecol. 2012;207(3):179.e1–6.

Gender Differences: Considerations for the Female Endurance Athlete

5

Scott Annett, Kyle Cassas, and Sean Bryan

Abbreviations

ACSM	American College of Sports Medicine
ADH	Antidiuretic hormone
ALP	Alkaline phosphatase
BMD	Bone mineral density
BMI	Body mass index
BMP	Basic metabolic panel
CAH	Congenital adrenal hyperplasia
CBC	Complete blood count
CO	Cardiac output
CPM	Central pontine myelinolysis
DEXA	Dual-energy X-ray absorptiometry
DHEA-S	Dehydroepiandrosterone sulfate
DSM-IV	Diagnostic and Statistical Manual of Mental Disorders 4th Edition
EAC	Exercise-associated collapse
EAH	Exercise-associated hyponatremia
EBV	Epstein-Barr virus
ESR	Erythrocyte sedimentation rate
FAT	Female athlete triad
FHA	Functional hypothalamic amenorrhea
FSH	Follicle-stimulating hormone
GnRH	Gonadotropin-releasing hormone
HcG	Human chorionic gonadotropin
ICP	Intracranial pressure
IV	Intravenous
LH	Luteinizing hormone
OCP	Oral contraceptive pill
PCOS	Polycystic ovary syndrome
PTH	Parathyroid hormone
RED-S	Relative energy deficiency in sport
SUI	Stress urinary incontinence
TFTs	Thyroid function tests
TIBC	Total iron binding capacity
TPR	Total peripheral resistance
TSH	Thyroid-stimulating hormone
UA	Urinalysis
$VO2_{max}$	Maximal oxygen consumption

S. Annett (✉)
Steadman Hawkins Clinic of the Carolinas, Heritage Internal Medicine and Pediatrics, Greenville Health System, 727 SE Main St., Suite 300, Simpsonville, SC 29681, USA
e-mail: scott.annett@gmail.com

K. Cassas
Steadman Hawkins Clinic of the Carolinas, Greenville Health System, 200 Patewood Dr. Ste C-100, Greenville, SC 29615, USA

S. Bryan
Family Medicine, Greenville Health System, 7 Independence Pointe, Suite 120, Greenville, SC 29615, USA

Historical Perspective

Women's participation in sport has made leaps and bounds in recent decades. In ancient Greek times, women were not allowed to even partake as spectators of the Olympics, and certainly they could not participate. Turn the clock forward, and in 2004, more than 4000 women participated in the majority of the events at the Olympics [1].

© Springer International Publishing Switzerland 2016
T.L. Miller (ed.), *Endurance Sports Medicine*, DOI 10.1007/978-3-319-32982-6_5

The adoption of Title IX in 1972 was an important legislative event in the United States that catapulted women's participation in athletics. Prior to this bill, 310,000 women were estimated to be participating in sports. In 2010, this number exceeded three million [2, 3].

Women participating in endurance events are an even newer phenomenon. Men have been running the marathon at the modern Olympics since London in 1908, while it wasn't until Beth Bonner made the leap in 1971 at the Philadelphia marathon that women even began competing in such distance events [4]. However, it did not take long for women to start excelling, as evident by Pamela Reed's accomplishment beating all comers at the 2003 Badwater 131 mile Ultramarathon. Triathlons did not begin until 1978 when 12 men battled the Hawaii Ironman Triathlon. By 1981, 20 women had completed this race, while in 2010, more than 470 women, or 27% of the participants, completed Hawaii Ironman. In fact, USA Triathlon's membership numbers had climbed to 38% women in 2011. In longer races, such as ultra-triathlons, women's participation remains relatively low, reported at <10% [5].

Anatomical and Physiological Differences in the Female Endurance Athlete

Male and female endurance athletes have different medical conditions, and some of these stem from some basic differences in their anatomy and physiology. These differences also play a role in training and performance. Anatomic differences in women such as smaller hearts pumping a smaller blood volume and lower muscle masses lead to different physiological adaptations. Muscle mass is greater in men than in women and certainly impacts performance. For example, male endurance cyclists have greater lower extremity muscle mass that seems to account for at least some of their peak and mean power output advantages compared to women [6]. Muscle fiber size seems to be the underlying principle behind this strength advantage [7]. Smaller lung volumes lead to a higher work of breathing in women, although these lung volumes are adaptable to endurance exercise [8, 9]. These changes in women are highlighted by a lower potential maximal oxygen consumption, or $VO2_{max}$, along with other physiological considerations such as their lactate threshold and muscle economy.

$VO2_{max}$

$VO2_{max}$, or maximal oxygen consumption, is widely accepted as the gold standard measure for assessing one's ability to perform endurance exercise, and strength training has little effect on this [10]. A 20–29-year-old male with fair fitness will have a $VO2_{max}$ between 36.5 and 40.9 ml/kg/min, while the same young, untrained female will be between 29 and 32.9 ml/kg/min. Even with significant endurance training, superior $VO2_{max}$ normative data indicate that a female in this same age range can top 41 ml/kg/min, while males will surpass 52.4 ml/kg/min [11]. Anatomic differences in body weight, body fat, and subsequently oxygen delivery with lower hemoglobin all drive this gap [12, 13]. We have already accounted for the differences in body weight with the above normative data, as it is a function of one's body weight. The difference in the true absolute $VO2_{max}$ would thus be even greater between the sexes, as men on average are taller and heavier than their female counterparts. Women also have higher percentages of body fat compared to men and thus less muscle mass that can contribute to oxygen delivery. The American Council on Exercise body fat chart shows that women require 10–13% body fat as essential fats compared to their male counterparts at 2–5%. Breast tissue, hormones, sexual organs, and ovulation account for the majority of this difference, as they require higher fat content for optimal physiology. Thus, high-level male athletes can have body fats in the 6–13% range, while women generally are in the 14–20% range [14]. As an aside, higher body fat content may be helpful as an insulator in cold water swimming endurance events and can add buoyancy [15, 16]. Multiple studies have also shown that a lower body fat does not necessarily correlate with faster race times in women as it does in men, but performance seems more dependent on training volume [17–21]. Once again, however, if we level the playing field and account for these differences, men would still hold a slight advantage in $VO2_{max}$.

Cardiac output (CO), oxygen carrying capacity, and pulmonary diffusion capacity are all principles that must be accounted for in determining one's $VO2_{max}$ based on the Fick principle. CO is a function of heart rate and stroke volume, while oxygen carrying capacity is influenced mainly by one's hemoglobin content and to a lesser extent one's oxygen saturation. Other smaller, peripheral factors such as muscle diffusion capacity, mitochondrial enzymes, and capillary density all play a role, but are less important. Stroke volume is a function mainly of fat-free mass [22], and thus males tend to have higher stroke volumes and thus a higher cardiac output. Women also on average tend to have a lower hemoglobin content (about 10 % less) than men and thus decreased oxygen delivery. This stems mainly from losses associated with menstruation and other hormonal differences.

Improvements in $VO2_{max}$ secondary to aerobic endurance training occur via different cardiac adaptations in younger and older women. Younger women have a greater change in their maximal cardiac output that drives their $VO2_{max}$, while older women rely more on the interactions of maximal arterial and venous oxygen differences [23]. This change in older women has been further delineated in that endurance-trained older women have better matching of oxygen delivery to oxygen utilization via increases in capillary density leading to an increased rate of adjustment for pulmonary oxygen uptake compared to their untrained peers [24]. Endurance training more so than sprint training can lead to myocardial wall thickening [25]. Furthermore, atrial remodeling seems to be more modest in female athletes in response to training [26].

Other Sex Differences

Hormones play a role in performance as well. There is certainly ample data on estrogen and its role in bone health and the development of stress fractures. The effects of progesterone and the menstrual cycle itself have to be analyzed as well. A woman's core body temperature threshold changes based on their menstrual cycle, and so what stage of the menstrual cycle a woman is in can affect heat loss and their training capacity [27]. Training capacity is even influenced by carbohydrate consumption based on the particular menstrual phase that a woman is in [28]. As a corollary, testosterone and its effect on one's recovery capacity may influence training volume and maximal output from one's training regimen [29]. Testosterone is important in building muscle mass and strength, and older women in particular may have limited gains in muscle strength with underlying low testosterone levels [13, 30].

Psychosocial factors have to be contemplated as well, and whether it's one's body image or passion for competition that drives one to succeed, these differences may alter the time it takes to cross the finish line. Mental fatigue can undermine performance, while imagery, self-talk, and goal setting can all help to improve performance [31]. Mirinda Carfrae's world record time of 8:52.14 in 2013 at the Kona Ironman World Championships was a phenomenal feat, but it was still 48 min slower than the fastest male time set in 2011. Most studies looking at sex differences in performance secondary to the aforementioned $VO2_{max}$ differences show a 10–15 % gap in endurance race times. A couple of studies, one in 100 km running and one in ultra open water swimming, have shown slightly smaller gaps in the 3.7–5.0 % range [32–35].

Medical Conditions in the Female Endurance Athlete

Endurance athletes often battle with a spectrum of injuries as well as medical conditions that are unique within the field of sports medicine. Overuse injuries such as patellofemoral pain syndrome and IT band syndrome are common, as well as stress fractures. However, there are medical conditions that are often seen in endurance athletes at a much higher prevalence than in non-endurance athletes. The female endurance athlete in particular seems to be at greater risk for certain conditions, such as anemia, stress urinary incontinence (SUI), and overtraining syndrome, all of which can adversely impact performance. Iron depletion and iron deficiency anemia have certainly come to light in recent years, and women endurance athletes are one of the groups at the highest risk. Stress urinary incontinence, once an idea revolving around elderly and parous women, has been shown to be quite the common condition in endurance-trained women. Overtraining syndrome is being recognized more and more as athletes are training harder than ever. Women are now facing this problem just as often as men given their increased participation in athletics. Even the most common medical conditions seen during endurance events, exercise-associated collapse (EAC) and hyponatremia (EAH), appear to have a higher prevalence among women endurance athletes. Medical conditions common in the female endurance athlete population are summarized in Table 5.1.

Iron Deficiency Anemia and Iron Depletion

Anemia is a common medical condition that is seen in both men and women, most often associated with iron deficiency. Women are at greater risk for anemia than men, and as many as 20–30 % of the general population of adolescent and young women have iron depletion. This rises to 40–50 % when discussing adolescent female athletes [3]. Iron deficiency with anemia can be seen with a prevalence of 3–5 % among 18–44-year-old women [36]. Other contributing causes such as dietary intake, hemolysis, increased losses from the GI or GU tract, as well as poor iron absorption can lead to anemia. Other risk factors besides female gender for anemia would include athletic activity, long-distance running, adolescence, and being a vegetarian.

In iron deficiency anemia, hemoglobin is reduced leading to less oxygen delivery to the peripheral tissues and thus a decrease in maximal oxygen consumption, or $VO2_{max}$. In fact, 65 % of body iron is incorporated into hemoglobin [37]. However, the impact of iron deficiency without anemia on performance is less clear. There are oxidative enzymes and respiratory proteins that are dependent upon iron, and thus one would hypothesize that iron deficiency itself would impair one's ability to sustain maximal performance during endurance exercise. Older studies, such as Klingshirn et al., showed that 8 weeks of iron supplementation in female endurance runners improved iron stores but did not affect endurance capacity [38]. More recently, multiple

Table 5.1 Common medical conditions in female endurance athletes

Clinical condition	Signs and symptoms	Female concerns	Treatment
Iron deficiency anemia and iron depletion	Poor performance and fatigue; reduced $VO2_{max}$	Increased prevalence, especially endurance athletes; up to 50 % female adolescent athletes are iron depleted	325 mg ferrous sulfate 1 tab 1–3 times daily Ensure adequate dietary intake Target ferritin of 60
Stress urinary incontinence (SUI)	Involuntary leakage of urine as a result of increased abdominal pressure	Up to 50 % of female endurance athletes report SUI	Pelvic floor exercises; electrical stimulation and surgery rarely needed
Overtraining syndrome	Decreased performance and fatigue; persist despite 2 weeks of rest	More susceptible to recurrent infection and upper respiratory symptoms	Rest for weeks to months; consider cross-training and short 5–10-min aerobic sessions
Exercise-associated collapse (EAC) and hyponatremia (EAH)	Collapse after vigorous exercise; weight gain from overhydration, weakness, vomiting, and possibly neurological symptoms with hyponatremia	Increased prevalence; may be more directly related to lower BMI and longer time-outs on the course in women	Oral hydration and Trendelenburg positioning for EAC; 3 % hypertonic saline for severe symptoms with hyponatremia; prevention drink based on athlete's thirst

studies have provided convincing data that iron depletion and not just anemia can have a negative impact on performance. Hinton et al. showed that iron-depleted, nonanemic women who underwent iron supplementation in conjunction with a training program did significantly improve their endurance capacity as evident by improved 15 km time trial times [36]. McClung et al. showed in a randomized control trial that daily supplementation with 100 mg of iron sulfate can attenuate iron depletion often observed during basic combat training as well as improving physical performance in those soldiers with iron deficiency anemia [39]. Dellavalle et al. investigated a cohort of female rowers and found that iron-depleted, nonanemic rowers' exertion and energy costs were increased to do the same workload [40]. They also showed that those that trained less hard had a more profound impact on their performance [41]. Thus, this growing body of evidence is certainly showing that athletes with iron depletion in the absence of anemia, in addition to athletes with anemia, will likely benefit from iron supplementation, especially in endurance events.

Treatment of iron depletion as well as iron deficiency anemia is with iron supplementation and a diet with highly bioavailable sources of iron. Meat, legumes, and seafood are good sources of dietary iron. Vitamin C intake in conjunction with dietary iron and/or iron supplements can help to enhance iron absorption, especially in those individuals taking histamine-2-blocking and proton pump-inhibiting medications, as the ascorbic acid helps chelate the iron making it more bioavailable. The American College of Sports Medicine in their joint position statement in 2009 recommended iron as a dietary supplement for endurance athletes, as they are at risk for depleting their stores of iron with training. Most studies have shown that treatment with 100 mg day^{-1} of heme iron in the form of ferrous sulfate can replenish iron stores within 2–3 months. A basal serum ferritin level <35 mg l^{-1} is often used as the cutoff to begin supplementation, with a target of 60 mg l^{-1}. Ferritin is usually checked on an annual or biannual basis depending on one's age and risk

factors [42]. Iron supplementation should be discontinued when serum ferritin values have reached their target to avoid adverse effects associated with iron toxicity [43]. Iron supplementation has not been shown to be helpful in those without iron depletion or iron deficiency anemia and may be harmful.

Stress Urinary Incontinence

Until recently, urinary incontinence was felt to affect primarily elderly and parous women. However, with more and more women participating in sport, including endurance sports and other high-impact activities, it has been shown that incontinence is more prevalent than once thought. Urinary incontinence is defined as involuntary loss of urine. This is usually characterized as stress, urge, or mixed. Stress urinary incontinence (SUI) is involuntary leakage of urine as a result of effort, exertion, sneezing, or coughing that increases one's intra-abdominal pressure. This is the most common form and occurs secondary to changes in the fascia and subcutaneous tissues as well as weakness of the pelvic floor muscles. Professional sport has been a known risk factor for SUI, along with pregnancy, surgery, and congenital anomalies. The prevalence of SUI in training athletes has been identified, and reported ranges are from a low of 10 % in studies where a large majority of the athletes are nulliparous to a high of 56 % [44]. Athletes participating in gymnastics seem to report the highest rates, reported at 56 %, and jumping is the activity with the highest association. In a study of female endurance athletes, Poświata et al. showed that 50 % of their study subjects reported incontinence, 45 % of these being of the stress variety [45]. The prevalence of urinary incontinence does not seem to be higher among former athletes than age-matched controls. However, athletes who report incontinence early in life, especially during competition, are at increased risk of incontinence later in life [46]. Studies are conflicting on whether or not elite female athletes have a higher prevalence of SUI than age-matched controls. One study that did show a difference was Caylet et al. who reported a prevalence of 28 % among elite female athletes while observing a rate of only 9.8 % in the general population [47].

The morbidity associated with SUI can have an impact on one's quality of life. For example, 27–30 % of athletes report avoiding sport or modifying activity when they have symptoms of incontinence [48]. The first line of treatment is generally pelvic floor muscle exercises. Randomized controlled trials have shown that pelvic floor exercises are superior to both placebo as well as electrical stimulation. It has been reported that only a week of practice where women voluntarily contract before and during coughing can significantly reduce urinary leakage [44]. Cure and improvement rates have been reported between 56 and 70 % for stress and mixed incontinence [49]. Theoretically, a combination of teaching women to precontract prior to an increase in abdominal pressure as well as performing strength training exercises of the pelvic floor muscles would lead to optimal improvement in symptoms. Electrical stimulation and surgery are other options as well, although rarely needed.

Overtraining Syndrome

Overtraining syndrome is a clinical entity where athletes are overwhelmed by their training regimen and their bodies are unable to adapt. There is a wide clinical spectrum for this condition, and it is essentially a systemic overuse injury. Burnout, staleness, and chronic fatigue in athletes are other terms that have been used to describe this condition. Decreased performance and fatigue are the hallmarks, but poor sleep, "heavy legs," and increased rates of other injuries and infections are often seen as well. In fact, more than 90 % of cases will have poor sleep associated with them [50]. Recurrent infections can occur as well when the athlete tries to return to training. This may be more problematic in women endurance athletes, as they seem to be a bit more susceptible to upper respiratory infections than their male counterparts [51]. Increased infections are often seen in overtraining syndrome, but this is likely associated

with impaired immune parameters secondary to prolonged high-intensity training. By definition, these symptoms persist despite 2 weeks of rest and time away from sport.

Overtraining results from under-recovery in the setting of prolonged and/or intense exercise. This may be in conjunction with a physical or psychological stress or a recent increase in training. Regardless, most athletes can recover within 2 weeks and the term overreaching is used. This can be quite helpful in building one's performance. But when an athlete cannot recover within 2 weeks, overtraining is present. Lab tests can be obtained to look for other causes of fatigue, but there are no labs that are specific for overtraining. For example, a complete blood count (CBC) may help to look for anemia, while Epstein-Barr viral (EBV) titers may show that they are suffering from a post viral syndrome. Sleep, nutrition, and social stressors are important diagnostic considerations. A sleep log can help to identify if poor sleep hygiene is contributing to their fatigue. Newer technologies such as the wearable fitness trackers often have sleep assessments built in that can aid a clinician in this assessment. A sports exercise test can be used if baseline data is available to show that the athlete is suffering from a decrease in performance. $VO2_{max}$ will be reduced and resting heart rate will be increased. Overtraining is typically a diagnosis of exclusion, thus making the diagnosis often requires evaluating for and ruling out other possible causes of fatigue. Table 5.2 summarizes some of the frequently encountered conditions to consider when entertaining the diagnosis of overtraining syndrome.

Training intensity and the spacing of the training sessions seem to be the most critical in optimizing performance while decreasing the risk of overtraining. Rest, tapering, and periodization are all important components to a training program, especially because many athletes compete year round and do not have an "off season" [52]. Treatment is vital and consists of rest and time away from sport. This can require several weeks or even several months. Often compliance is an issue as no athlete wants to be told that they cannot train. Therefore, cross-training and utilizing

Table 5.2 Common diagnostic considerations in the evaluation of overtraining syndrome

Clinical condition	Historical clues	Evaluation and diagnostic work-up
Nutritional deficiency	Increased training volume without increasing caloric intake; losing weight while training	25-OH vitamin D, basic metabolic panel, magnesium, phosphorus Food diary
Anemia	Exertional fatigue; inadequate iron intake, heavy menstrual periods	CBC, iron studies (iron, ferritin, TIBC, transferrin, % saturation)
Psychological problems	Morning fatigue, impaired mental performance, apathy, disinterest, performance anxiety	No specific laboratory work-up is useful
Hyper-/hypothyroidism	Hypothyroidism: cold intolerance, weight gain, constipation, and periorbital edema Hyperthyroidism: heat intolerance, warm skin, weight loss, diarrhea, urinary frequency, and exophthalmos	TSH (thyroid-stimulating hormone) with reflex free T4
Post-viral syndrome	Fever, lymphadenopathy, myalgias, pharyngitis, cough, and rash 2–12 weeks prior	Viral-specific testing (Heterophile antibody or EBV titers for mononucleosis)

short training sessions of 5–10 min of aerobic activity a day may be helpful while the symptoms abate. These sessions can be increased over a 6–12-week period. Antidepressants may have a transient role if the athlete is suffering from concurrent depression, although no specific medications have been shown to be helpful for overtraining alone.

Exercise-Associated Collapse and Hyponatremia

EAC is a common entity seen at the end of endurance events, comprising 59–85 % of all visits after marathons and ultramarathons to the medical tent [53]. The majority of these cases are a benign form of transient hypotension secondary to venous pooling in the lower extremities after cessation of exercise with an inadequate baroreflex response. During the recovery phase immediately after endurance exercise, skin and arm blood flow is increased along with blood flow back to the visceral organs, while one's active muscles maintain their increased blood flow initially. Post-exercise hypotension occurs equally in both men and women, but this may occur via different mechanisms. Total peripheral resistance (TPR) is reduced and is not completely offset by an increased CO, thus leading to post-exercise hypotension in women [54, 55]. In endurance-

trained men, vasodilation occurs more as a result of decreased CO, while there is little change in TPR [56].

The diagnostic challenge for clinicians is sorting out this benign cause versus potentially more severe causes such as hyponatremia, heat-related illness, or cardiovascular events. The athlete with EAC is unable to stand or walk unaided secondary to syncope or dizziness after completion of an event. Treatment consists of elevation of the athlete's legs and feet along with oral rehydration, and this should lead to resolution of symptoms. Skin surface cooling has shown some evidence as a supplemental therapy as well. Runners who are prone to this condition may even benefit from wearing compression hose while running [53]. Compression socks have also been shown in some studies to improve performance [57]. Should symptoms persist, one must search for other causes as mentioned above.

Exercise-associated hyponatremia (EAH) occurs secondary to overhydration with hypotonic fluids during an endurance event. This is defined by a serum sodium less than 135 mEq/l during or within 24 h post-race. Overdrinking, antidiuretic hormone (ADH) secretion, and a failure to mobilize sodium are felt to be the main factors causing this [58]. The latter of the three, related to losses from sweat, is probably the most controversial and contributes the least. EAH is seen more commonly in female endurance athletes, as well as those that are slower runners who are subsequently out on the course longer or competing in longer events [59]. The prevalence of EAH in the literature has been quite variable, with ranges as high as 50 % [60]. One study in marathoners showed the prevalence to be around 12–13 % for elite marathoners, as opposed to 22 % in non-elite marathoners. Even longer races, such as Ironman triathlons, have reported prevalence rates as high as 29 % [58]. Female athletes also tend to have higher prevalence rates as compared to males. The effects of progesterone and estrogen on one's thirst threshold as well as on ADH secretion may help to explain why females seem to be at greater risk for developing EAH. However, when adjusted for time-out on the course and body mass index (BMI), gender does not seem to make as much of a difference [60].

Athletes may have gained weight during the endurance event secondary to excess fluid intake. These athletes may also complain of bloating, weakness, weight gain, and vomiting. In severe cases, altered mental status, seizures, and respiratory distress from pulmonary edema can occur. This can progress to cerebral edema and death if not recognized and treated promptly. These athletes are typically not hyperthermic, in contrast to collapse associated with heat illness.

Treatment of exercise-associated hyponatremia consists of hypertonic saline. A 100 ml intravenous (IV) bolus of 3 % hypertonic saline can usually reverse severe symptoms from hyponatremia within a few minutes, while oral rehydration solutions may be more appropriate for mild symptoms. Three IV boluses spaced at 10 min apart can be given to relieve severe symptoms. Central pontine myelinolysis (CPM) is always a fear when reversing hyponatremia rapidly, but an acute drop in sodium that occurs during an endurance event suggests that one will tolerate quick normalization of the sodium. In fact, there have not been any cases of CPM in athletes reported to date [61]. Both isotonic saline (0.9 %) and lactated Ringer's have been shown to prolong recovery and are not recommended.

Avoiding overhydration and thus prevention are key. Consuming 400–800 ml of fluid per hour instead of 800–1000 ml/h in events longer than 4 h may help prevent hyponatremia [62]. It has been shown that hyponatremic marathoners consume on average 0.84 L/h [60]. Other studies have suggested that athletes who drink only in response to thirst have not developed EAH [58]. Spacing out drink stations every 3 km can help mitigate this problem as well.

The Female Athlete Triad and the Relative Energy Deficiency in Sport

With the increase in sports participation by women after Title IX was passed in the United States in the 1970s, several medical conditions became more apparent in women. It started with the recognition that professional ballet dancers suffered from a high incidence of stress fractures as well as amenorrhea. Soon thereafter, an association was identified between disordered eating, amenorrhea, and musculoskeletal injuries. In 1992, the Task Force on Women's Issues of the American College of Sports Medicine (ACSM) coined the term the female athlete triad (FAT). By definition, disordered eating, amenorrhea, and osteoporosis had to be present to qualify for the diagnosis. Over the next 15 years, it was concluded that the condition was being underreported and under-recognized. Then in 2007, the ACSM updated its definition as a spectrum of dysfunction in energy availability, menstrual function, and bone mineral density (BMD). No longer did an athlete have to suffer from all three conditions to qualify for the diagnosis, but having one condition should prompt clinicians to search for the other components. This dramatically increased the prevalence and recognition of the disorder. Then in 2012 and 2013, the Female Athlete Triad Coalition convened. The goals of this convention were to address screening, treatment, and return to play. They identified 11 risk factors that should be screened. Each risk factor was assigned a different point, and if the athlete was identified as having six or more points, they should be restricted from participation. Screening

Table 5.3 Medical conditions associated with the female athlete triad. When one condition is present, the clinician should evaluate for the other ones

Clinical condition	Signs and symptoms	Diagnostic work-up	Treatment
Low energy availability	Restricting calories or excessive exercise; BMI <17.5; eating disorders	Labs to consider: CBC, ESR, TSH, ferritin, Mg, Phos, 25OH vitamin D, vitamin B12; may require EKG or DEXA scan	Multidisciplinary approach; increase caloric intake to gain weight
Menstrual dysfunction	No menarche by age 15; 3 consecutive months without periods	Initial labs to consider: pregnancy test, LH, FSH, TSH, prolactin; may require pelvic US	Varies depending on etiology; if FHA, need to increase calories; OCPs falling out of favor
Poor bone health	Consider with stress fracture and after 6 months of amenorrhea, oligomenorrhea, disordered eating, or an eating disorder	Labs to consider: CBC, BMP, TSH, PTH, ALP, 24-h urine calcium, cortisol, and celiac antibodies; requires a DEXA scan	1200–1500 mg of elemental calcium and 400–800 IU of vitamin D; assess risk factors (e.g., cessation of tobacco use)
Stress fractures	Pain over bony structure, worse with weight bearing; can progress to pain at rest	Plain radiographs often negative within first 2–4 weeks and then may show periosteal reaction or fracture line; MRI and bone scan are more sensitive	Relative rest; stiff soled plate for metatarsal stress fractures; high-risk stress fractures usually require orthopedic referral

is recommended at the pre-participation exam or annual health exam. The 2014 IOC consensus statement took the female athlete triad one step further adapting a broader term called relative energy deficiency in sport or RED-S. This syndrome encompasses the components of the female athlete triad but also includes metabolic rate, immunity, protein synthesis, cardiovascular health, and psychological health and can be applied to male athletes as well [63]. Melin et al. showed that hypotension, hypoglycemia, and hyperlipidemia are common clinical features along with female athlete triad conditions [64]. Table 5.3 summarizes the medical conditions surrounding the female athlete triad (Fig. 5.1).

Energy Availability

Formerly called disordered eating, energy availability is the new term identifying the spectrum of nutritional optimization of a female athlete. Eating disorders such as anorexia nervosa and bulimia fall under this umbrella, but are not essential for diagnosis. These disorders are 10 times more likely in women than in men and far more common in athletes than non-athletes. Sports that emphasize low body weights and thinness such as ballet, gymnastics, figure skating, and

distance running have even higher rates. The prevalence of this disorder is difficult to calculate and currently unknown, but some estimates have ranged from 15 to 62 % in female athletes [3]. In one study, 5.4 % of athletes with eating disorders had suicide attempts, emphasizing the significant morbidity of the condition [65]. There are two main causes of poor energy availability: one, the athlete is restricting calories or not consuming enough calories, such as in bulimia or anorexia nervosa, and two, they are burning more calories than the body is designed to handle. Calculating energy availability is simple in principle but is often difficult clinically. It is obtained by subtracting the calories expended from those consumed divided by lean body weight. Low energy availability is seen with <45 kcal/kg of lean body mass, with most symptoms developing with <30 kcal/kg. Perhaps a better screening tool is looking at BMI. A BMI <17.5 kg/m^2 usually represents an athlete with low energy stores. However, triad-associated conditions are commonly seen in elite endurance athletes despite a normal BMI [64]. A detailed diet and exercise history is essential to help identify those athletes that are not so clear cut.

Eating disorders represent the spectrum of energy availability with the most severe pathology. Anorexia nervosa is defined as refusal to

Fig. 5.1 Medical considerations of relative energy deficiency in sport (RED-S) and the incorporation of the female athlete triad into this concept [63]

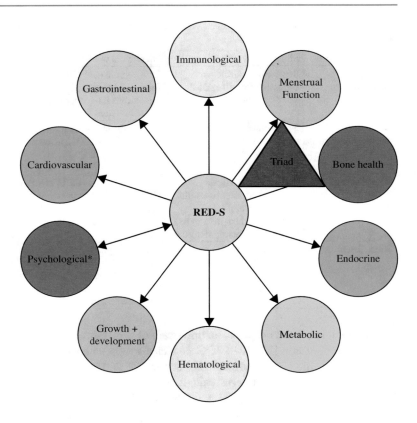

maintain minimal body weight for height (<85 % of expected weight), intense fear of weight gain, disturbed body image, and 3 months of consecutive secondary amenorrhea or primary amenorrhea at the age of 16. Bulimia is defined as recurrent binge eating, overeating, compensatory behavior from overeating (such as vomiting or laxative abuse), or fasting. This is often associated with excessive exercise with a negative body image. Binge eating and purging occur at least twice weekly for 3 months. Examination can be helpful in identifying those who may be battling low energy availability and an eating disorder. Bradycardia, lanugo, orthostatic hypotension, poor dentition, chipmunk cheeks (swollen parotid glands), and Russell's sign (callus on dorsum of finger) may be present. In addition to a low BMI, clinicians who are adept at recognizing the above exam findings can help to identify those with possible low energy availability. Laboratory work-up should include electrolytes, a CBC, erythrocyte sedimentation rate (ESR),

thyroid-stimulating hormone (TSH), and urinalysis (UA) [65]. Other labs to consider would include ferritin, magnesium, phosphorus, vitamin D, and vitamin B12. An EKG is often done to evaluate for bradycardic arrhythmias, while a dual-energy X-ray absorptiometry (DEXA) scan can assist in evaluating bone health.

Treatment of low energy availability is also simple in principle and difficult in practice. The athlete needs more calories and increased weight. This typically requires a multidisciplinary team including a dietician, primary care physician with expertise in the field, and a mental health professional. Antidepressants may have a role, especially if an eating disorder is concurrent by DSM-IV definitions. Identifying those athletes with low energy availability early on may help prevent associated conditions such as amenorrhea and osteoporosis as well as stress fractures. Those athletes with disordered eating are at a two- to fourfold increase likelihood of developing a sports injury [2].

Menstrual Dysfunction

Menstrual dysfunction can come in a variety of shapes and sizes and is also quite frequent in female endurance athletes. Amenorrhea can be primary or secondary where primary is defined as an absence of menarche after the age of 15 while secondary occurs with the cessation of menses for three consecutive cycles. Oligomenorrhea can also occur, with cycles longer than 35 days or fewer than 9 per year. The prevalence of amenorrhea among female athletes has ranged from 18 to 54 % in studies, with most of these focusing on the high school athlete [2]. That of the general population is 2–5 %.

Prolonged exertion and weight loss have been shown to affect gonadotropin-releasing hormone (GnRH), although the exact mechanism remains unclear. This leads to downstream effects of luteinizing hormone (LH) and follicle-stimulating hormone (FSH), which disrupts estrogen release from the ovaries. This produces a functional hypothalamic amenorrhea or FHA. When evaluating an athlete for menstrual dysfunction, it is critical to consider other causes besides FHA such as thyroid abnormalities, structural anomalies, pregnancy, polycystic ovary syndrome, or even pituitary masses. Work-up of these conditions often includes a pregnancy test, FSH, LH, prolactin, and TSH. If signs of androgen excess are apparent, free testosterone and DHEA sulfate can be checked. Estradiol and progesterone challenge test may be needed as well (Fig. 5.2).

Estrogen plays an important role in bone health. It has been shown that estrogen deficiency leads to loss of bone mass, and thus amenorrheic women have lower bone mineral density than eumenorrheic women. Athletes have higher BMD than their non-athletic peers as well [66]. Estrogen also helps to mediate vascular adaptations in postmenopausal women who are engaged in endurance exercise and may have a cardioprotective role [67].

Treatment of FHA begins with a focus on increasing one's energy availability, as this is typically the driving force. As long as energy expenditure is relatively controlled, increasing caloric intake will cause weight gain and resumption of normal menses. Oral contraceptive pills (OCPs) have been traditionally used as second-line agents in athletes over 16 years of age. However, they should only be instituted after caloric intake is increased, bone mineral density continues to decrease, and amenorrhea persists. The data is inconclusive on the benefits of OCPs for treating FHA, and long-term OCP use may cause a reduction in bone mineral density if used for more than 2 years, thus this practice is falling out of favor [2].

Poor Bone Health

Ninety to ninety-five percent of peak bone mineral density (PMD) is reached by 18 years of age, with the greatest accrual during puberty between the ages of 11 and 14. Optimal nutrition and adequate caloric intake are vital, even at such young ages. Moderate physical activity with weight-bearing exercise is another crucial component to building BMD. However, high training volumes with high-intensity exercise may have a detrimental effect on bone health [68]. Once an athlete reaches peak bone mass into their 20s and 30s, the rest of life is geared toward maintaining and preventing losses. An amenorrheic runner at age 25 may have comparable bone density to that of a 50-year-old woman [69]. Low BMD is defined as a history of nutritional deficiencies, hypoestrogenism, stress fractures, or other clinical risks for fracture in conjunction with a Z score <1.0 [70]. The prevalence of poor bone health in athletes is difficult to accurately assess, and ranges for low bone mineral density are from 16 to 34 %, with the higher values being identified in elite endurance athletes [2]. Multiple studies have shown that there is a positive association between high training volume, low BMI, and BMD reduction in elite endurance runners [71, 72].

A DEXA scan is the diagnostic procedure of choice when evaluating an athlete's bone mineral density. The Z score along with a PA of the lumbar spine is often used when looking at bone mineral density in premenopausal female athletes. Z scores are used to compare subjects with controls of the same age and sex. In premenopausal

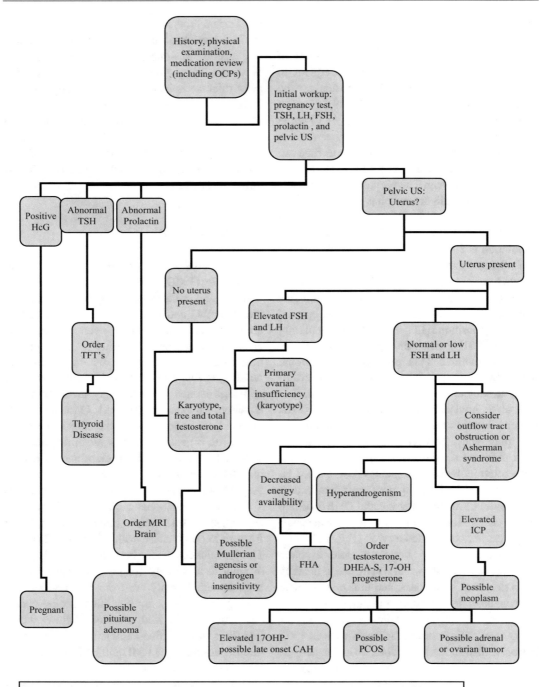

FHA = Functional Hypothalamic Amenorrhea; TSH = thyroid stimulating hormone;
LH = luteneizing hormone; FSH = follicle-stimulating hormone; OCPs = oral
contraceptive pills; DHEA-S = dehydroepiandrosterone sulfate; HcG = human
chorionic gonadotropin; TFTs = thyroid function tests; ICP = intracranial pressure;
CAH = congenital adrenal hyperplasia; PCOS = polycystic ovary syndrome

Fig. 5.2 Algorithm showing the diagnostic considerations when evaluating a patient with primary or secondary amenorrhea

female athletes, a Z score more than 1.0 standard deviation below the mean is considered abnormal and requires further work-up and/or treatment. DEXA should be obtained after a stress or low impact fracture and after 6 months of amenorrhea, oligomenorrhea, disordered eating, or an eating disorder. Vitamin D and calcium should be checked at a minimum, and other possible labs would include CBC, basic metabolic panel (BMP), TSH, parathyroid hormone (PTH), alkaline phosphatase (ALP), 24-h urine calcium, cortisol, and celiac antibodies [70].

Treatment once again starts with optimizing nutrition and ensuring adequate and appropriate exercise. Weight-bearing and dynamic exercises seem to have the most positive effect on bone health. Calcium and vitamin D intake are also important. 1200–1500 mg of elemental calcium and 400–800 IU of vitamin D per day are the recommended daily intakes [73]. Bisphosphonates are not approved to treat bone loss in young athletes. As mentioned previously, maintaining normal menstrual function is important as estrogen is vital for bone health. However, menstrual dysfunction is likely a secondary component to low energy availability, and thus this needs to be addressed first along with identifying high training volumes [74]. Other medical conditions that have to be considered in the work-up of poor bone health would include cigarette smoking, alcohol consumption, corticosteroid use, hyperthyroidism, renal disease, and hyperparathyroidism [75].

Stress Fractures

Stress fractures occur when bone is subjected to repetitive loading and microtrauma develops. Bony remodeling cannot keep pace with these changes, and a stress injury ensues. Athletes with poor bone health have even less capacity to keep up and thus are more susceptible to injury. Female athletes have a higher incidence of stress fractures than their male counterparts. They also seem to have stress fractures at different sites than males. They occur more commonly in amenorrheic women than normally menstruating women, 2–4 times more commonly in fact [1, 65].

Compulsive exercise and lower leg lean tissue mass in female endurance athletes have been identified as risk factors as well [76]. Fractures of the femoral neck, tarsal navicular, metatarsals, and pelvis are seen more commonly in women than in men.

Treatment consists of rest and cross-training when possible and a gradual return to activity. High-risk stress fractures at the superior femoral neck (tension side), patella, middle third of the anterior tibia (tension side), medial malleolus, talus, tarsal navicular, fifth metatarsal, and great toe sesamoids often require more aggressive treatment and frequently are managed by orthopedic surgeons who may advise surgical management.

References

1. Ivković A, Franić M, Bojanić I, Pećina M. Overuse injuries in female athletes. Croat Med J. 2007;48:767–78. doi:10.3325/cmj.2007.6.767.
2. Matzkin E, Curry EJ, Whitlock K. Female athlete triad: past, present, and future. J Am Acad Orthop Surg. 2015;23:424–32.
3. Ireland ML, Ott SM. Special concerns of the female athlete. Clin Sports Med. 2004;23:281–98.
4. Linderman JK. The women's marathon: historical perspective for exercise physiologists. Prof Exerc Physiol Online. 2007;10(11):1–7.
5. Lepers R, Knechtle B, Stapley P. Trends in triathlon performance: effects of sex and age. Sports Med. 2013;43:851–63.
6. Perez-Gomez J, Rodriguez GV, Ara I, Olmedillas H, Chavarren J, González-Henriquez JJ, et al. Role of muscle mass on sprint performance: gender differences? Eur J Appl Physiol. 2008;102(6):685–94.
7. Hunter SK. Sex differences in human fatigability: mechanisms and insight to physiological responses. Acta Physiol (Oxf). 2014;210(4):768–89. doi:10.1111/apha.12234.
8. Layton AM, Garber CE, Thomashow BM, Gerardo RE, Emmert-Aronson BO, Armstrong HF, et al. Exercise ventilatory kinematics in endurance trained and untrained men and women. Respir Physiol Neurobiol. 2011;178:223–9.
9. Guenette JA, Witt JD, McKenzie DC, Road JD, Sheel AW. Respiratory mechanics during exercise in endurance-trained men and women. J Physiol. 2007;581(3):1309–22.
10. Cesar Mde C, Borin JP, Gonelli PR, Simões RA, de Souza TM, Montebelo MI. The effect of local muscle endurance training on cardiorespiratory capacity in young women. J Strength Cond Res. 2009;23(6):1637–43.

11. Heyward VH. VO2$_{Max}$ normative data tables - the physical fitness specialist certification manual. Dallas, TX: Cooper Institute for Aerobics Research. Revised 1997, printed in Advanced fitness assessment and exercise prescription. 3rd ed; 1998. p. 48.

12. Baumgart C, Hoppe MW, Freiwald J. Different endurance characteristics of female and male German soccer players. Biol Sport. 2014;31(3):227–32. doi:10.5604/20831862.1111851.

13. Gender differences in endurance performance and training. http://novellaqalive2.mhhe.com/sites/dl/free/0072461667/38472/Gender_Differences_in_Performance_and_Training.doc.

14. Exercise AC. Ace lifestyle and weight management consultant manual, the ultimate resource for fitness professionals. San Diego, CA. American Council on Exercise; 2009.

15. Knechtle B, Baumann B, Knechtle P. Speed during training and anthropometric measures in relation to race performance by male and female open-water ultra-endurance swimmers. Percept Mot Skills. 2010;111(2):463–74.

16. Rüst CA, Rosemann T, Knechtle B. Performance and sex differences in ultra-triathlon performance from ironman to double deca iron ultra-triathlon between 1978 and 2013. SpringerPlus. 2014;3:219. http://www.springerplus.com/content/3/1/219.

17. Knechtle B, Wirth A, Baumann B, Knechtle P, Rosemann T. Personal best time, percent body fat, and training are differently associated with race time for male and female ironman triathletes. Res Q Exerc Sport. 2010;81(1):62–8.

18. Garcin M, Fleury A, Ansart N, Mille-Hamard L, Billat V. Training content and potential impact on performance. Res Q Exerc Sport. 2006;77(3):351–61. doi:10.1080/02701367.2006.10599369.

19. Knechtle B, Wirth A, Baumann B, Knechtle P, Rosemann T, Oliver S. Differential correlations between anthropometry, training volume, and performance in male and female Ironman triathletes. J Strength Cond Res. 2010;24(10):2785–93.

20. Rüst CA, Knechtle B, Wirth A, Knechtle P, Ellenrieder B, Rosemann T, et al. Personal best times in an Olympic distance triathlon and a marathon predict an Ironman race time for recreational female triathletes. Chin J Physiol. 2012;55(3):156–62.

21. Knechtle B, Rüst CA, Rosemann T, Lepers R. Age and gender interactions in half-Ironman triathlon performances – the Ironman 70.3 Switzerland from 2007 to 2010. Open Access J Sports Med. 2012;3:59–66.

22. Collis T, Devereux RB, Roman MJ, de Simone G, Yeh JL, Howard BV, et al. Relations of stroke volume and cardiac output to body composition: the strong heart study. Circulation. 2001;103:820–5. doi:10.1161/01.CIR.103.6.820.

23. Murias JM, Kowalchuk JM, Paterson DH. Mechanisms for increase VO2max with endurance training in older and young women. Med Sci Sports Exerc. 2010. doi:10.1249/MSS.0b013e3181dd0bba.

24. Dogra S, Spencer MD, Murias JM, Paterson DH. Oxygen uptake kinetics in endurance-trained and untrained postmenopausal women. Appl Physiol Nutr Metab. 2013;38:154–60.

25. Venckunas T, Raugaliente R, Mazutaitiene B, Ramoskeviciute S. Endurance rather than sprint running training increases left ventricular wall thickness in female athletes. Eur J Appl Physiol. 2008;102:307–11. doi:10.1007/s00421-007-0586-5.

26. Mosén H, Steding-Ehrenborg K. Atrial remodeling is less pronounced in female endurance-trained athletes compared with that in male athletes. Scand Cardiovasc J. 2014;48:20–6.

27. Ichinose TK, Inoue Y, Hirata M, Shamsuddin AKM, Kondo N. Enhanced heat loss responses induced by short-term endurance training in exercising women. Exp Physiol. 2008;94(1):90–102. doi:10.1113/expphysiol.2008.043810.

28. McLay RT, Thomson CD, Williams SM, Rehrer NJ. Carbohydrate loading and female endurance athletes: effect of menstrual-cycle phase. Int J Sport Nutr Exerc Metab. 2007;17:189–205.

29. Taipale RS, Häkkinen K. Acute hormonal and force responses to combined strength and endurance loadings in men and women: the "order effect". PLoS One. 2013;8(2), e55051. doi:10.1371/journal.pone.0055051.

30. Sillanpää E, Häkkinen A, Laaksonen DE, Karavirta L, Kraemer WJ, Häkkinen K. Serum basal hormone concentrations, nutrition and physical fitness during strength and/or endurance training in 39–64-year-old women. Int J Sports Med. 2010;31:110–7.

31. McCormick A, Meijen C, Marcora S. Psychological determinants of whole-body endurance performance. Sports Med. 2015;45:997–1015.

32. Zingg MA, Karner-Rezek K, Rosemann T, Knechtle B, Lepers R, Rüst CA. Will women outrun men in ultra-marathon road races from 50 km to 1,000 km? SpringerPlus. 2014;3:97.

33. Rüst CA, Knechtle B, Rosemann T, Lepers R. Women reduced the sex difference in open-water ultra-distance swimming—La Traversée Internationale du Lac St-Jean, 1955–2012. Appl Physiol Nutr Metab. 2014;39:270–3.

34. Lepers R, Stapley PJ. Differences in gender and performance in off-road triathlon. J Sports Sci. 2010;28(14):1555–62.

35. Lepers R, Maffiuletti NA. Age and gender interactions in ultraendurance performance: insight from the triathlon. Med Sci Sports Exerc. 2011;43(1):134–9.

36. Hinton PS, Giordano C, Brownlie T, Haas JD. Iron supplementation improves endurance after training in iron-depleted, nonanemic women. J Appl Physiol. 2000;88:1103–11.

37. Deldicque L, Francaux M. Recommendations for healthy nutrition in female endurance runners: an update. Front Nutr. 2015;2(17). doi:10.3389/fnut.2015.00017.

38. Klingshirn L, Pate RR, Bourque SP, Davis JM, Sargent RG. Effect of iron supplementation on endur-

ance capacity in iron-depleted female runners. Med Sci Sports Exerc. 1992;24(7):819–24.

39. McClung JP, Karl JP, Cable SJ, Williams KW, Nindl BC, Young AJ, et al. Randomized, double-blind, placebo-controlled trial of iron supplementation in female soldiers during military training: effects on iron status, physical performance, and mood. Am J Clin Nutr. 2009;90:124–31.

40. Dellavalle DM, Haas JD. Iron supplementation improves energetic efficiency in iron-depleted female rowers. Med Sci Sports Exerc. 2014. doi:10.1249/MSS.0000000000000208.

41. Dellavalle DM, Haas JD. Iron status is associated with endurance performance and training in female rowers. Med Sci Sports Exerc. 2012. doi:10.1249/MSS.0b013e3182517ceb.

42. Zourdos MC, Sanchez-Gonzalez MA, Mahoney SE. A brief review: the implications of iron supplementation for marathon runners on health and performance. J Strength Cond Res. 2015;29(2):559–65.

43. Haymes EM, Lamanca JL. Iron loss in runners during exercise. Sports Med. 1989;7:277–85.

44. Bø K, Sundgot-Borgen J. Prevalence of stress and urge urinary incontinence in elite athletes and controls. Med Sci Sports Exerc. 2001;33(11):1797–802.

45. Poświata A, Socha T, Opara J. Prevalence of stress urinary incontinence in elite female endurance athletes. J Hum Kinet. 2014;44:91–6. doi:10.2478/hukin-2014-0114.

46. Bø K, Sundgot-Borgen J. Are former female elite athletes more likely to experience urinary incontinence later in life than non-athletes? Scand J Med Sci Sports. 2010;20:100–4.

47. Caylet N, Fabbro-Peray P, Marès P, Dauzat M, Prat-Padal D, Corcos J. Prevalence and occurrence of stress urinary incontinence in elite women athletes. Can J Urol. 2006;13(4):3174–9.

48. Salvatore S, Serati M, Laterza R, Uccella S, Torella M, Bolis PF. The impact of urinary stress incontinence in young and middle-age women practising recreational sports activity: an epidemiological study. Br J Sports Med. 2009;43:1115–8.

49. Bø K. Pelvic floor muscle training is effective treatment of female stress urinary incontinence, but how does it work? Int Urogynecol J. 2004;15:76–84.

50. Budgett R. Fatigue and underperformance in athletes: the overtraining syndrome. Br J Sports Med. 1998;32:107–10.

51. He CS, Bishop NC, Handzlik MK, Muhamad AS, Gleeson M. Sex differences in upper respiratory symptoms prevalence and oral-respiratory mucosal immunity in endurance athletes. Exerc Immunol Rev. 2014;20:8–22.

52. Vetter RE, Symonds ML. Correlations between injury, training intensity, and physical and mental exhaustion among college athletes. J Strength Cond Res. 2010;24(3):587–96.

53. Asplund CA, O'Connor FG, Noakes TD. Exercise-associated collapse: an evidence-based review and primer for clinicians. Br J Sports Med. 2011;45:1157–62. doi:10.1136/bjsports-2011-090378.

54. Cote AT, Bredin SSD, Phillips AA, Koehle MS, Warburton DER. Greater autonomic modulation during post-exercise hypotension following high-intensity interval exercise in endurance-trained men and women. Eur J Appl Physiol. 2015;115:81–9.

55. Rossow L, Yan H, Fahs CA, Ranadive SM, Agiovlasitis S, Wilund KR, et al. Postexercise hypotension in an endurance-trained population of men and women following high-intensity interval and steady-state cycling. Am J Hypertens. 2010;23(4):358–67.

56. Senitko AN, Charkoudian N, Halliwill JR. Influence of endurance exercise training status and gender on postexercise hypotension. J Appl Physiol. 2002;92:2368–74.

57. Chlíbková D, Knechtle B, Rosemann T, Žákovská A, Tomášková I, Shortall M, et al. Changes in foot volume, body composition, and hydration status in male and female 24-hour ultra-marathon bikers. J Int Soc Sports Nutr. 2014;11:12.

58. Wagner S, Knechtle B, Knechtle P, Rüst CA, Rosemann T. Higher prevalence of exercise-associated hyponatremia in female than in male open-water ultra-endurance swimmers: the 'Marathon-Swim' in Lake Zurich. Eur J Appl Physiol. 2012;112:1095–106.

59. Weikunat T, Knechtle B, Knechtle P, Rüst CA, Rosemann T. Body composition and hydration status changes in male and female open-water swimmers during an ultra-endurance event. J Sports Sci. 2012;30(10):1003–13.

60. Urso C, Brucculeri S, Caimi G. Physiopathological, epidemiological, clinical and therapeutic aspects of exercise-associated hyponatremia. J Clin Med. 2014;3(4):1256–75.

61. Hew-Butler T, Boulter J, Bhorat R, Noakes TD. Avoid adding insult to injury—correct management of sick female endurance athletes. S Afr Med J. 2012;102(12):927–30.

62. Cosca DD, Navazio F. Common problems in endurance athletes. Am Fam Physician. 2007;76:237–44.

63. Mountjoy M, Sundgot-Borgen J, Burke L, Carter S, Constantini N, Lebrun C, et al. The IOC consensus statement: beyond the female athlete triad—relative energy deficiency in sport (RED-S). Br J Sports Med. 2014;48:491–7.

64. Melin A, Tornberg AB, Skouby S, Møller SS, Sungot-Borgen J, Faber J, et al. Energy availability and the female athlete triad in elite endurance athletes. Scand J Med Sci Sports. 2014. doi:10.1111/sms.12261.

65. Nattiv A, Loucks AB, Manore MM, Sanborn CF, Sundgot-Borgen J, Warren MP. American College of Sports Medicine position stand. The female athlete triad. Med Sci Sports Exerc. 2007. doi:10.1249/mss.0b013e318149f111.

66. Duckham RL, Pierce N, Bailey CA, Summers G, Cameron N, Brooke-Wavell K. Bone geometry according to menstrual function in female endurance

athletes. Calcif Tissue Int. 2013;92:444–50. doi:10.1007/s00223-013-9700-3.

67. Moreau KL, Stauffer BL, Kohrt WM, Seals DR. Essential role of estrogen for improvements in vascular endothelial function with endurance exercise in postmenopausal women. J Clin Endocrinol Metab. 2013;98:4507–15. doi:10.1210/jc.2013-2183.

68. Braam L, Knapen M, Geusens P, Brouns F, Vermeer C. Factors affecting bone loss in female endurance athletes. Am J Sports Med. 2003;31(6):889–95.

69. O'Brien M. Problems of high performance female athletes. In: FISA Level 3 Coaching Development Programme Course. p. 145–8. http://www.worldrowing.com/mm//Document/General/General/10/85/59/3Chapter5_English.pdf. Accessed 3 Aug 2015.

70. Scofield KL, Hecht S. Bone health in endurance athletes: runners, cyclists, and swimmers. Curr Sports Med Rep. 2012;11(6):328–34.

71. Pollock N, Grogan C, Perry M, Pedlar C, Cooke K, Morrissey D, et al. Bone-mineral density and other features of the female athlete triad in elite endurance runners: a longitudinal and cross-sectional observational study. Int J Sport Nutr Exerc Metab. 2010;20:418–26.

72. Hind K, Truscott JG, Evans JA. Low lumbar spine bone mineral density in both male and female endurance runners. Bone. 2006;39:880–5.

73. American Diabetic Association and Dietitians of Canada. ACSM Joint Position Statement: nutrition and athletic performance. Med Sci Sports Exerc. 2009. doi:10.1249/MSS.0b013e318190eb86.

74. Micklesfield LK, Hugo J, Johnson C, Noakes TD, Lambert EV. Factors associated with menstrual dysfunction and self-reported bone stress injuries in female runners in the ultra- and half-marathons of the two oceans. Br J Sports Med. 2007;41:679–83. doi:10.1136/bjsm.2007.037077.

75. Herring SA, Bergfeld JA, Boyajian-O'Neill LA, Duffey T, Griffin L, Hannafin J, et al. Female athlete issues for the team physician: a consensus statement. Med Sci Sports Exerc. 2003. doi:0195-9131/03/3510-1785.

76. Duckham RL, Peirce N, Meyer C, Summers GD, Cameron N, Brooke-Wavell K. Risk factors for stress fracture in female endurance athletes: a cross sectional study. BMJ Open. 2012;2, e001920. doi:10.1136/bmjopen-2012-001920.

Considerations for the Pediatric Endurance Athlete

Kelsey Logan and Gregory Walker

Background

Similar to more traditional sports for children and adolescents, endurance sports are increasing in popularity. Even though half of running race finishers 5 K distance and longer in 2014 were aged 25–44, the 6–17 age group accounted for 10 % of overall US timed race finishers [1]. Specifically for the marathon distance, over 550,000 people finished marathons in 2014, which was an all-time high; 2 % of those finishers were "juniors" (under 20 years of age) [2]. That percentage of junior finishers has remained steady at about 2 % since 1995, as the number of finishers overall has nearly doubled since then. The Asics LA event annually has the most junior finishers, with nearly 4000 in 2014. Junior finishers accounted for 4 % of over two million half-marathon finishers in 2014 [3]. Again, that percentage is stable, even as the number of finishers nearly doubled since 2009. Even though we may consider junior endurance athletes to be the exception rather than the rule, it appears that tens of thousands of adolescent runners are training for, and completing, half-marathon and marathon distances. In addition, according to data collected by the National Federation of High Schools, Associations, over 472,000 students competed in cross-country in the 2014–2015 season; this is an increase of over 30,000 runners from five seasons prior [4, 5]. We should expect to see endurance athletes in our clinics, needing injury treatment and counseling about training.

Is Long-Distance Running Safe?

There is little written about long-distance running for children and adolescents. There is no published research on safety or evidence-based training guidelines. However, there is injury data on high school cross-country participation. The injury rate is low. Additionally, it is easy to understand that since the majority of stress in running occurs in the legs, this is where most injuries will present. In the 2013–2014 school year, the injury rate for boys' cross-country (ages 14–18) was 0.72 per 1000 athlete exposures; the girls' cross-country (ages 13–18) injury rate was 0.76 for the same school year. In boys, the most common site of injury was the lower leg (27 %), followed by the hip/thigh/upper leg (21.6 %). The knee was specifically injured in 16.2 % of cases, and the ankle accounted for 14.4 % of injuries. The vast majority of injuries were categorized as "sprain/strain" or "other." Girls had similar injury characteristics, with most being "sprain/strain" or "other" (not fracture). A quarter of the injuries were

K. Logan • G. Walker (✉)
Sports Medicine, Cincinnati Children's Hospital Medical Center, 3333 Burnett Ave., MLC 10001, Cincinnati, OH 45249, USA
e-mail: Gregory.walker@cchmc.org

© Springer International Publishing Switzerland 2016
T.L. Miller (ed.), *Endurance Sports Medicine*, DOI 10.1007/978-3-319-32982-6_6

lower leg, 18.3 % were ankle, 18.3 % were of the knee, 17.3 % were of the hip/thigh/upper leg, and 14.4 % were foot. Only one injury in both groups required surgery [6]. Races in high school cross-country are 5000 m, or 3.1 miles, for both boys and girls. In junior high (grades 7 and 8), the maximum distance is 2 miles. Training for these distances varies greatly based on desire and coaching. If less-experienced or poorly trained runners are required to do high-mileage training before they are ready, injuries may be more likely to occur, as they would in any sport. The practice of doing high-mileage training programs before and during cross-country seasons, even for relatively short races, seems to be part of the culture of cross-country; whether this leads to higher injury rates is not clear. From the RIO high school data, the injury rate appears to be very low in school runners and involves largely nonsurgical injuries to the legs.

The discussion of safety for longer distance events (10 K, half-marathon, marathon, and longer) becomes much more controversial. The few articles that have been written on the topic are not recent and are not research studies; they are review and policy statements. The American Academy of Pediatrics (AAP), in its clinical report "Overuse Injuries, Overtraining, and Burnout in Child and Adolescent Athletes" [7], briefly discusses endurance events. It rightly reports "There is, at present, no scientific evidence that supports or refutes the safety of children who participate in marathons." The clinical report recommends a "clearly devised weekly plan" that involves education on nutrition, hydration, and environmental conditions; it also recommends allowing participation of a willing young runner "as long as the athlete enjoys the activity and is asymptomatic." Some authors have argued passionately for the safe inclusion of young runners in long-distance races, recognizing that risk for injury at any age is likely to increase as training volume increases; this occurs at any age, not just in youth [8, 9].

It is important to acknowledge that several characteristics of the immature skeleton may make endurance running more stressful than in an adult: shorter stride length leads to more rep-

etitions; immature articular cartilage is at higher risk for damage relative to that of an adult; repetitive trauma to the growth plate has been implicated in hip arthritis; rapid periods of growth place muscles, tendons, and apophyses under additional stress [10]. Again, while recognizing these potential problems, long-distance running, while understudied, appears to be safe for young athletes. Any running program should be carefully planned and monitored while initiated and motivated by the child. External stressors should not be driving the child to run. Education should be provided to the athlete and the family about common injuries, nutrition, and hydration. Female runners should be educated about the female athlete triad; there is clear connection between running and negative energy balance, leading to disturbances in menstruation and bony health [11].

Endurance Training Physiology

As youth sports competition grows, so too does the quest for performance benefits linked to training. Numerous preadolescent youth participate in sports-specific training programs. However, the profits of such efforts are unclear [12, 13]. Designing and implementing research studies to better understand aerobic fitness in youth has proved difficult. The equipment and protocols used to test aerobic fitness in adults may not be well suited for youth. Compared to adults, youth tend to have a greater baseline physical activity, which may serve as a confounder for aerobic performance gains with training. Still, there are factors worth illustrating. Youth have physiologic adaptations through growth and puberty that afford gains in aerobic fitness. Additionally, youth do appear to show gains in aerobic fitness through training.

The two well-recognized determinants of aerobic fitness in humans are maximal oxygen uptake (VO_{2max}) and anaerobic threshold (AT). VO_{2max} describes the maximal uptake of oxygen during incremental exercise. Originally described by exercise physiology pioneers A. V. Hill H. Lupton in the 1920s [14], VO_{2max} correlates to a plateau or upper limit for any individual to take in and utilize oxygen despite increases in workload. Children, however, do not classically exhibit this plateau in oxygen consumption. Rather, peak VO_2, which is the utmost VO_2 reached during an exercise test to exhaustion, is a much better predictor of VO_{2max} in children [15]. First thought to represent the threshold level of work where metabolic acidosis would ensue causing resultant Bohr effect, AT is better recognized as the balance between lactate production and elimination [13]. In adults, the reference commonly used is 4.0 mM. However, this may not be appropriate for youth as exercising at the same relative intensity produces lower lactate levels compared with adults. It has been recommended that a reference threshold of 2.5 mM be used in children and adolescents [16]. Increases in VO_{2max} and/or AT will afford an athlete to maintain enhanced rates of aerobic energy expenditure.

Growth

Growth and maturation appear to play a large role on aerobic performance. Growth is relatively stable in preadolescence [17]. However, the onset of puberty contributes to marked hormonal changes, particularly increases in growth hormone and testosterone, along with growth of the cardiorespiratory and musculoskeletal systems [18]. Testosterone appears to be a key hormonal factor related to gains in VO_2. A study linking resting testosterone pre- and post-training of prepubescent males (aged 11–12 years old) illustrated testosterone levels almost three times higher than controls after a year of training [19]. Additionally, there appears to be sex differences in the trainability of aerobic fitness in children. Boys appear to have greater capacity for training-induced gains in aerobic performance. In a 2003 study, Obert et al. was able to illustrate 15 and 8 % gains in peak VO_2 in boys and girls, respectively [20]. One could infer that a training-induced rise in testosterone, preferentially affecting males, is at least partially responsible for such gains in aerobic performance.

Training

It has been shown that training can cause an increase in exercise performance. The extent of such training-induced increases is not clear. Improvements in VO_2 have most commonly been reported to be minimal at 5–6 %, with higher gains correlating to elevated exercise intensities greater than 80 % of maximal heart rate (HR_{max}) [12, 21]. Banquet et al. wrote that when studies not reporting significant changes were excluded, VO_2 improvements rose to 8–10 % [12]. Rowland and Boyajian were able to demonstrate a 6 % average increase VO_{2max} from baseline with the training intervention consisting of three 30-min exercise sessions per week with participants exercising at an intensity of 80–85 % of their HR_{max} [21]. Interestingly, this is significantly less than the current physical activity recommendations of 60 min of moderate to vigorous physical activity [22, 23]. It is possible that youth exhibit a higher baseline level of fitness when compared to adults, who are relatively more sedentary [24]. Thus, training responses may be more attenuated in youth.

Cardiac Changes

The cardiovascular composition of athletes has been studied at length. In adults, gains in VO_{2max} are related to increases in maximal cardiac output (Q_{max}) and maximal arteriovenous oxygen difference ($AVO\text{-}D_{max}$) [25, 26]. Cardiac output is directly proportional to stroke volume (SV) and HR. Adults show a gradual decline in HR_{max} with age. However, exercise has been shown as a way to attenuate such declines. In adults, it is possible that gains in Q_{max} are partially attributable to exercise-induced attenuation of HR_{max} [27]. In children, however, HR appears to have less of an impact on cardiovascular adaptations associated with performance gains in exercise. Early studies pointed only to SV as the etiology for increased VO_{2max} in exercise-trained children [28]. Ventricular size and SV gains are found in exercise-trained youth [29]. Together these have a profound effect on the cardiac output in exercise-trained youth [25]. Obert et al., through the use of echocardiography, corroborated significantly elevated SV, with concomitant gains in VO_{2max}, in trained prepubertal cyclists aged 10–11 years old vs age-matched controls [20]. These authors concluded that the gains in VO_{2max}, reported at 10 % from pre-training values, in their study cohort, were attributable primarily to their elevated SV. Overall, Q_{max} changes secondary to aerobic exercise are mediated by inotropic principles rather than chronotropic principles.

AVO-D is a measure of the difference in arterial oxygen content versus venous oxygen content. Simply, it is a measure of how efficient the body is in extracting oxygen from blood within capillaries. Factors affecting diffusion are thought to include capillary density, myoglobin concentration, mitochondrial concentration, and pH. In adults, submaximal aerobic exercise has been shown to increase the AVO-D [23]. The AVO-D is felt to be most beneficial at submaximal efforts. In children, no difference in AVO-D has been reported. It is possible that the greater proportion of slow-twitch (oxidative) muscle fibers vs fast-twitch glycolytic muscle fibers in children is responsible for this finding.

References

1. Running USA. 2015 State of the sport – U.S. race trends. 2015. http://www.runningusa.org/2015-state-of-sport-us-trends?returnTo=annual-reports. Accessed 27 Aug 2015.
2. Running USA. 2014 Running USA annual marathon report. 2015. www.runningusa.org/marathon-report-2015?returnto+annual-reports. Accessed 27 Aug 2015.
3. Running USA. 2015. 2014 Running USA annual half marathon report. www.runningusa.org/half-marathon-report-2015?returnTo=main. Accessed 27 Aug 2015.
4. The National Federation of State High School Associations. 2014–2015 High school athletics participation survey. 2015. http://www.nfhs.org/ParticipationStatistics/PDF/2014-15_Participation_Survey_Results.pdf. Accessed 27 Aug 2015.
5. The National Federation of State High School Associations. 2009–2010 High school athletics survey. 2010. http://www.nfhs.org/ParticipationStatistics/PDF/2009-10%20Participation%20Survey.pdf. Accessed 27 Aug 2015.
6. National High School Sports-Related Injury Surveillance Study. Convenience sample summary report, 2013–2014. 2014. http://www.ucdenver.edu/academics/colleges/PublicHealth/research/ResearchProjects/piper/projects/RIO/Documents/2013-14%20Convenience%20Report.pdf. Accessed 27 Aug 2015.
7. Brenner JS. American Academy of Pediatrics Council on Sports M, Fitness. Overuse injuries, overtraining, and burnout in child and adolescent athletes. Pediatrics. 2007;119(6):1242–5.
8. Roberts WO. Children and running: at what distance safe? Clin J Sport Med. 2005;15(2):109–10. Author reply 10–1.
9. Roberts WO. Can children and adolescents run marathons? Sports Med. 2007;37(4–5):299–301.
10. Rice SG, Waniewski S. Children and marathoning: how young is too young? Clin J Sport Med. 2003;13(6):369–73.
11. De Souza MJ, Nattiv A, Joy E, Misra M, Williams NI, Mallinson RJ, et al. 2014 Female Athlete Triad Coalition consensus statement on treatment and return to play of the female athlete triad: 1st International Conference held in San Francisco, CA, May 2012, and 2nd International Conference held in Indianapolis, IN, May 2013. Clin J Sport Med. 2014;24(2):96–119.
12. Baquet G, van Praagh E, Berthoin S. Endurance training and aerobic fitness in young people. Sports Med. 2003;33(15):1127–43.
13. Baxter-Jones A, Maffulli N. Endurance in young athletes: it can be trained. Br J Sports Med. 2003;37(2):96–7.
14. Hill AV, Long CNH, Lupton H. Muscular exercise, lactic acid, and the supply and utilisation of oxygen. Proc R Soc Lond Ser B. 1924;96(679):438–75.
15. Armstrong N, Welsman J, Winsley R. Is peak VO2 a maximal index of children's aerobic fitness? Int J Sports Med. 1996;17(5):356–9.
16. Armstrong N, Welsman JR. Assessment and interpretation of aerobic fitness in children and adolescents. Exerc Sport Sci Rev. 1994;22:435–76.
17. Rogol AD, Roemmich JN, Clark PA. Growth at puberty. J Adolesc Health. 2002;31 Suppl 6:192–200.
18. Naughton G, Farpour-Lambert NJ, Carlson J, Bradney M, Van Praagh E. Physiological issues surrounding the performance of adolescent athletes. Sports Med. 2000;30(5):309–25.
19. Mero A, Jaakkola L, Komi PV. Serum hormones and physical performance capacity in young boy athletes during a 1-year training period. Eur J Appl Physiol Occup Physiol. 1990;60(1):32–7.
20. Obert P, Mandigouts S, Nottin S, Vinet A, N'Guyen LD, Lecoq AM. Cardiovascular responses to endurance training in children: effect of gender. Eur J Clin Invest. 2003;33(3):199–208.
21. Rowland TW, Boyajian A. Aerobic response to endurance exercise training in children. Pediatrics. 1995;96(4 Pt 1):654–8.
22. American Heart Association. The AHA's recommendations for physical activity in children. 2013. http://www.heart.org/HEARTORG/HealthyLiving/

HealthyKids/ActivitiesforKids/The-AHAs-Recommendationsfor-Physical-Activity-in-Children_UCM_304053_Article.jsp#.VzXfg5MwjJw.

23. Centers for Disease Control and Prevention. How much physical activity do children need? 2015. http://www.cdc.gov/physicalactivity/basics/children/.

24. Haskell WL, Lee IM, Pate RR, Powell KE, Blair SN, Franklin BA, et al. Physical activity and public health: updated recommendation for adults from the American College of Sports Medicine and the American Heart Association. Med Sci Sports Exerc. 2007;39(8):1423–34.

25. Wilmore JH, Stanforth PR, Gagnon J, Rice T, Mandel S, Leon AS, et al. Cardiac output and stroke volume changes with endurance training: the HERITAGE Family Study. Med Sci Sports Exerc. 2001;33(1):99–106.

26. Saltin B, Blomqvist G, Mitchell JH, Johnson Jr RL, Wildenthal K, Chapman CB. Response to exercise after bed rest and after training. Circulation. 1968;38 Suppl 5:Vii1–78.

27. Ogawa T, Spina RJ, Martin 3rd WH, Kohrt WM, Schechtman KB, Holloszy JO, et al. Effects of aging, sex, and physical training on cardiovascular responses to exercise. Circulation. 1992;86(2):494–503.

28. Eriksson BO, Koch G. Effect of physical training on hemodynamic response during submaximal and maximal exercise in 11-13-year old boys. Acta Physiol Scand. 1973;87(1):27–39.

29. Faria IE, Faria EW, Roberts S, Yoshimura D. Comparison of physical and physiological characteristics in elite young and mature cyclists. Res Q Exerc Sport. 1989;60(4):388–95.

Part II

Musculoskeletal Conditions

Treatment of Stress Fractures

Timothy L. Miller

Stress fractures are not a single consistent injury. They occur along a spectrum of severity which can impact treatment and prognosis [1–3]. Not only does the extent of these injuries vary, but the clinical behavior of these injuries varies by location and causative activity [4, 5]. An understanding of common sports-specific stress injuries can help the clinician in the diagnosis, prevention, and treatment of these sports-related stress injuries given that certain sports are more commonly associated with stress fractures, including running (69 %), fitness class/cross-fit (8 %), racket sports (5 %), and basketball (4 %) [6]. The most frequently reported anatomic sites of stress fractures in the literature involve the tibia, metatarsals, and fibula [7].

When treating these injuries, it should be borne in mind that no two stress fractures behave exactly alike. Treatment protocols should be individualized to the patient, the causative activity, the anatomical site, and the severity of the fracture. As athletes become more competitive and focus solely on one sport, the incidence of stress fractures continues to increase. A holistic approach to the treatment of these injuries should be taken by orthopedists and sports medicine

specialists. This is reflected in the treatment algorithm employed by the authors and presented later in this manuscript.

Pathophysiology

Stress fractures are a fatigue failure of the bone [8–10]. These stress injuries result from an overuse mechanism. Repeated episodes of bone strain can result in the accumulation of enough microdamage to become a clinically symptomatic stress fracture [9, 11]. Any stress or load causes some strain of or deformation to the bone, and any strain of the bone results in some microdamage [9, 12]. Healthy bone is in homeostasis between microcrack creation and repair.

Fatigue failure of the bone has three stages: crack initiation, crack propagation, and complete fracture. Crack initiation typically occurs at sites of stress concentration during bone loading [13]. Stress concentration occurs at sites of differential bone consistency such as lacunae or canaliculi [13]. Crack propagation occurs if loading continues at a frequency or intensity above the level at which the new bone can be laid down and microcracks repaired. Propagation, or extension of a microcrack, typically occurs along the cement lines of the bone. Continued loading and crack propagation allow for the coalescence of multiple cracks to the point of becoming a clinically symptomatic stress fracture [10, 14]. If the loading episodes are not modified or the reparative response is

T.L. Miller (✉)
Department of Orthopaedic Surgery, Ohio State University Wexner Medical Center,
920 North Hamilton Road, Suite 600, Gahanna, OH 43230, USA
e-mail: timothy.miller@osumc.edu

© Springer International Publishing Switzerland 2016
T.L. Miller (ed.), *Endurance Sports Medicine*, DOI 10.1007/978-3-319-32982-6_7

not increased, crack propagation can continue until structural failure or complete fracture occurs [2, 15]. Through the adaptive process of remodeling, the bone is able to respond to crack initiation and propagation such that the loaded bone is strengthened in preparation for future loading [16]. This positive adaptive response is known as Wolff's law and is an essential part of bone health [9, 10].

Risk Factors for Stress Fractures

A variety of biological and mechanical factors are thought to influence the body's ability to remodel the bone and therefore impact an individual's risk for developing a stress fracture. These include, but are not limited to, sex, age, race, hormonal status, nutrition, neuromuscular function, and genetic factors. Other predisposing factors to consider include abnormal bony alignment, improper technique/biomechanics, poor running form, poor blood supply to specific bones, improper or worn-out footwear, and hard training surfaces [11, 17, 18]. It is important to remember that the cause of stress fractures is multifactorial, and individual athletes will vary in their susceptibility to stress injuries.

The key modifiable risk factors in the development of overuse injuries of the bone relate to the pre-participation condition of the bone and the frequency, duration, and intensity of the causative activity. Without preconditioning and acclimation to a particular activity, athletes are at significantly increased risk for the development of overuse and fatigue-related injuries of the bone [19–21]. Multiple intrinsic and extrinsic factors can influence the balance between the creation/propagation of microcracks and the body's ability to repair them (Table 7.1).

Intrinsic Factors

Anatomic alignment and kinematics can predispose a particular area to stress fracture and must be considered in the treatment of these injuries (e.g., a patient with a fifth metatarsal or navicular stress fracture) [3]. Without consideration of the

Table 7.1 Etiologic factors for stress fractures (Reproduced from Kaeding et al. [3])

Intrinsic factors
Muscle imbalance muscle weakness
Alignment/anatomic abnormalities
Tibial torsion flexibility
Leg length discrepancy
Aging/hormonal
Extrinsic factors
Improper training
Improper equipment
Improper technique
Varied training surfaces (terrain, hills)
Environmental
Extrinsic pressure

surrounding anatomy, poor outcomes may result. Some stress fractures are affected by delayed or nonunion because of insufficient blood supply to the region. Proximal fifth metatarsal and tarsal navicular fractures are particularly difficult to heal because they occur within the vascular "watershed" region at the metaphyseal-diaphyseal junction [3].

Muscle strength can also affect an individual's susceptibility to stress fractures. Proper neuromuscular function can dissipate the energy of externally applied impact loads on bones and joints that can occur during running and jumping [3]. Muscle fatigue may be an important factor in fatigue fractures. This is referred to as the *neuromuscular hypothesis*. As muscle fatigues, its capacity to dissipate the energy of an externally applied load diminishes, resulting in higher peak stresses and thus more rapid accumulation of microdamage [2]. Overall, general fitness is protective, and studies have shown that military recruits with higher activity levels before enlistment had fewer stress fractures during basic training [22, 23].

Recent studies have also looked at the association between vitamin D levels and the formation of stress fractures in military personnel. A prospective study of Finnish military recruits found that the average serum vitamin D concentration was significantly lower in the group that had sustained a stress fracture. This suggests that a lower level of serum vitamin D may be a predisposing factor for the development of stress fractures. Another randomized, double-blind, placebo-controlled study examined whether calcium and vitamin D intervention could reduce the incidence of stress fractures in female recruits during basic training. Their study suggested that calcium and vitamin D supplementation could have prevented a significant percentage of their recruits from sustaining a stress fracture, which would have been associated with a significant decrease in morbidity and financial costs [24]. As these studies highlight, supplementation of vitamin D to prevent stress fractures is a subject of ongoing and future research [25].

Additionally, certain endocrine and nutritional conditions can impair the delicate balance between bone formation and resorption, thus predisposing one to stress fractures. Oligomenorrheic or amenorrheic female athletes are at increased risk for stress fractures. This may be secondary to decreased estrogen levels and increased osteoclastic activity. Stress fractures are also associated with lower fat intake, lower calorie intake, eating disorders, and body weight of <75 % ideal body weight. The female athlete triad (menstrual irregularity, disordered eating, and osteopenia) has been associated with increased susceptibility to stress fractures and may contribute to the increased stress fracture risk seen in female athletes and female military recruits compared with their male counterparts. High-intensity training may suppress menses, which can exacerbate these risk factors [26].

Extrinsic Factors

It has been estimated that up to 60 % of running injuries are associated with training errors [9]. Training and technique errors include rapidly escalating frequency, duration, or intensity of training or perform a task with poor form, posture, or footstrike. Stress fractures are increased in the first 2 weeks after increased training of less than 30 % in duration or intensity over a single season and in college freshman runners adjusting to demands of collegiate training regimens [5]. Stress fractures are often associated with changes in footwear or training surfaces, which can increase focal stresses in the lower extremity. Poorly fitting shoes (particularly those that have poor heel counters), poor cushioning, or poor midfoot stability may lead to excessive heel motion, overload of the metatarsals, or poor shock absorption. The use of appropriate sports-specific equipment including shoes or custom insoles may be valuable in preventing overload and stress [2].

Clinical Presentation

Pain that is initially present only during activity is common in patients presenting with a stress fracture. Symptom onset is usually insidious, and typically patients cannot recall a specific injury or trauma to the affected area. If activity level is not decreased or modified, symptoms persist or worsen. Those who continue to train without modification of their activities may develop pain with normal daily activity and potentially sustain a complete fracture [26]. Physical examination reveals reproducible point tenderness with direct palpation of the affected bone site. There may or may not be swelling or a palpable soft tissue or bone reaction.

Imaging Evaluation

Radiography

Plain X-rays are usually negative early on in the course of a stress fracture, especially in the first 2–3 weeks [27, 28]. Two-thirds of initial X-rays are negative, but half ultimately prove positive once healing begins to occur making standard radiographs specific but not sensitive [29]. Even after healing has begun to occur, radiographic findings can be subtle and may be easily overlooked if the images are not thoroughly scrutinized [30]. Figure 7.1 shows the anteroposterior radiograph of a healing nondisplaced distal fibular stress fracture. Likewise, diagnostic ultrasound imaging has not been shown to be reliable for diagnosing stress injuries of the bone [31].

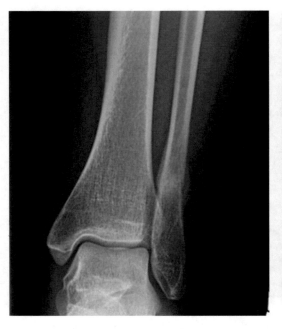

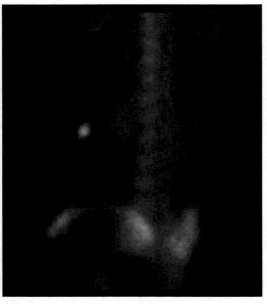

Fig. 7.1 Anteroposterior radiograph of a healing nondisplaced Grade 3 distal fibular stress fracture in a 19-year-old female collegiate lacrosse player. Callus formation is evident after 6 weeks of activity modification

Fig. 7.2 Nuclear bone scintigraphy image of a 20-year-old female rower with ongoing left rib pain. A Grade 2 stress fracture is present of the left tenth rib

Bone Scintigraphy

Bone scintigraphy had for many years been regarded as the gold standard for evaluating stress-induced injuries, and although recently supplanted by MRI, it continues to be widely utilized in many situations. It measures bone response to injury by depicting areas of increased osseous metabolism through the localization of radionuclide tracers, particularly Tc-99m-MDP. The degree of uptake depends on the rate of bone turnover and local blood flow, and abnormal uptake may be seen within 6–72 h of injury [19, 32, 33]. Whole body bone scans can be performed with relatively low cost and have the advantage of being able to image the entire skeletal system at once, which is useful in cases when more than one area is symptomatic. The sensitivity of bone scintigraphy is nearly 100 % [32].

The characteristic scintigraphic appearance of a stress fracture in delayed static images is intense, fusiform cortical uptake along the long axis of the bone at the level of the fracture

(Fig. 7.2) [34]. However, there can be a wide spectrum of findings representative of the pathophysiologic continuum of the process and the variations in the orientation of the fracture such as in a longitudinal fracture. A stress reaction is manifested by an area of less intense radionuclide uptake along the cortex corresponding to areas of remodeling the bone during the period that radiographs are typically normal.

Ultrasound

Ultrasonography has a very limited role in the evaluation of stress fractures and is not recommended as a stand-alone study [35]. However, studies have shown that this modality may occasionally be used to assess the superficial surface of the cortex in bones that are located close to the skin such as in the ankle/feet and tibia [36]. Cortical irregularities such as periostitis and callus formation can be depicted as well as muscular edema around the bone, and compression of the probe is useful in confirming pain. Color Doppler imaging can demonstrate areas of hyperperfusion at and near the stress fracture. Recent studies have demonstrated a sensitivity of 82 % and a specificity of 67–76 %, but predictive values offer a wide range with studies reporting a 59–99 % positive predictive value and a 14–92 % negative predictive value [37, 38].

SPECT Scan

Single-photon emission computed tomography (SPECT) scan is a more specific nuclear medicine scanning technique than planar bone scan. Using analysis of the metabolic rate of cells, it is especially helpful in detecting stress fractures of the vertebral pars interarticularis, pelvis, and femoral neck [39].

Computed Tomography

Computed tomography (CT) delineates the bone well and is useful when the diagnosis of a stress injury is difficult, particularly in the case of tarsal navicular stress fractures (Fig. 7.3) as well as those of the pars interarticularis or linear stress fractures. CT scanning is useful for demonstrating evidence of healing by clearly showing the periosteal reaction and the absence of a discrete lucency or sclerotic fracture line [27, 39–41]. It is also helpful in determining if the fracture is complete or incomplete [42, 43].

MRI

MRI is an effective diagnostic technique in patients who show strong clinical manifestations of a stress fracture but have normal initial radiographs [44, 45]. Like scintigraphy, MRI depicts changes in the bone and periosteum weeks before any radiographic abnormality develops. The early stages of a stress fracture are characterized by focal hyperemia and bone marrow edema that correlates with the development of microfractures and osseous resorption (Fig. 7.4). Endosteal reactive changes, periostitis, and peri-osseous edema are important early observations on STIR

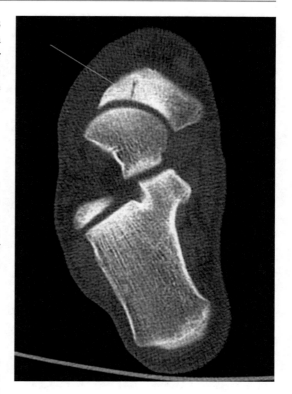

Fig. 7.3 Axial CT scan of a Grade 5 tarsal navicular stress fracture in an 18-year-old high school football player. Evidence of a nonunion is present

or T2-weighted spin-echo images and are characteristic of stress reactions [46, 47]. The most common patterns of a fatigue stress fracture on MRI are a linear, uni-cortically based abnormality of low signal intensity surrounded by a larger, ill-defined region of marrow edema or a linear cortical abnormality with adjacent muscular or soft tissue edema [48–50]. Callus formation indicates a more chronic stress fracture.

MRI has comparable sensitivity to nuclear scintigraphy. Specificity, accuracy, positive predictive value, and negative predictive value are all superior at 100 %, 90 %, 100 %, and 62 %, respectively [51]. Additionally, MRI has a distinct advantage by depicting the surrounding soft tissue structures thus permitting concomitant evaluation of muscular, tendinous, or ligamentous structures. In the athletic population, injuries to any of these structures may mimic the symptoms of a stress fracture, which are sources that reduce the specificity of nuclear scintigraphic

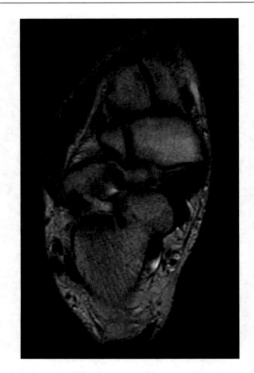

Fig. 7.4 Axial T2 MRI of a 19-year-old female middle distance runner with midfoot pain. A Grade 4 stress fracture is present at the midbody of the tarsal navicular

Table 7.2 Anatomic sites for high-risk stress fractures [5]

Femoral neck (tension side)
Patella (tension side)
Anterior tibial cortex
Medial malleolus
Talar neck
Dorsal tarsal navicular cortex
Fifth metatarsal proximal metaphysis
Sesamoids of the great toe

studies. Another feature of MRI that should be underscored is its ability to assess regions of the skeleton that are challenging with other imaging modalities.

Classification/Grading

Stress fractures are classified in multiple ways but most commonly by the size of the fracture line seen on imaging, the severity of pain or disability, the biologic healing potential of the particular injury or location, the natural history of the particular fracture, or some combination of these parameters [52, 53]. The classification of stress fractures as either "high risk" or "low risk" has been suggested by multiple authors [4, 5, 54]. High-risk stress fractures have at least one of the following characteristics: risk of delayed or nonunion, risk of refracture, and significant long-term consequences if they progress to complete fracture [2, 5]. Table 7.2 shows a list of anatomic

locations considered high-risk for stress fractures. This distinction allows clinicians to quickly determine if they can be aggressive or conservative with the decision to return an athlete to training or competition.

In addition to knowing the classification of whether a stress fracture is high risk or low risk as determined by its anatomic site, the extent of the fatigue failure or "grade" of the stress fracture is also needed to completely describe the injury and make appropriate treatment plans [2, 3, 26, 55]. As described above, stress injuries to the bone occur on a continuum from simple bone marrow edema (stress reaction) to a small microcrack with minor cortical disruption to a complete fracture with or without nonunion. The management of bony stress injuries should be based on the location and grade of the injury.

Recently, Kaeding and Miller proposed a comprehensive descriptive system for stress fractures [56]. This includes a grading scale for classifying the extent of structural failure from Grade 1 to Grade 5. Grade 1 injuries are asymptomatic, usually incidental findings on imaging studies. Grade 2 injuries have imaging evidence of fatigue failure of the bone but no fracture line (Fig. 7.3). Grade 3 injuries have a fracture line with no displacement (Fig. 7.1). Grade 4 fractures are displaced (Figs. 7.4 and 7.5), and Grade 5 stress fractures are chronic having gone onto nonunion (Fig. 7.3). This system is summarized in Table 7.3.

Two key features of the Kaeding–Miller system are that it is generalizable and has been validated with intra- and interobserver reliability. This classification system has been shown to have high inter- and intra-observer reliability [56]. Coupling this fracture grade with the location of

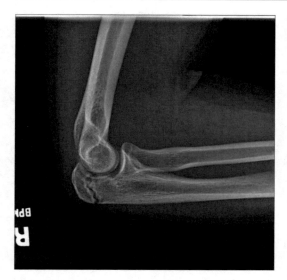

Fig. 7.5 Lateral radiograph of the elbow of a 25 year-old baseball pitcher with a displaced (Grade 4) olecranon stress fracture

Table 7.3 Kaeding–Miller stress fracture classification system [56]

Grade	Pain	Radiographic findings (CT, MRI, bone scan, or X-ray)
I	–	Imaging evidence of stress FX No fracture line
II	+	Imaging evidence of stress FX No fracture line
III	+	Nondisplaced fracture line
IV	+	Displaced fracture (>2 mm)
V	+	Nonunion

Shown is a combined clinical and radiographic classification system for stress fractures that has shown high intra- and interobserver reliability

the fracture provides a more comprehensive description of the injury that takes into account both the extent of structural failure and healing potential of the injury. When reporting the stress fracture grade in this system, the imaging modality used should be reported. Almost perfect intraobserver agreement was found among 15 evaluators of the classification system which included orthopedists, primary care sports medicine specialists, and physician assistants. Substantial to almost perfect interobserver reliability was observed for the classification grades among the same evaluators.

High-Risk Stress Fractures Versus Low-Risk Stress Fractures

Low-risk stress fractures include the femoral shaft, medial tibia, ribs, ulnar shaft, and first through fourth metatarsals, all of which have a favorable natural history. These sites tend to be on the compressive side of the bone and respond well to activity modification. Low-risk stress fractures are less likely to reoccur, develop nonunion, or have a significant complication should it progress to complete fracture [4].

High-risk stress fracture locations are noted in Table 7.2. Not only do fractures at these anatomical sites have a predilection to progress to complete fracture, delayed union, or nonunion, have a refracture, or have significant long-term consequences should they progress to a complete fracture, but they also often have worsening prognosis if they have a delay in diagnosis. A delay in treatment may prolong the patient's period of complete rest of the fracture site and potentially alter the treatment strategy to include surgical fixation with or without bone grafting. Due to their location on the tension side of the respective bones, these fractures possess common biomechanical properties regarding propagation of the fracture line. In comparison to low-risk stress fractures, high-risk stress fractures do not have an overall favorable natural history. With delay in diagnosis or with less aggressive treatment, high-risk stress fractures tend to progress to nonunion or complete fracture, require operative management, and recur in the same location [5, 57].

Rib and Upper Extremity Stress Fractures

Though over 90 % of stress fractures occur in the lower extremities as a result of impact loading [7, 29, 30], athletes who perform repetitive tasks with the shoulder and upper extremity may also develop stress injuries of the bone. Rib and shoulder girdle stress fractures are most commonly reported in rowers and throwing athletes along with those requiring repetitive rotation of the torso. The most common mechanisms for these injuries involve repetitive bony torsion, weight bearing, and muscle contraction overload [58–60]. Any athlete complaining of the nontraumatic onset of pain in the ribs or upper extremity that occurs during or shortly after the repetitive activity should raise concern for a possible stress fracture [58, 60].

In recent years, there has been increased attention focused on upper extremity stress fractures, and case reports of these injuries have increased in athletes such as baseball players who train continuously for one sport. Incidence has also paralleled the increase in popularity of cross-fit sports. In 2012, Miller and Kaeding reviewed 70 cases of stress fractures of the ribs and upper extremity, the largest series in the literature [60]. The authors noted that individuals performing weight-bearing activities of the upper extremity (e.g., gymnastics, cheerleading) developed nearly all of their stress fractures at or distal to the elbow, indicating that with such activities significant bony overload occurs in the distal upper extremity as opposed to the proximal portion [60].

The great majority of rib and upper extremity stress injuries are considered low risk and usually require only activity modification to heal. One of the few exceptions to this that may require surgical intervention is the olecranon stress fracture in a competitive thrower (Fig. 7.5). Though this injury has the potential to heal with conservative management, when a fracture line (Grade 3 injury) is discovered in a throwing athlete's olecranon process, internal fixation is the ideal treatment [61–63].

General Treatment Principles

Treatment principles for stress fractures include reestablishing the normal balance between the creation and repair of microcracks in the bone. In order to decrease the creation of microcracks, one must evaluate the patient's training regimen, biomechanics, and equipment. In order to maximize the patient's biologic capacity to repair

microcracks, one must evaluate the general health of the patient, including nutritional status, hormonal status, and medication use. The clinician should be aware of the female athletic triad and its potential detrimental effect on healing potential [17, 18, 26, 64]. A treatment algorithm employed by the authors and based on the Kaeding–Miller classification systems is presented in Fig. 7.6.

Management of High-Risk Stress Fractures

Treatment decision-making for high-risk stress fractures should be based on radiographic findings with less consideration given to symptom severity. The immediate goal of treatment of a high-risk stress fracture is to avoid progression and get the fracture to heal. Typically, this requires either complete elimination of loading of the site or surgical stabilization. Ideally, while the fracture is healing, one works to avoid deconditioning of the athlete while minimizing the risk of a significant complication of fracture healing [1, 26]. While overtreatment of a low-risk stress fracture may result in unnecessary deconditioning and loss of playing time, undertreatment of a high-risk injury puts the athlete at risk of significant complications. In this case, relative rest may be achieved with alternative training options such as aquatic training which may include an aquatic treadmill (Fig. 7.7) or suspended treadmill training.

The presence of a visible fracture line on a plain radiograph in a high-risk stress fracture should prompt serious consideration of operative management. Depending on injury classification, patients with stress injuries in high-risk locations may require immediate immobilization and/or restriction from weight-bearing activities with close monitoring. If an incomplete fracture is present on plain films with evidence of fracture on MRI or CT in a high-risk location, immobilization and strict non-weight bearing is indicated. Worsening symptoms or radiographic evidence

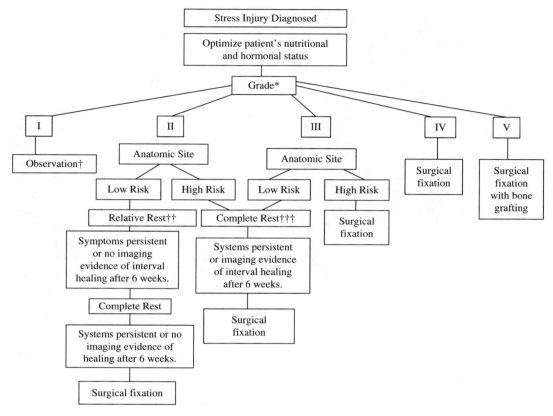

Fig. 7.6 Author's recommended treatment algorithm for stress injuries of the bone (Reproduced from Rockwood and Green's Fractures in Adults, 2012). *Grading based on the Kaeding–Miller classification system presented in Table 7.2 [56]. †*Observation* return to activity with close follow-up. Consider relative rest and cross-training. ††*Relative rest* decrease frequency or intensity of inciting activity. May cross-train. Gradual return to full pain-free activity. †††*Complete rest* discontinuation of any activity that places stress at fracture site. May include immobilization

of fracture progression despite nonoperative treatment is an indication for surgical fixation.

All complete fractures at high-risk sites should receive serious consideration for surgical treatment. In summary, surgical fixation should be considered for high-risk stress fractures for several reasons. These include expediting healing of the fracture to allow earlier return to full activity as well as to minimize the risk of nonunion, delayed union, and refracture. Finally, surgical intervention may be necessary to prevent catastrophic fracture progression such as in the case of a tension-sided femoral neck fracture [5, 15].

Return to Sports Participation

Generally in athletes, return to play should only be recommended after proper treatment and complete healing of the injury. Because of the significant complications associated with progression to complete fracture, it is not recommended that an individual be allowed to continue to participate in their activity with evidence of a high-risk stress fracture [1]. Return to play decision-making for a low-grade injury at a high-risk location should be predicated on the patient's compliance level,

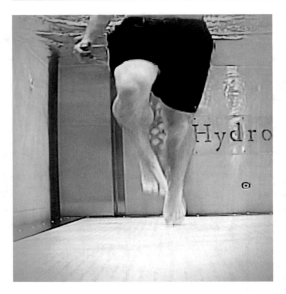

Fig. 7.7 Underwater view of 23-year-old male professional sprinter/long jumper running on an aquatic treadmill during recovery from a tarsal navicular stress fracture

healing potential, and risk of worsening of the injury. A key difference between a low-grade stress fracture at a high-risk location and a low-risk location is that with the low-risk site, the athlete or patient can be allowed to continue to train, whereas the high-risk site needs to heal prior to full return to activity.

Regardless of the grade and location, the risk of continued participation should be discussed with each athlete, and the management of each fracture should be individualized. Cross-training while resting from the inciting activity allows maintenance of cardiovascular fitness while decreasing stresses at the healing fracture site [26, 65]. Return to participation should be a joint decision between the physician, athletic trainer, coach, and athlete. If a stress fracture is diagnosed in the noncompetitive season, most athletes seek to achieve complete healing prior to return to training or competition. If the injury occurs at mid-season or in the championship season, elite athletes may limit the volume and intensity of their training while continuing to compete. Complete healing of the fracture is then sought once the season is over.

Prevention of Stress Injuries

Prevention is the ideal treatment of stress injuries of the bone. An assessment of the athlete's risks should be made at pre-participation evaluations, especially in those with a history of previous stress fractures [1, 26]. Correction of amenorrhea in females and calcium and Vitamin D supplementation is recommended in addition to general nutritional optimization. If biomechanical abnormalities are encountered, the use of appropriately designed orthotic devices should be considered as an initial corrective measure. However, gait analysis and appropriate running form and technique changes may be necessary to prevent future injuries. Additionally, bone density with body composition evaluation (iDEXA) may be required in individuals with recurrent bony stress injuries. An example report of an iDEXA evaluation is shown in Fig. 7.8. Keys to preventing stress fractures are listed in Table 7.4.

Summary

Stress fractures are common injuries particularly in endurance athletes and military recruits. The Kaeding-Miller classification system for stress fractures characterizes these injuries based on the patient's symptoms as well as their position on a radiographic continuum of severity. The treatment algorithm included in this chapter further stratifies these injuries as either high-risk or low-risk based upon the biomechanical environment in which they are located. Stress fracture management should employ a holistic approach and should be individualized to the patient taking into consideration injury site (low vs. high risk), grade (extent of microdamage accumulation), the individual's activity level, competitive situation, and risk tolerance.

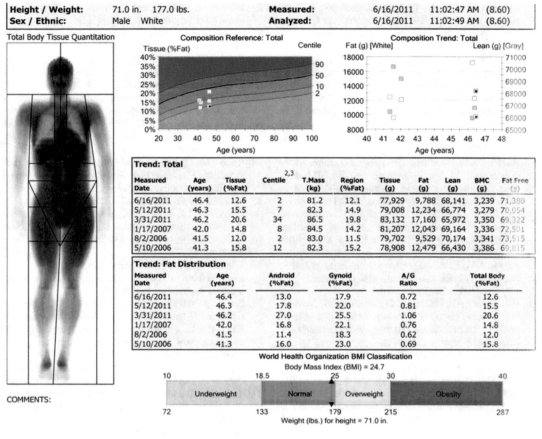

| Height / Weight: | 71.0 in. | 177.0 lbs. | | Measured: | 6/16/2011 | 11:02:47 AM | (8.60) |
| Sex / Ethnic: | Male | White | | Analyzed: | 6/16/2011 | 11:02:49 AM | (8.60) |

Trend: Total

Measured Date	Age (years)	Tissue (%Fat)	Centile 2,3	T.Mass (kg)	Region (%Fat)	Tissue (g)	Fat (g)	Lean (g)	BMC (g)	Fat Free (g)
6/16/2011	46.4	12.6	2	81.2	12.1	77,929	9,788	68,141	3,239	71,380
5/12/2011	46.3	15.5	7	82.3	14.9	79,008	12,234	66,774	3,279	70,054
3/31/2011	46.2	20.6	34	86.5	19.8	83,132	17,160	65,972	3,350	69,322
1/17/2007	42.0	14.8	8	84.5	14.2	81,207	12,043	69,164	3,336	72,501
8/2/2006	41.5	12.0	2	83.0	11.5	79,702	9,529	70,174	3,341	73,515
5/10/2006	41.3	15.8	12	82.3	15.2	78,908	12,479	66,430	3,386	69,815

Trend: Fat Distribution

Measured Date	Age (years)	Android (%Fat)	Gynoid (%Fat)	A/G Ratio	Total Body (%Fat)
6/16/2011	46.4	13.0	17.9	0.72	12.6
5/12/2011	46.3	17.8	22.0	0.81	15.5
3/31/2011	46.2	27.0	25.5	1.06	20.6
1/17/2007	42.0	16.8	22.1	0.76	14.8
8/2/2006	41.5	11.4	18.3	0.62	12.0
5/10/2006	41.3	16.0	23.0	0.69	15.8

World Health Organization BMI Classification
Body Mass Index (BMI) = 24.7

Fig. 7.8 Bone density/body composition report (iDEXA) of a 20-year-old male collegiate middle distance runner with recurrent lower extremity stress fractures

Table 7.4 Keys to prevention of stress fractures

Appropriate equipment, technique, and coaching
Optimization of nutrition and hormonal status
Optimization of body composition, lean mass to non-lean mass
Bone density evaluation (DEXA/iDEXA)
Cross-training
Adequate rest
Off seasons

References

1. Kaeding C, et al. Management and return to play of stress fractures. Clin J Sport Med. 2005;15(6):442–7.
2. Kaeding C, et al. Management of troublesome stress fractures. Instr Course Lect. 2004;53:455–69.
3. Kaeding C, et al. Stress fractures: classification and management. Phys Sportsmed. 2010;38(3):45–54.
4. Boden B, et al. Low-risk stress fractures. Am J Sports Med. 2001;29(1):100–11.
5. Boden B. High-risk stress fractures: evaluation and treatment. J Am Acad Orthop Surg. 2000;8:344–53.
6. Bennell KL, Malcolm SA, Wark JD, Brukner PD. Models for the pathogenesis of stress fractures in athletes. Br J Sports Med. 1996;30(3):200–4.
7. Matheson GO, Clement DB, McKenzie DC, Taunton JE, Lloyd-Smith DR, MacIntyre JG. Stress fractures in athletes: a study of 320 cases. Am J Sports Med. 1987;15:46–58.
8. Baker J, Frankel VH, Burstein A. Fatigue fractures: biomechanical considerations. J Bone Joint Surg. 1972;54:1345–6.
9. Jones BH, Harris JM, Vinh TN, Rubin C. Exercise-induced stress fractures and stress reactions of bone: epidemiology, etiology, and classification. Exerc Sport Sci Rev. 1989;17:379–422.

10. Keaveny TM, Hayes WC. Mechanical properties of cortical and trabecular bone. In: Hall BK, editor. Bone, vol. 7. Boca Raton, FL: CRC Press; 1993. p. 285–344.

11. Korpelainen R, Orava S, Karpakka J, et al. Risk factors for recurrent stress fractures in athletes. Am J Sports Med. 2001;29:304–10.

12. Morris JM, Blickenstaff LD. Fatigue fractures: a clinical study. Springfield, IL: Charles C. Thomas; 1967. p. 3–6.

13. Koch JC. The laws of bone architecture. Am J Anat. 1917;21:177–298.

14. Blickenstaff LD, Morris JM. Fatigue fractures of the femoral neck. J Bone Joint Surg. 1966;48:1031–47.

15. Bennell K, Brukner P. Epidemiology and site specificity of stress fractures. Clin Sports Med. 1997;16:179–96.

16. Li GP, Zhang SD, Chen G, Chen H, Wang AM. Radiographic and histologic analyses of stress fracture in rabbit tibias. Am J Sports Med. 1985; 13:285–94.

17. Barrow GW, Saha S. Menstrual irregularity and stress fractures in collegiate female distance runners. Am J Sports Med. 1988;16:209–16.

18. Drinkwater BL, Nilson K, Chesnut III CH, Bremner WJ, Shainholtz S, Southworth MB. Bone mineral content of amenorrheic and eumenorrheic athletes. N Engl J Med. 1984;311:277–81.

19. Greaney RB, Gerber FH, Laughlin RL, et al. Distribution and natural history of stress fractures in U.S. Marine recruits. Radiology. 1983;146:339–46.

20. Milgrom C, Giladi M, Stein M, et al. Stress fractures in military recruits: a prospective study showing an unusually high incidence. J Bone Joint Surg (Br). 1985;67:732–5.

21. Sormaala M, et al. Bone stress injuries of the talus in military recruits. Bone. 2006;39:199–204.

22. Winfield AC, Moore J, Bracker M, Johnson CW. Risk factors associated with stress reactions in female Marines. Mil Med. 1997;162(10):698–702.

23. Hoffman JR, Chapnik L, Shamis A, Givon U, Davidson B. The effect of leg strength on the incidence of lower extremity overuse injuries during military training. Mil Med. 1999;164(2):153–6.

24. Lappe J, Cullen D, Haynatzki G, Recker R, Ahlf R, Thompson K. Calcium and vitamin d supplementation decreases incidence of stress fractures in female navy recruits. J Bone Miner Res. 2008;23(5):741–9.

25. Ruohola JP, Laaksi I, Ylikomi T, et al. Association between serum 25(OH) D concentrations and bone stress fractures in Finnish young men. J Bone Miner Res. 2006;21(9):1483–8.

26. Diehl JJ, Best TM, Kaeding CC. Classification and return-to-play considerations for stress fractures. Clin Sports Med. 2006;25(1):17–28. vii.

27. Coughlin MJ, Grimes JS, Traughber PD, Jones CP. Comparison of radiographs and CT scans in the prospective evaluation of the fusion of hindfoot arthrodesis. Foot Ankle Int. 2006;27(10):780–7.

28. Whitelaw G, Wetzler M, Levy A, et al. A pneumatic leg brace for the treatment of tibial stress fractures. Clin Orthop. 1991;270:301–5.

29. Brukner P, et al. Stress fractures: a review of 180 cases. Clin J Sport Med. 1996;6(2):85–9.

30. Fredericson M, et al. Stress fractures in athletes. Top Magn Reson Imaging. 2006;17(5):309–25.

31. Romani W, et al. Identification of tibial stress fractures using therapeutic continuous ultrasound. J Orthop Sports Phys Ther. 2000;30(8):444–52.

32. Anderson MW, Greenspan A. Stress fractures. Radiology. 1996;199:1–12.

33. Moran DS, Evans RK, Hadad E. Imaging of lower extremity stress fracture injuries. Sports Med. 2008;38:345–56.

34. Roub LW, Gumerman LW, Hanley EN, Clark MW, Goodman M, Herbert DL. Bone stress: a radionuclide imaging perspective. Radiology. 1979;132:431–8.

35. Schneiders AG, Sullivan SJ, Hendrick PA, Hones BD, McMaster AR, Sugden BA, et al. The ability of clinical tests to diagnose stress fractures: a systematic review and meta-analysis. J Orthop Sports Phys Ther. 2012;42:760–71.

36. Bianchi S, Luong DH. Stress fractures of the ankle malleoli diagnosed by ultrasound: a report of 6 cases. Skeletal Radiol. 2014;43:813–8.

37. Banal F, Gandjbakhch F, Foltz V, Goldcher A, Etchepare F, Rozenberg S, et al. Sensitivity and specificity of ultrasonography in early diagnosis of metatarsal bone stress fractures: a pilot study of 37 patients. J Rheumatol. 2009;36:1715–9.

38. Papalada A, Malliaropoulos N, Tsitas K, Kiritsi O, Padhiar N, Del Buono A, et al. Ultrasound as a primary evaluation tool of bone stress injuries in elite track and field athletes. Am J Sports Med. 2012;40:915–9.

39. Bryant L, et al. Comparison of planar scintigraphy alone with SPECT for the initial evaluation of femoral neck stress fractures. Am J Roentgenol. 2008;191: 1010–5.

40. Bradshaw C, Khan K, Brukner P. Stress fracture of the body of the talus in athletes demonstrated with computer tomography. Clin J Sport Med. 1996;6:48–51.

41. Gaeta M, et al. High-resolution CT grading of tibial stress reactions in distance runners. Am J Roentgenol. 2006;187:789–93.

42. Pavlov H, Torg J, Freiberger R. Tarsal navicular stress fractures: radiographic evaluation. Radiology. 1983;148(3):641–5.

43. Torg JS, Pavlov H, Cooley LH, et al. Stress fractures of the tarsal navicular: a retrospective review of twenty-one cases. J Bone Joint Surg. 1982;64:700–12.

44. Nachtrab O, Cassar-Pullicino VN, Lalam R, Tins B, Tyrrell PN, Singh J. Role of MRI in hip fractures, including stress fractures, occult fractures, avulsion fractures. Eur J Radiol. 2012;81:3813–23.

45. Behrens SB, Deren ME, Matson A, Fadale PD, Monchik KO. Stress fractures of the pelvis and legs in athletes: a review. Sports Health. 2013;5:165–74.

46. Lee JK, Yao L. Stress fractures: MR imaging. Radiology. 1988;169:217–20.

47. Swischuk LE, Jadhay SP. Tibial stress phenomena and fractures: imaging evaluation. Emerg Radiol. 2013;21:173–7.

48. Gaeta M, Mileto A, Ascenti G, Bernava G, Murabito A, Minutoli F. Bone stress injuries of the leg in athletes. Radiol Med. 2013;118:1034–44.
49. Navas A, Kassarjian A. Bone marrow changes in stress injuries. Semin Musculoskelet Radiol. 2011;15:183–97.
50. Dixon S, Newton J, Teh J. Stress fractures in the young athlete: a pictorial review. Curr Probl Diagn Radiol. 2011;40:29–44.
51. Gaeta M, Minutoli F, Scribano E, Ascenti G, Vicni S, Bruschetta D, et al. CT and MR imaging findings in athletes with early tibial stress injuries: comparison with bone scintigraphy findings and emphasis on cortical abnormalities. Radiology. 2005;235: 553–61.
52. Arendt EA, Griffiths HJ. The use of MR imaging in the assessment and clinical management of stress reactions of bone in high-performance athletes. Clin Sports Med. 1997;16:291–306.
53. Dutton J. Clinical value of grading the scintigraphic appearances of tibial stress fractures in military recruits. Clin Nucl Med. 2002;27(1):18–21.
54. Brukner P, et al. Management of common stress fractures. Phys Sportsmed. 1998;26(8):39–47.
55. Miller T, Kaeding C. Stress fractures: a new classification system. Seattle, WA: Podium Presentation at the American College of Sports Medicine; 2009.
56. Kaeding CC, Miller TL. The comprehensive description of stress fractures: a new classification system. J Bone Joint Surg Am. 2013;95:1214–20.
57. Noakes TD, Smith JA, Lindenberg G, et al. Pelvic stress fractures in long distance runners. Am J Sports Med. 1985;13:120–3.
58. Jones GL. Upper extremity stress fractures. Clin Sports Med. 2006;25(1):159–74, xi.
59. Verma R, et al. Athletic stress fractures: Part III. The upper body. Am J Orthop. 2001;20(12):848–60.
60. Miller TL, Kaeding CC. Upper-extremity stress fractures: distribution and causative activities in 70 patients. Orthopedics. 2012;35(9):789–93.
61. Ahmad C, et al. Valgus extension overload syndrome and stress injury of the olecranon. Clin Sports Med. 2004;23(4):665–76.
62. El Attrache NS, Ahmed CS. Valgus extension overload syndrome and olecranon stress fractures. Sports Med Arthroscopy Rev. 2003;11:25–9.
63. Schickendantz M, Ho C, Koh J. Stress injury of the proximal ulna in professional baseball players. Am J Sports Med. 2002;30:737–41.
64. Hod N, et al. Characteristics of skeletal stress fractures in female military recruits of the Israel Defense Forces on bone scintigraphy. Clin Nucl Med. 2006;31:742–9.
65. Jensen J. Stress fracture in the world class athlete: a case study. Med Sci Sports Exerc. 1998;30:783–7.

Evaluation and Treatment of Soft Tissue Overuse Injuries

8

Bryant Walrod

Achilles Tendinosis

Introduction

Achilles tendon pain is common in endurance athletes. Injuries to this tendon are often the result of repetitive stress from excessive activity; however, symptoms of pain can also be noted in sedentary individuals. Patients may have pain at the midportion of the tendon with palpation and/or activity.

Terminology

Often termed Achilles tendinitis, this may not most accurately describe the condition. While a true tendinitis can be seen, most often, inflammation is not seen on histopathologic specimens of painful Achilles. Instead, one notes collagen disarray, increased proteoglycans, and disordered healing, more accurately reflecting a tendinosis (Fig. 8.1). Tendinosis is often thought to be the result of overuse, causing microtrauma to the tendon such that it cannot adequately repair itself. Leadbetter defined tendinosis as a failure of the cell matrix to adapt to repetitive trauma caused by an imbalance between the degeneration and synthesis of the matrix [1]. Maffulli described Achilles tendinopathy as a clinical syndrome characterized by three elements: pain, swelling, and functional impairment corresponding to the histopathologic pattern of tendinosis [2].

Anatomy

The Achilles tendon represents the distal combination of the medial and lateral gastrocnemius with the soleus. It is approximately 15 cm long. As it descends, it twists approximately 90° (30°–150°) on itself, and then the tendon inserts onto the calcaneus (Fig. 8.2). Thus, the tendon has two junctional regions, the myotendinous junction and the osteotendinous junction. The vascular supply for the Achilles tends to occur at both of these junctions which may leave the midportion vulnerable for potential vascular compromise. There is no true synovial sheath, but there is a paratendon which assists with gliding of the tendon. This paratendon also contributes to the vascular supply of the Achilles. Contraction of this muscle will cause plantar flexion of the foot and generate power for locomotion. The Achilles tendon can generate power up to 12 times one's body weight during fast running. The predominant collagen in the Achilles tendon is type 1 with the fibers being arranged in a parallel manner. Ground substance, proteoglycans, and glycosaminoglycan chains surround the collagen.

B. Walrod (✉)
Family Medicine, Ohio State University,
2050 Kenny Road., Suite 3100, Columbus,
OH 43221, USA
e-mail: Bryant.walrod@osumc.edu

© Springer International Publishing Switzerland 2016
T.L. Miller (ed.), *Endurance Sports Medicine*, DOI 10.1007/978-3-319-32982-6_8

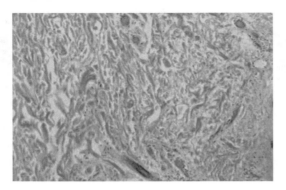

Fig. 8.1 Histologic picture revealing tendinosis

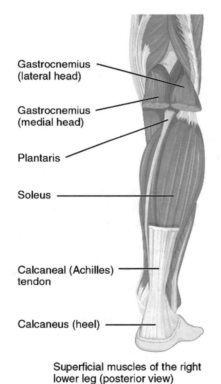

Gastrocnemius
(lateral head)

Gastrocnemius
(medial head)

Plantaris

Soleus

Calcaneal (Achilles)
tendon

Calcaneus (heel)

Superficial muscles of the right
lower leg (posterior view)

Fig. 8.2 Anatomic picture of Achilles tendon

Pathophysiology of Tendinosis

Overuse and improper loading of a tendon may damage tissue and cause breakdown. Inadequate repair of this breakdown initiates the process of tendinosis. Biopsies of tendinotic tendons reveal increased cell numbers, ground substance, colla-

gen disarray, and neovascularization. Typical prostaglandin-mediated inflammatory mediators are absent. Often, however, neurogenic mediators accompany this increased neovascularization and contribute to the pain associated with Achilles tendinosis. In fact, substance P and calcitonin gene-related peptides have been isolated.

Epidemiology

Achilles tendinosis is often associated with land-based endurance-type activities such as running. There are variable reports of incidence in the literature [3]. The annual incidence of Achilles tendinosis is 7–9 % in top-level runners. However, Kujala noted lifetime incidence of Achilles tendinosis to be up to 24 % in competitive athletes and up to 40–50 % in competitive runners. The majority of individuals tend to have midportion issues. In fact, Kvist looked at 698 athletes and noted 66 % of these athletes had midportion Achilles tendinopathy, and 23 % of them had insertional issues [4].

Etiology

The etiology of Achilles tendon disorders is multi-factorial with some discrepancies noted in the literature. Common thinking is that abnormal stresses on the Achilles tendon, its midportion, or insertion may lead to microtrauma with resultant poor healing and subsequent tendinosis. Kvist revealed that poor alignment of the lower extremity leads to Achilles issues [5]. Common malalignment issues were overpronation, over-supination, hindfoot varus or valgus, leg length discrepancy, decreased flexibility, and joint laxity. In addition to mechanical risk for the development of Achilles tendinosis, there are general factors that may increase the risk: male gender, increased age, and obesity. Certain training habits have also been associated with increased risk. These include excessive training, training errors, hill training, and specialized training (i.e., only running) [6].

Fluoroquinolones have frequently been implicated in risk for developing Achilles tendon problems. Sode noted 12 episodes of Achilles tendon rupture per 100,000 fluoroquinolone treatment episodes [7]. Another study by Van der Lin looked at 46,776 patients treated with fluoro-quinolones and noted 3.2 cases of tendon problems for every 1000 years of exposure [8]. Symptoms occurred within 1 month of initiating treatment and resolved within 2 months of discontinuing treatment. Concomitant use of systemic glucocorticoids with fluoroquinolones also increased the risk.

Oral glucocorticoids and cortisone injections also increase the risk of the development of Achilles rupture and tendinosis [8, 9].

Physical Exam

Individuals will typically describe an area of pain 2–6 cm proximal to the insertion of the Achilles tendon on the calcaneus. The pain is typically described as burning and achy and worse with activity, especially stairs and hills. However, the pain is sometimes also present in the morning. Individuals may have cut back or ceased activities that worsen their symptoms like running. Passive range of motion is typically full, but plantar flexion may be decreased secondary to pain. Affected side single-leg heel raise strength and endurance are also compromised. Provocation of pain with palpation at the midportion of the Achilles is also present. Oftentimes, there are a concomitant thickening of the Achilles or a painful palpable nodule (Fig. 8.3). Observation of the patient's gait may reveal some of the abnormalities listed above as risk factors for Achilles tendinosis like overpronation. Always compare the injured, symptomatic limb with the unaffected, contralateral limb.

Imaging

Imaging may be helpful, but often the diagnosis can be made from history and physical exam. Imaging may contribute to the workup if the diagnosis is not clear. Plain films may reveal a bony prominence such as Haglund's deformity which may contribute to Achilles tendon pain (Fig. 8.4). Ultrasound is a modality with increas-

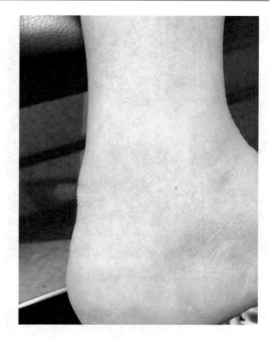

Fig. 8.3 Achilles tendon thickening

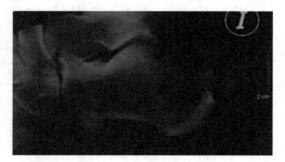

Fig. 8.4 X-ray of Haglund's deformity

ing usefulness in evaluating tendinopathies. It is inexpensive and can clearly define pathology. Common findings on ultrasound are thickened Achilles tendon, hypoechogenic areas, collagen disarray, and tendon sheath swelling or fluid. Ultrasound can also be used to determine partial from complete Achilles tendon tears (Fig. 8.5). MRI can be used for further detail of the anatomy of the Achilles tendon and for preoperative planning. Common MRI findings for those with chronic Achilles tendinosis are tendon thickening and increase uptake or signal intensity within the tendon on the T1 images (Fig. 8.6).

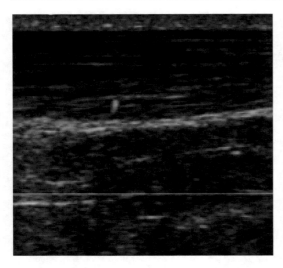

Fig. 8.5 Ultrasound picture of Achilles tendinosis

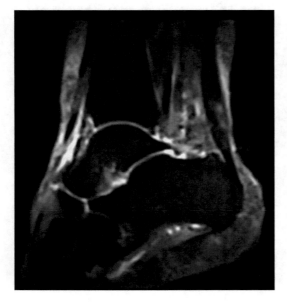

Fig. 8.6 MRI with Achilles tendinosis

Treatment

Relative rest and activity modification are initially recommended for treatment. Avoidance of painful activities such as running and jumping also should be discussed with the patient. If specific biomechanical abnormalities are noted on physical examination, certain methods may be

employed to correct these issues. These may include heel lifts, arch supports, orthotics, motion control running shoes, stretching tight calves, changing training surfaces, or decreasing the intensity of training. If the patient's pain is severe with simple ambulation, temporary immobilization in a CAM walking boot may be effective. Night-time splints pulling the foot into dorsiflexion may also help to reduce morning symptoms.

Medications

Nonsteroidal anti-inflammatory drugs (NSAIDs) are also frequently used to treat Achilles tendinosis. However, since the bulk of midportion Achilles pain is not secondary to an inflammatory process, patients may find a decrease in their pain simply from the analgesic component of these medications. Thus, acetaminophen is also a reasonable choice for pain relief for midportion Achilles pain. Astrom and Westllin compared piroxicam to placebo for patients with Achilles tendinosis in a randomized placebo-controlled trial of 70 individuals and found that the medication was not superior for treatment of Achilles tendinosis for pain, range of motion, and strength [10].

Rehabilitation

Rehabilitation should be a cornerstone of treatment for Achilles tendinosis. In fact, treatment should be considered early in the symptom presentation. Harnessing the body's own reparative ability during a controlled exercise regimen can be helpful. Eccentric exercises have been studied as a treatment for this condition. Alfredson studied 15 recreational individuals with chronic Achilles tendinosis and found improvement in symptoms when treated with a heavy eccentric loading exercise regimen for twice daily for 12 weeks [11]. These patients were then followed for 2 years, and 14/15 are still running pain free. Multiple other studies have further supported the use of eccentric exercise chronic tendinopathic conditions [12]. However, it has also been noted that eccentric exercises may be more effective for

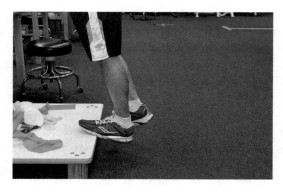

Fig. 8.7 Individual doing an eccentric heel drop

midportion Achilles tendinosis rather than insertional tendinosis with a treatment success rate of 89 and 32% [13]. In addition, Magnussen et al. performed a systematic review that revealed eccentric exercises to be effective for treatment of midportion Achilles tendinosis but not insertional tendinosis [12]. These exercises need to be performed in a slow and controlled manner to assist in allowing the collagen to form parallel to the lines of stress. Mild discomfort is allowed in the rehabilitation process (Fig. 8.7).

Rehabilitation for insertional Achilles tendinosis has less robust evidence and may be more difficult to treat. Again, Fahlstrom demonstrated improvement with midportion Achilles tendinosis of 89% versus only 32% improvement for insertional Achilles tendinosis. A variation in rehabilitation was proposed by Jonsson and Alfredson in 2008 for the treatment of insertional Achilles tendinosis. Eccentric exercises were performed, but the patient was limited to stay out of dorsiflexion. At 4 months, 67% were satisfied and back to their activity [14]. Despite all of this, a systematic review in 2006 by Woodley questioned the quality of evidence supporting eccentric exercises for chronic tendinosis and called for better studies to evaluate their effectiveness [15].

Extracorporeal Shock Wave Therapy (ESWT)

ESWT has demonstrated some promise in treatment of chronic Achilles tendinosis. A systematic review by noted ESWT to be an effective

treatment for chronic insertional and non-insertional Achilles tendinosis [16]. A large RCT revealed the shock wave therapy was superior to eccentric exercises in the treatment of chronic insertional Achilles tendinopathy [17]. Finally, Furia also looked at ECWT plus eccentric exercises versus eccentric exercises alone for chronic non-insertional Achilles tendinosis and found that the combination was superior [18]. A systematic review published by Kearney et al. in 2010 for treatment of insertional Achilles tendinosis concluded that conservative treatment should be attempted first. Conservative treatment for insertional achilles tendinosis should start with eccentric loading and shock wave therapy before surgical intervention is considered [19].

Injection Therapies

There are a multitude of injection options for the treatment of Achilles tendinosis with varying degrees of effectiveness.

Cortisone injections are frequently employed by Sports Medicine providers to treat endurance medicine maladies. As stated earlier, typically Achilles pain is secondary to an overused, poorly healing tendon, rather than an acutely inflamed tendon. As expected, studies are conflicting with respect to effectiveness. Short-term benefit has been seen in one study [20]. But another one revealed no significant improvement [21]. Risk of rupture is a concern, and this should preclude consideration for cortisone injections as early therapy in the treatment of Achilles tendinosis.

Pro-inflammatory injections have also demonstrated effectiveness in the treatment of chronic Achilles tendinosis. Injecting any substance into or around a tendon will cause an inflammatory response, which when paired with appropriate physical therapy will hopefully lead to proper and permanent healing. Some concerns with pro-inflammatory injection are the lack of standardized injections as well as standardized rehabilitation protocols. There is also variability as to whether or not ultrasound guidance is used.

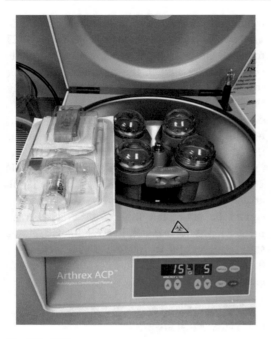

Fig. 8.8 PRP

Ultrasound-guided injection of hyperosmolar dextrose into the Achilles tendon decreased pain for both insertional and midportion Achilles pain in 99 patients [22]. In addition, dextrose injections and dextrose injections plus eccentric exercises demonstrated a greater improvement in pain for midportion Achilles pain when compared to eccentric exercises alone [23].

Platelet-rich plasma (PRP) has also been studied for the treatment of chronic Achilles tendinosis. Injecting concentrated platelets into the Achilles tendon is thought to stimulate inflammation and promote proper healing (Fig. 8.8). However, de Vos et al. followed 54 people with midportion Achilles tendinosis for 1 year after randomizing to either receive a PRP injection or a saline injection in addition to the a program of eccentric exercises. Both groups improved, but there was no significant difference between the two groups. These patients were then followed for a year and still no significant difference was noted [24]. Small studies have revealed varying response to midportion Achilles pain from an autologous blood injection as well [25, 26].

The idea of injecting sclerosing agents into an area of a tendon with painful neovascularization has also been studied for chronic Achilles tendon pain. Alfredson performed a small double-blinded randomized controlled trial of injections of either polidocanol or lidocaine and noted decreased pain in the polidocanol group [27]. Ohberg also found similar improvements after injections of polidocanol in a prospective study of 11 patients [28]. And finally, Clemetson noted similar improvement for polidocanol injections in a retrospective review of 25 patients [29].

Topical Treatment

Topical glyceryl nitrate patches have also been studied to treat chronic Achilles tendinosis. Paoloni et al. conducted a double-blinded placebo-controlled randomized controlled trial (DBPCRT) that revealed that topical glyceryl nitrate was superior to placebo in reducing pain from chronic Achilles tendinosis [30]. Hunte also came to a similar conclusion noting that topical glyceryl nitrate was superior to placebo in a DBPCRT [31]. However, mild controversy exists because Kane et al. preformed a randomized controlled trial comparing topical glyceryl nitrate plus physical therapy to physical therapy alone and found no significant difference [32].

Surgery

About 25 % of patients will continue to have symptoms despite conservative care; thus, various surgical options are available for recalcitrant cases of chronic midportion Achilles tendinosis. Typically, an open surgical approach will involve resection of posterior superior calacaneal prominence, retrocalcaneal bursa, and intratendinous calcifications and extensive debridement of fibrotic adhesions. However, there has also been some evidence of percutaneous needle tenotomy as an effective surgical treatment [33]. Endoscopic debridement of the tendon is another surgical option with good outcomes [34]. Typically, those individuals who present with an acute full thickness Achilles tendon tear are recommended to have surgical repair. However, recently there has been some evidence for conservative treatment of full thickness tears with reasonable outcomes [35–37].

Patellar Tendinosis

Introduction

Patellar tendinosis is a relatively common finding in athletes with repetitive activities like running and jumping and typically is an overuse injury presenting with anterior knee pain. There can be significant disability secondary to this condition resulting in chronic pain.

Terminology

Similar to other chronic tendon pain issues, chronic patellar pain is also more correctly described as a tendinosis or a tendinopathy, not a tendinitis secondary to the absence of inflammatory changes on histopathologic specimens of chronically painful patella tendons. Rather, one often sees a failure of a proper healing response to mechanical overuse with resultant collagen disarray and painful neovascularization (Fig. 8.9). Specific histologic changes include increased glycosaminoglycans and decreased expression of type I collagen with increased type III collagen expression. This condition is often

termed "jumper's knee" but also should possibly be more accurately labeled "lander's knee" as the tendon experiences greater eccentric forces during landing over jumping. This increased force is thought to contribute to the development of this condition.

Anatomy

The patella tendon is the tendon that stretched from its origin on the distal pole of the patella to its insertion on the tibial tuberosity (Fig. 8.10). It may be more accurately termed a ligament as it stretches from bone to bone. The tendon assists in the lever motion of the knee for leg extension. In adults, the tendon is typically 5–6 cm long, 2–3 cm wide, and 0.5 cm thick. A fat pad is also located posterior to the patella tendon.

Epidemiology

Between 2001 and 2009, Hagglund et al. looked at 2229 elite soccer players and noted an incidence of 0.12 injuries/1000 h. In each season, 2.4 % of the players were affected [38].

A questionnaire was completed by 891 male and female nonelite athletes from seven popular sports in the Netherlands: basketball, volleyball, handball, korfball, soccer, field hockey, and track and field. The overall prevalence of jumper's knee was 8.5 % (78 of 891 athletes), showing a significant difference between sports with different

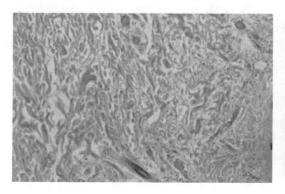

Fig. 8.9 Tendinosis

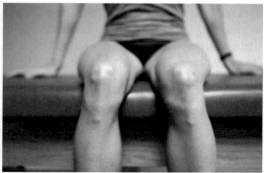

Fig. 8.10 Anatomic picture of patella tendon

loading characteristics. Prevalence was highest among volleyball players (14.4 %) and lowest among soccer players (2.5 %); it was significantly higher among male athletes (10.2 %) than female athletes (6.4 %). The mean duration of symptoms was 18.9 months [39].

Lian et al. also looked at 50 Norwegian male and female athletes at the national elite level from each of the following nine sports: sprinting, basketball, ice hockey, volleyball, orienteering, road cycling, soccer, team handball, and wrestling. They found the overall prevalence of patellar tendinitis was 14.2 %. The prevalence of current symptoms was highest in volleyball (44.6 %) and basketball (31.9 %), whereas there were no cases in cycling or orienteering [40].

Risk Factors

In elite soccer players, high total exposure hours and increased body mass increased the risk of developing patellar tendinosis.

Hagglund also noted increased risk for the development of patellar tendinosis in athletes who were significantly younger, taller, and heavier than those without jumper's knee, and Lian noted increased incidence in males over females.

Patellar tendinopathy was also more common in females with specialization in only one sport [41].

An older study looked at risk factors for patellar tendinopathy and found that poor quadriceps and hamstring flexibility were also risk factors [42].

History and Physical Exam

Symptomatic individuals will often report anterior knee pain with jumping, running, and explosive movements. The pain is typically worse with repetitive knee flexion movements and lessens with rest. The pain is often described as achy. Its occurrence is insidious without a specific trauma or twist that precludes symptom presentation. Provocative maneuvers are squatting on a decline. The pain can also be worse with palpation. The location of pain associated with anterior patella pain is typically at the distal patella pole/origin of

patella tendon (70 %), quad tendon insertion on the proximal patella (20 %), or at the patella tendon insertion at the tibial tuberosity (10 %). The remainder of the knee exam is typically unremarkable, with no laxity on provocative maneuvers.

Workup

Laboratory studies are typically not useful in the workup of chronic patellar tendinosis.

Imaging

Although radiographic evaluation is not universally needed in the workup and diagnosis of patellar tendinosis, it can be helpful in differentiation and confirmation of a patient's symptoms. Plain film radiographs are rarely useful. Plain radiographs may reveal enthesopathic changes at the origin or insertion of the patella tendon (Fig. 8.11). Plain radiographs may also reveal lateral subluxation of the patella which can be a risk factor for developing tendinosis. Sports ultrasound is emerging as an excellent tool to aid in the diagnosis and also treatment of patellar tendi-

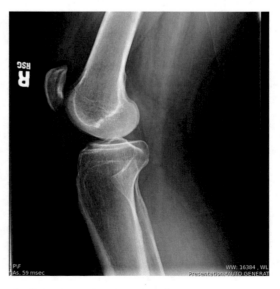

Fig. 8.11 Plain film of patella enthesopathy

Fig. 8.12 Ultrasound with hypoechogenic and thickened patella tendon

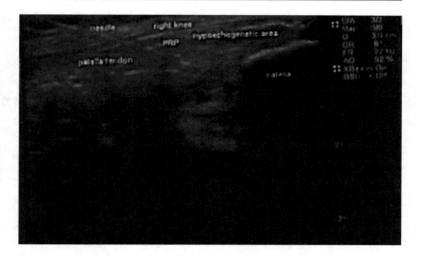

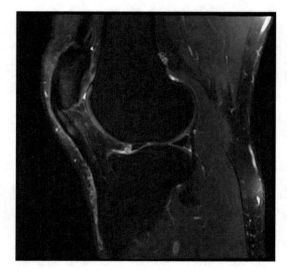

Fig. 8.13 MRI with increased TI signal intensity

nosis. Ultrasound will typically reveal a thickening of the tendon with area of hypoechogenic signal and evidence of neovascularization on color Doppler flow (Fig. 8.12).

MRI is also a useful tool to assist in the diagnosis and management of chronic patellar tendinosis. MRI reveals a thickened tendon with increased T1 signal intensity at the area of tendinosis (Fig. 8.13). Ultrasound and MRI can also be helpful in evaluating for patella tendon tears.

A recent study looked at the accuracy of imaging for clinically diagnosed patella tendinosis and found that color Doppler and gray scale ultrasound had an accuracy of 83 % each, while MRI had an accuracy of 70 % [43].

Treatment

Medication

Nonsteroidal anti-inflammatory (NSAIDs) medications may have a role in the treatment of acute patellar tendinitis; however, their role on chronic poorly healing tendinosis may be limited to simply analgesia as no inflammation is present in this condition. As a result, analgesic medications such as acetaminophen may also be a reasonable option for individuals with chronic patellar tendon pain.

Rehabilitation

Rest and/or relative rest is often employed as an initial treatment option for chronic patellar tendinosis, but typically the symptoms return after resuming their previous level of activity.

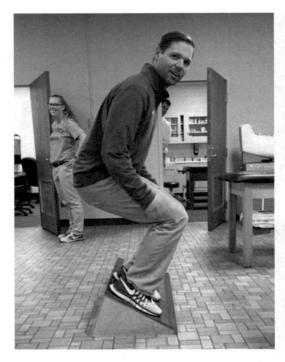

Fig. 8.14 25° Decline eccentric squat

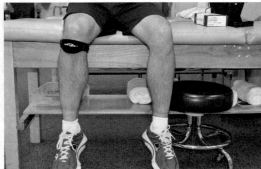

Fig. 8.15 Infrapatellar strap

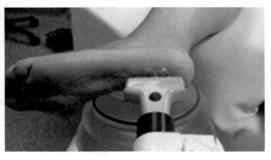

Fig. 8.16 ESWT

Physical therapy should be employed as first-line treatment for chronic patellar tendinosis. Eccentric rehabilitation has been a mainstay in the treatment of patellar tendinosis with a large body of evidence supporting its effectiveness. Common thoughts as to the rationale for eccentric training being effective for the treatment of chronic tendon pain is the idea that it reduces blood flow through the neovessels causing them to collapse which would in turn decrease to pain that accompanies these neovessels. The 25° decline eccentric squat seems to be the most effective [44] (Fig. 8.14). Eccentric training was also found to be superior to concentric training for the treatment of chronic patellar tendinosis. Eccentric training was also compared with surgical treatment, and there was no significant difference in outcome [45]. Multiple reviews have found eccentric exercises to be effective for the treatment of chronic patellar tendinosis [46, 47]. However, Visnes noted that eccentric training was not as effective for treatment when employed during the competitive season [48]. Eccentric training when used as a prophylaxis for the devel-

opment of patella tendinosis was not found to be effective in reducing risk of injury [49].

Much of the evidence for the effectiveness of patellar tendon straps (Fig. 8.15) has been anecdotal. There have been reported decrease in general anterior knee pain with an infrapatellar straps, but studies specifically looking at treatment of chronic patellar tendinosis with an infrapatellar strap have been lacking. One recent study however did note that infrapatellar straps decreased patella tendon strain [50].

Extracorporeal Shock Wave Therapy (ESWT)

ESWT is a procedure where acoustic waves are focused on a specific site on the body. Subsequent dissipation of energy is thought to cause alterations in tissue and stimulate healing and decrease pain receptor activation (Fig. 8.16). A small randomized controlled study revealed a benefit for treatment of chronic patellar tendinosis versus conservative treatment [51]. Some other studies reveal a benefit of treatment with ESWT for chronic patellar tendinosis, but many of these studies are limited by lack of a control group or prospective study design [52, 53]. A review of seven studies with differing protocols in 2007 concluded that ESWT is an effective treatment for chronic patellar tendinosis [54].

However, it is important to note that if one applies ESWT during the competitive season, the results (similar to eccentric exercises) do not demonstrate any benefit [55].

Peers compared ESWT to surgical intervention for chronic patellar tendinopathy and found similar outcomes [56].

Injections

Numerous injection therapies with varying evidence and effectiveness have been proposed to treat chronic patellar tendinosis. Corticosteroid injections are commonly considered in the treatment of tendon pain. However, as previously elucidated, chronic patellar tendinosis is more of a poorly healing response rather than an acute inflammatory response, thus limiting the potential effectiveness of cortisone injections. Available studies are weak to support cortisone injections for chronic patellar tendinosis for long-term pain relief [57]. One also needs to be cautious of an increased risk of tendon rupture after the injection of cortisone around a tendon and especially into a tendon.

Hyperosmolar dextrose has also been used to treat chronic tendon pain. Ryan et al. prospectively treated patients who had chronic patellar tendinosis pain with a series of four injections of hyperosmolar dextrose. This treatment yielded a significant decrease in pain and also neovascularization and hypoechogenicity on ultrasound [58].

Simultaneous dry needling and autologous blood injection were effective in a prospective study of refractory chronic patellar tendinosis when the individuals also followed a prescribed rehabilitation protocol after the injection [59]. A very recent double-blinded randomized controlled trial evaluated ultrasound-guided autologous blood injection versus saline injection for chronic patellar tendinosis. Both groups reported a significant decrease in symptoms with no significant difference between the two groups [60].

Platelet-rich plasma (PRP) injections have generated a lot of interest in the treatment of soft tissue injuries over the past decade. Injection of concentrated platelets is thought to induce inflammation and promote healing with the presence of various bioactive growth factors. Thus, PRP injections have been studied for the treatment of chronic patellar tendinosis. Two prospective studies revealed improvement in pain after a PRP injection and a standardized rehabilitation protocol [61, 62]. A recent double-blinded study compared ultrasound-guided injection of PRP to dry needling alone followed by an eccentric exercise regimen for individuals with chronic patellar tendinosis. At 12 weeks, both groups had improved, but the PRP group had improved significantly more than the dry needling group alone. This benefit was diminished at 26 weeks, however [63]. When comparing PRP injection to ESWT, Vetrano noted both groups demonstrated improvement, but the PRP group had a significantly greater improvement in pain at 6- and 12-month follow-up [64]. Smith noted that in athletes with chronic patellar tendinopathy, both groups responded positively to PRP injection and ESWT. However, the PRP-treated patients demonstrated significantly greater improvements in VISA-P and pain scores by 6 months and significantly better functional outcomes and satisfaction based on a modified Blazina scale at 12 months [65]. A systematic review by Liddle stated that the superiority of PRP to other treatments is unproven, and further study is needed [66]. Another systematic review by Di Matteo revealed that PRP is an effective treatment for chronic patellar tendinosis [67].

Sclerosing injections are another option often cited to treat chronic patellar tendinosis. Typically, this entails ultrasound-guided injections of a sclerosing substance like polidocanol. When compared with ultrasound-guided injections of lidocaine and epinephrine, polidocanol was more effective in reducing pain and restoring function in high-level individuals with chronic patellar tendinosis [68]. The same authors completed a prospective study looking at over a 100 individuals with chronic patellar pain and noted reduced pain and improved function at 24 and 44 months. However, while two thirds of the patients did well, one third of the patients went on to surgery at the 44-month mark [69, 70]. Alfredson treated individuals with chronic patellar tendinosis with polidocanol injections with ultrasound guidance targeting neovessels and found improvements in pain and neovessels in 80 % tendons at 6 months [71]. However, when comparing injections of polidocanol to arthroscopic shaving, individuals who underwent shaving reported less pain and were more satisfied with treatment. There was no structured rehabilitation after either intervention in this study [72].

Surgery should be considered after an appropriate trial of conservative care, eccentric exercises, injection, or ESWT treatments. One RCT looked at eccentric training versus open surgery and found no difference in pain scores between the two groups at 12 months [73]. There have also been variable outcomes with various surgical approaches outlined in the literature [74]. However, a recent systematic review revealed that minimally invasive, arthroscopically assisted, or all arthroscopic procedures may lead to a significantly faster return to sporting activities and may, therefore, be the preferred method of surgical treatment [45].

Greater Trochanteric Pain Syndrome (GTPS) or Gluteal Tendinopathy

Definition

This condition encompasses a broad spectrum of conditions, and the etiologies are various. Often termed greater trochanteric bursitis, this specific description does not accurately identify the typical pathophysiology underlying a patient's complaints of lateral hip pain. In fact, when looking at patients with lateral hip pain, MRI and ultrasound revealed an inflamed greater trochanteric bursa in less than 10 % of individuals [75]. More often, the cause of lateral hip pain is secondary to hip abductor and external rotator weakness with resultant tendinopathy.

Epidemiology

Gluteal tendinopathy is more common in females with a 4:1 ratio and in individuals 40–60 years of age. It affects about 10–25 % of individuals in general.

Anatomy

The gluteus medius originates on the superior half of the ilium and inserts superiolaterally on the greater trochanter of the femur. The function of the gluteus medius is to abduct to the hip and also to assist with hip internal rotation and with pelvic stability while running. The gluteus minimus also originates on the ilium between the anterior and inferior gluteal lines and inserts just inferior and anterior to the medius on the greater trochanter. It functions similar to the gluteus medius assisting with abduction, internal rotation, and pelvis stability. Other important muscles in this area are the hip external rotators, the piriformis, superior and inferior gemelli, and the obturator internus. These muscles can share a conjoined tendon that will insert on the greater trochanter and can confound and contribute to lateral hip pain in the endurance athlete (Fig. 8.17). However, there can also be some variability in the insertion of the various muscles on the greater trochanter adding to some confusion. Understanding this basic anatomy is crucial in understanding the pathophysiology of lateral hip pain in endurance athletes. Often described as a bursitis or a tendinitis, the underlying mechanism is more often gluteal tendinopathy or a tendinosis. Characteristic findings in tendinosis are a lack of inflammatory cells. One also observes disordered healing, increased proteoglycans, and angiofibroblastic neovascularization in the tendon. In tendinosis, there is also often a change from type I collagen to type III. These tendinopathic

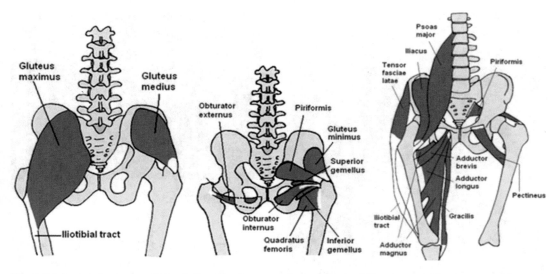

Fig. 8.17 Anatomic picture of lateral hip with gluteus medius, minimus, piriformis, gemelli, obturator, and greater trochanter

areas are traditionally difficult to treat secondary to a relatively poor blood supply. Compressive forces in this area contribute to the development of tendinosis of the gluteal tendons. The subgluteus maximus bursa is the bursa typically implicated in greater trochanteric bursitis, but there are also subgluteal medius and minimus bursae in this area.

Risk Factors/History

Gluteal tendinopathy is more common on individuals who are obese and sedentary individuals; however, it can also affect endurance athletes. This condition is common in runners with increased hip adduction when running. It is also seen in runners who run on a domed road affecting the hip that is closest to the side of the road. Patients typically report an increase in pain when sleeping on the affected side at night but also may report pain on the contralateral side secondary to excessive adduction of the affected hip at night. Pain is also noted with going up and downstairs and when training on hills. Patients may also complain of increased pain after prolonged sitting, epically when rising after the hip has been flexed to greater than 90°, like when sitting low in a car.

Physical Examination

Begin with inspection. Examine for leg length discrepancy by measuring the distance from the anterior superior iliac spine (ASIS) to the medial malleolus of each side. The shorter leg side will have increased adduction and thus stress the lateral hip and may contribute to the development of GTPS. Also observe the patient walk and have them stand on one leg to look for a positive Trendelenburg sign: This test is considered positive when standing on one leg; the pelvis tilts down toward the raised foot. This is a result of weakness of the abductor muscles of the hip on which they are standing (Fig. 8.18). One will also often note valgus deviation or adduction of the knee when single-leg squatting (Fig. 8.19). All of these abnormalities increase the stress and compressive forces on the lateral hip contributing to greater trochanteric pain syndrome.

Pain with palpation over the greater trochanteric area is also a common but insensitive finding. In addition, there may be pain along the bodies of the gluteus medius, minimus and piriformis muscles, and at their insertion. Patients may also have pain with resisted active abduction and with full passive adduction. A positive flexion

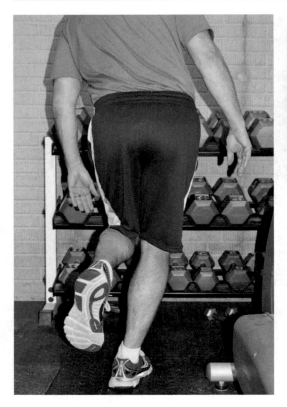

Fig. 8.18 Trendelenburg sign

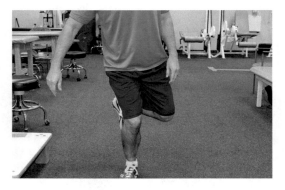

Fig. 8.19 Valgus deviation with single-leg squatting

abduction and external rotation (FABER) may be noted for pain in the lateral hip area (Fig. 8.20). Limitation of range of motion or deep groin pain with this test should raise concern for intra-artic-ular hip issues, not GTPS. Typically, GTPS pain may be noted on resisted internal rotation of the hip. Affected patients may also report a stretch-ing or pulling sensation with flexion adduction

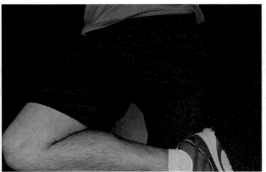

Fig. 8.20 FABER test

and internal rotation (FADIR). A tight iliotibial band with a positive Ober's test may also contrib-ute to pain at the lateral hip. Bird looked at the sensitivities and specificities of some of these tests and found a positive Trendelenburg test to be the most sensitive at 72.7 %, and it had a speci-ficity of 76.9 %. This was followed by pain with resisted hip abduction (sensitivity 72.7 % and specificity 46.2 %) and pain on resisted hip inter-nal rotation (sensitivity 54.5 % and specificity at 69.2 %) [76].

In addition, Lequesne noted that lateral hip pain with single-leg standing for 30 s was 100 % sensitive and 97.3 % specific for GTPS. Pain with resisted hip external derotation was 88 % sensi-tive and 97 % specific [77].

One study noted that the absence of difficulty with manipulating shoes and socks along with pain with palpation of the greater trochanter and lateral hip pain with FABER testing are likely to have greater trochanteric pain syndrome [78].

Examining the athletes' running gait can also uncover some potential contributing factors to GTPS or gluteal tendinopathy. Increased hip adduction during running will increase pressure on the greater trochanteric area. Weak hip abduc-tors obviously contribute to this condition and are easily identifiable on physical examination or gait analysis. Thus, strengthening these muscles should be a focus of treatment. Further analysis of gait reveals that a slow cadence and a longer stride length are both associated with greater hip adduction. This could be an area on which to focus rehabilitative treatment.

Laboratory Studies

Laboratory studies are generally not helpful in the diagnosis and management of gluteal tendinopathy.

Radiographic Workup

Plain film radiographs can be helpful to rule in or out other potential contributing factors to hip pain. Advanced hip degenerative arthritis can be seen on X-rays. In the setting of gluteal tendinopathy, one would expect normal appearing femoral acetabular articulation and joint space; however, calcific changes near the gluteal tendons and enthesopathic changes may be evident (Fig. 8.21). Plain film radiographs can also assess for femoral neck stress fractures and femoral acetabular impingement (FAI).

MRI can be helpful in the evaluation of lateral hip pain. It can better identify the potentially variable anatomy. Some characteristic findings on MRI in GTPS are edema at the insertion of the gluteus medius and minimus tendons (Fig. 8.22). MRI can also evaluate for partial tears and tendinosis of these tendons. On one study, Bird et al. examined 24 patients with clinical features consistent with GTPS and found 83% of those individuals had gluteus medius pathology with only 8% of cases having bursal distension consistent with bursitis [76].

Ultrasound is emerging as an excellent and possibly could be considered the initial radiographic evaluation of lateral hip pain. Ultrasound is significantly cheaper than an MRI and is better at detecting calcifications in the tendon. It is also readily available and can be done in the office on the same day as the office visit. However, it should be noted that MRI is still considered the gold standard at this time. Ultrasound can reveal heterogenous echogenicity and increased vascularity on color Doppler [79] (Fig. 8.23). Ultrasound can

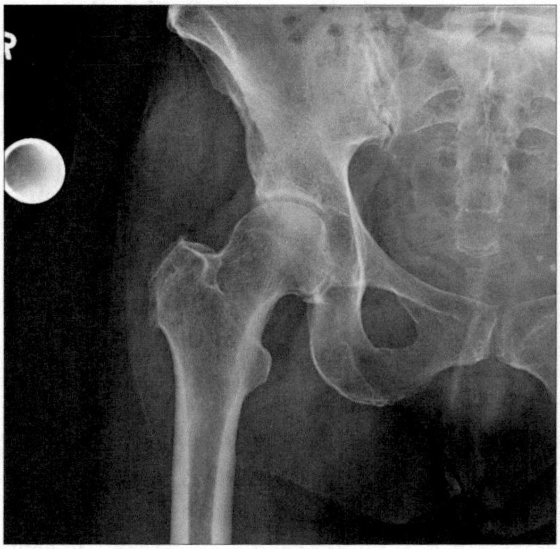

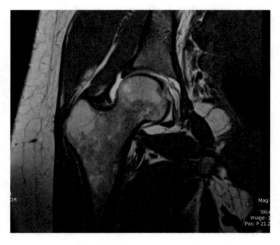

Fig. 8.22 MRI with edema at insertion of gluteus medius

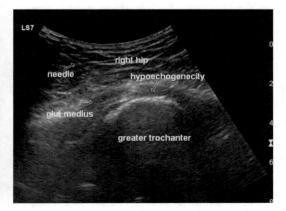

Fig. 8.23 Ultrasound with heterogenous echogenicity and thickening of gluteal tendons

Fig. 8.21 X-ray with enthesopathic changes at greater trochanter

also demonstrate tendon thickening in chronic tendinosis and is also helpful in evaluating partial tears from full thickness tears. Bursal fluid and calcific tendinitis can also be evaluated on ultrasound, and this modality may assist with image-guided procedures like aspiration. A recent study by Long evaluated 877 patients with GTPS, almost 80 % did not have bursitis on ultrasound, 50 % had gluteal tendinosis, 29 % had a thickened iliotibial band, and only 20 % had bursitis [75].

Management

Gluteal tendinopathy can progress into a chronic and difficult to treat condition. There are various treatment options available to consider.

Relative rest and avoidance of painful activities should be considered as initial treatment. Endurance athletes may need to temporarily stop running and consider cross-training pain with free activities like swimming, cycling, weight training, and elliptical training as tolerated. One may also need to gradually return to running but avoid activities like hill running and speed work until the symptoms abate.

Medications

It is not unreasonable to treat lateral hip pain with a temporary course of an analgesic like acetaminophen or an NSAID like ibuprofen. Again, secondary to the fact that lateral hip pain is often the result of a poorly healing tendinosis and not an acutely inflamed condition, analgesia is the property of these medications that will hopefully decrease symptoms.

Physical Therapy

The goal of physical therapy should be to identify and correct biomechanical abnormalities that lead to the development of this condition. Decreasing pressure and the lateral hip and greater trochanteric areas is an important concept. Strengthening the hip abductors and rotators can take some of

the pressure off of this area. Also addressing muscle imbalance and/or tightness in the pelvic ring and targeting core strength can be helpful. Assisting with gait in endurance athletes can also decrease symptoms. Decreasing stride length and limiting hip adduction with running can decrease the load on the lateral hip.

Injection Therapy

Cortisone injections are also widely used in the management of greater trochanteric pain syndrome. As previously stated, it is uncommon to find an inflamed bursa in individuals with lateral hip pain. However, injections into the lateral hip area can be effective. It is thought that decreasing the pain with an injection of cortisone will have an analgesic not anti-inflammatory effect on lateral hip pain. This will then allow for increased tolerance to strengthening relatively weak muscles in physical therapy. A systematic review by Del Buono et al. revealed consistently positive responses of treating GTPS with cortisone injections [80] although, as is typically seen with corticosteroid injections, some of the improvements were temporary [81]. It is thought that if patients do not address the underlying tendinopathy and weakness, the improvement with cortisone injections will be short-lived. Interestingly, Cohen et al. compared fluoroscopically guided greater trochanteric injections to landmark-guided injections and found no intergroup difference [82]. Another consideration with respect to injection of a combination of a local anesthetic like lidocaine in addition to cortisone is an immediate improvement in symptoms. Pain relief from a local anesthetic into an area confirms that area to be the source of pain. Thus, these injections can be somewhat diagnostic as well as therapeutic.

Extracorporeal Shock Wave Therapy (ESWT)

ESWT has been frequently employed to treat chronic tendon issues and is thought to have an analgesic and potentially healing effect. ESWT has been studied in the treatment of GTPS in various studies.

Multimodal approaches to lateral hip pain have also been proposed and thus evaluated. Furia compared two groups of patients with GTPS. One group had ESWT and the other had conservative care consisting of rest, PT, and ultrasound-guided cortisone injection. Both groups had statistical improvement with the ESWT group demonstrating statistical improvement over the control group of conservative therapy [83]. Rompe et al. compared home training to cortisone injection and ESWT treatments. After 4 months, 64% of those in the SWT group were able to return to their previous sports compared with 49% in the cortisone injection group and 34% in the home training group [84].

Surgical Intervention

In individuals who have failed conservative care in the form of medications, injections, physical therapy, and other modalities, surgical intervention may be considered. Surgical techniques are variable and often depend on the underlying pathology, i.e., bursectomy versus tendon repair. Surgical treatment has demonstrated success in the patients as noted by a systematic review by Lustenburger et al. [85].

Newer Considerations

Supporting that concept that often lateral hip pain is not secondary to an inflamed bursa but rather a disordered healing process like a tendinosis, consideration for pro-inflammatory injections may be entertained. Common injections that need more rigorous study include but are not limited to prolotherapy, autologous blood, and platelet-rich plasma (PRP) injections.

References

1. Leabetter WB. Cell matrix response in tendon injury. Clin Sports Med. 1992;11(3):533–78.
2. May VDC. Terminology for Achilles tendon related disorders. Knee Surg Sports Traumatol Arthrosc. 2001;19(5):835–41.
3. Kujala UM. Cumulative incidence of Achilles tendon rupture and tendinopathy in male former elite athletes. Clin J Sport Med. 2005;15(3):133–5.
4. Kvist M. Achilles tendon injuries in athletes. Sports Med. 1994;18(3):173–201.
5. Järvinen TA. 2005. Achilles tendon disorders: etiology and epidemiology. Foot Ankle Clin. 2005;10(2):255–66.
6. Sode J. Use of fluoroquinolone and risk of Achilles tendon rupture: a population-based cohort study. Eur J Clin Pharmacol. 2007;63(5):499–503.
7. Van der Lin PD. Fluoroquinolone use and the change in incidence of tendon ruptures in the Netherlands. Pharm World Sci. 2001;23(3):89–92.
8. Newnham DM. Achilles tendon rupture: an underrated complication of corticosteroid treatment. Thorax. 1991;46(11):853–4.
9. Kleinman M. Achilles tendon rupture following steroid injection. Report of three cases. J Bone Joint Surg Am. 1983;65(9):1345–7.
10. Aström M. No effect of piroxicam on Achilles tendinopathy. A randomized study of 70 patients. Acta Orthop Scand. 1992;63(6):631–4.
11. Alfredson H. Heavy-load eccentric calf muscle training for the treatment of chronic Achilles tendinosis. Am J Sports Med. 1998;26(3):360–6.
12. Fahlstrom MF. Chronic Achilles tendon pain treated with eccentric calf-muscle training. Knee Surg Sports Traumatol Arthrosc. 2003;11(5):327–33.
13. Magnussen RA. Nonoperative treatment of midportion Achilles tendinopathy: a systematic review. Clin J Sport Med. 2009;19(1):54–64.
14. Jonsson PAH. New regimen for eccentric calf-muscle training in patients with chronic insertional Achilles tendinopathy: results of a pilot study. Br J Sports Med. 2008;42(9):746–9.
15. Woodley BL. Chronic tendinopathy: effectiveness of eccentric exercise. Br J Sports Med. 2007;41(4):188–98.
16. Al-Abbad H. The effectiveness of extracorporeal shock wave therapy on chronic Achilles tendinopathy: a systematic review. Foot Ankle Int. 2013;34(1):33–41.
17. Rompe JD. Eccentric loading compared with shock wave treatment for chronic insertional Achilles tendinopathy. A randomized, controlled trial. J Bone Joint Surg Am. 2008;90(1):52–61.
18. Rompe JD. Eccentric loading versus eccentric loading plus shock-wave treatment for midportion achilles tendinopathy: a randomized controlled trial. Am J Sports Med. 2009;37(3):463–70.
19. Kearney R. Insertional Achilles tendinopathy management: a systematic review. Foot Ankle Int. 2010;31(8):689–94.
20. Fredberg U. Ultrasonography as a tool for diagnosis, guidance of local steroid injection, and together with pressure algometry, monitoring of the treatment of athletes with chronic jumper's knee and Achilles tendinitis: a randomized, double-blind, placebo-controlled. Scand J Rheumatol. 2004;33(2):94–101.

21. DaCruz D. Achilles paratendonitis: an evaluation of steroid injection. Br J Sports Med. 1988;22(2):64–5.
22. Ryan M. Favorable outcomes after sonographically guided intratendinous injection of hyperosmolar dextrose for chronic insertional and midportion Achilles tendinosis. AJR Am J Roentgenol. 2010;194(4): 1047–53.
23. Yelland MJ. Prolotherapy injections and eccentric loading exercises for painful Achilles tendinosis: a randomised trial. Br J Sports Med. 2011;45(5):421–8.
24. de Vos RJ. Platelet-rich plasma injection for chronic Achilles tendinopathy: a randomized controlled trial. JAMA. 2010;303(2):144–9.
25. Bell K. Impact of autologous blood injections in treatment of mid-portion Achilles tendinopathy: double blind randomised controlled trial. BMJ. 2013; 18(34)346.
26. Pearson J. Autologous blood injection to treat Achilles tendinopathy? A randomized controlled trial. J Sport Rehabil. 2012;21(3):218–24.
27. Alfredson H. Sclerosing injections to areas of neovascularisation reduce pain in chronic Achilles tendinopathy: a double-blind randomised controlled trial. Knee Surg Sports Traumatol Arthrosc. 2005;13(4): 338–44.
28. Ohberg L. Sclerosing therapy in chronic Achilles tendon insertional pain-results of a pilot study. Knee Surg Sports Traumatol Arthrosc. 2003;11(5):339–43.
29. Clemetson M. Sclerosing injections in midportion Achilles tendinopathy: a retrospective study of 25 patients. Knee Surg Sports Traumatol Arthrosc. 2008;16(9):887–90.
30. Paoloni JA, Appleyard RC, Nelson J, Murrell GA. Topical glyceryl trinitrate treatment of chronic noninsertional Achilles tendinopathy. A randomized, double-blind, placebo-controlled trial. J Bone Joint Surg Am. 2004;86-A(5):916–22.
31. Kane TP. Topical glyceryl trinitrate and noninsertional Achilles tendinopathy: a clinical and cellular investigation. Am J Sports Med. 2008;36(6):1160–3.
32. Hunt G. Topical glyceryl trinitrate for chronic Achilles tendinopathy. Clin J Sport Med. 2005;15(2):116–7.
33. Maffulli N. Multiple percutaneous longitudinal tenotomies for chronic Achilles tendinopathy in runners: a long-term study. Am J Sports Med. 2013;41(9): 2151–7.
34. Maquirriain J. Endoscopic Achilles tenodesis: a surgical alternative for chronic insertional tendinopathy. Knee Surg Sports Traumatol Arthrosc. 2007;15(7): 940–3.
35. Weber M. Nonoperative treatment of acute rupture of the Achilles tendon: results of a new protocol and comparison with operative treatment. Am J Sports Med. 2003;31(5):685–91.
36. Soroceanu A. Surgical versus nonsurgical treatment of acute Achilles tendon rupture: a meta-analysis of randomized trials. J Bone Joint Surg Am. 2012;94(23): 2136–43.
37. Willits KA. Operative versus nonoperative treatment of acute Achilles tendon ruptures: a multicenter randomized trial using accelerated functional rehabilitation. J Bone Joint Surg Am. 2010;92(17): 2767–75.
38. Hagglund M. Epidemiology of patellar tendinopathy in elite male soccer players. Am J Sports Med. 2011;39(9):1906–11.
39. Zwerver J. Prevalence of jumper's knee among non-elite athletes from different sports: a cross-sectional survey. Am J Sports Med. 2011;39(9):1984–8.
40. Lian ØB. Prevalence of jumper's knee among elite athletes from different sports: a cross sectional study. Am J Sports Med. 2005;33(4):561–7.
41. Hall R. Sport specialization's association with an increased risk of developing anterior knee pain in adolescent female athletes. J Sport Rehabil. 2015;24(1):31–5.
42. Witvrouw E. Intrinsic risk factors for the development of patellar tendinitis in an athletic population. A two-year prospective study. Am J Sports Med. 2001;29(2):190–5.
43. Warden S. Comparative accuracy of magnetic resonance imaging and ultrasonography in confirming clinically diagnosed patellar tendinopathy. Am J Sports Med. 2007;35(3):427–36.
44. Jonsson P. Superior results with eccentric compared to concentric quadriceps training in patients with jumper's knee: a prospective randomised study. Br J Sports Med. 2005;39(11):847–50.
45. Bahr RF. Surgical treatment compared with eccentric training for patellar tendinopathy (jumper's knee). A randomized, controlled trial. J Bone Joint Surg Am. 2006;88(8):1689–98.
46. Young MA. Eccentric decline squat protocol offers superior results at 12 months compared with traditional eccentric protocol for patellar tendinopathy in volleyball players. Br J Sports Med. 2005;39(2):102–5.
47. Gaida J. Treatment options for patellar tendinopathy: critical review. Curr Sports Med Rep. 2011;10(5): 255–70.
48. Visnes H. No effect of eccentric training on jumper's knee in volleyball players during the competitive season: a randomized clinical trial. Clin J Sport Med. 2005;15(4):227–34.
49. Fredberg UB. Prophylactic training in asymptomatic soccer players with ultrasonographic abnormalities in Achilles and patellar tendons: the Danish Super League study. Am J Sports Med. 2008;36(3):451–60.
50. Lavagnino M. Infrapatellar straps decrease patellar tendon strain at the site of the jumper's knee lesion. Sports Health. 2011;3(3):296–302.
51. Wang CJ. Extracorporeal shockwave for chronic patellar tendinopathy. Am J Sports Med. 2007;35(6): 972–8.
52. Zwerver J. Patient guided piezo-electric extracorporeal shockwave therapy as treatment for chronic severe patellar tendinopathy: a pilot study. J Back Musculoskelet Rehabil. 2010;23(3):111–5.
53. Vulpiani MC. Jumper's knee treatment with extracorporeal shock wave therapy: a long-term follow-up

observational study. J Sports Med Phys Fitness. 2007;47(3):323–8.

54. Van Leeuwen MT. Extracorporeal shockwave therapy for patellar tendinopathy: a review of the literature. Br J Sports Med. 2009;43(3):163–8.

55. Zwerver J. No effect of extracorporeal shockwave therapy on patellar tendinopathy in jumping athletes during the competitive season: a randomized clinical trial. Am J Sports Med. 2011;39(6):1191–9.

56. Peers K. Cross-sectional outcome analysis of athletes with chronic patellar tendinopathy treated surgically and by extracorporeal shock wave therapy. Clin J Sport Med. 2003;13(2):79–83.

57. Kongsgaard M. Corticosteroid injections, eccentric decline squat training and heavy slow resistance training in patellar tendinopathy. Scand J Med Sci Sports. 2009;19(6):790–802.

58. Ryan M. Ultrasound-guided injections of hyperosmolar dextrose for overuse patellar tendinopathy: a pilot study. Br J Sports Med. 2011;45(12):972–7.

59. James S. Ultrasound guided dry needling and autologous blood injection for patellar tendinosis. Br J Sports Med. 2007;41(8):518–21.

60. Resteghini P. Double-blind randomized controlled trial: injection of autologous blood in the treatment of chronic patella tendinopathy—a pilot study. Clin J Sport Med. 2015. Jan 26(1)

61. Filardo G. Platelet-rich plasma for the treatment of patellar tendinopathy: clinical and imaging findings at medium-term follow-up. Int Orthop. 2013;37(8): 1583–9.

62. Kaux JF. One-year follow-up of platelet-rich plasma infiltration to treat chronic proximal patellar tendinopathies. Acta Orthop Belg. 2015;81(2):251–6.

63. Vetrano M. Platelet-rich plasma versus focused shock waves in the treatment of jumper's knee in athletes. Am J Sports Med. 2013;41(4):795–803.

64. Smith J. Comparing PRP injections with ESWT for athletes with chronic patellar tendinopathy. Clin J Sport Med. 2014;24(1):88–9.

65. Dragoo J. Platelet-rich plasma as a treatment for patellar tendinopathy: a double-blind, randomized controlled trial. Am J Sports Med. 2014;42(3):610–8.

66. Liddle AD. Platelet-rich plasma in the treatment of patellar tendinopathy: a systematic review. Am J Sports Med. 2015;43(10):2583–90.

67. Dimetto B. Platelet-rich plasma: evidence for the treatment of patellar and Achilles tendinopathy—a systematic review. Musculoskelet Surg. 2015;99(1):1–9.

68. Hoksrud A. Ultrasound-guided sclerosis of neovessels in painful chronic patellar tendinopathy: a randomized controlled trial. Am J Sports Med. 2006; 34(11):1738–46.

69. Hoksrud A. Ultrasound-guided sclerosing treatment in patients with patellar tendinopathy (jumper's knee). 44-month follow-up. Am J Sports Med. 2011;39(11): 2377–80.

70. Hoksrud A. Ultrasound-guided sclerosis of neovessels in patellar tendinopathy: a prospective study of 101 patients. Am J Sports Med. 2012;40(3):542–7.

71. Alfredson H. Neovascularisation in chronic painful patellar tendinosis—promising results after sclerosing neovessels outside the tendon challenge the need for surgery. Knee Surg Sports Traumatol Arthrosc. 2005;13(2):74–80.

72. Willberg L. Sclerosing polidocanol injections or arthroscopic shaving to treat patellar tendinopathy/jumper's knee? A randomised controlled study. Br J Sports Med. 2011;45(5):411–5.

73. Larsson ME. Treatment of patellar tendinopathy—a systematic review of randomized controlled trials. Knee Surg Sports Traumatol Arthrosc. 2012;20(8): 1632–46.

74. Brockmeyer M. Results of surgical treatment of chronic patellar tendinosis (jumper's knee): a systematic review of the literature. Arthroscopy. 2015;42(10) 2583–90

75. Long SS. Sonography of greater trochanteric pain syndrome and the rarity of primary bursitis. AJR Am J Roentgenol. 2013;201(5):1083–6.

76. Bird PA. Prospective evaluation of magnetic resonance imaging and physical examination findings in patients with greater trochanteric pain syndrome. Arthritis Rheum. 2001;44(9):2138–45.

77. Lequesne M. Gluteal tendinopathy in refractory greater trochanter pain syndrome: diagnostic value of two clinical tests. Arthritis Rheum. 2008;59(2):241–6.

78. Fearson AM. Greater trochanteric pain syndrome: defining the clinical syndrome. Br J Sports Med. 2013;47(10):649–53.

79. Kong A. MRI and US of gluteal tendinopathy in greater trochanteric pain syndrome. Eur Radiol. 2007;17(7):1772–83.

80. Del Buono A. Management of the greater trochanteric pain syndrome: a systematic review. Br Med Bull. 2012;102(June):115–31.

81. Brinks A. Corticosteroid injections for greater trochanteric pain syndrome: a randomized controlled trial in primary care. Ann Fam Med. 2011;9(3): 226–34.

82. Cohen SP. Comparison of fluoroscopically guided and blind corticosteroid injections for greater trochanteric pain syndrome: multicentre randomised controlled trial. BMJ. 2009;338:986–8.

83. Furia JP. Low-energy extracorporeal shock wave therapy as a treatment for greater trochanteric pain syndrome. Am J Sports Med. 2009;37(9):1806–13.

84. Rompe JD. Home training, local corticosteroid injection, or radial shock wave therapy for greater trochanter pain syndrome. Am J Sports Med. 2009; 37(10):1981–90.

85. Lustenburger L. Efficacy of treatment of trochanteric bursitis: a systematic review. Clin J Sport Med. 2011;21(5):447–53.

Chronic Exertional Compartment Syndrome

9

Robin West, Joseph Ferguson,
and Alexander Butler

Introduction

For those involved in endurance sports, such as distance runners or soccer athletes, pain in the lower leg can be a debilitating issue. When the athlete has pain with activity and there is no history of a traumatic incident, this should narrow the differential diagnosis. The diagnoses can be grouped into disorders of the bone, such as tibial stress fracture or posteromedial tibial stress syndrome; disorders of nerves, such as nerve entrapment disorders or radiculopathy; and disorders of vessels, such as intermittent claudication or popliteal artery entrapment syndrome. Chronic exertional compartment syndrome (CECS) is a physiologic phenomenon primarily of soft tissue, but in extreme cases may involve vessels and nerves as well.

R. West (✉)
Sports Medicine, Inova Health System,
8110 Gatehouse Road, Suite 200E, Falls Church, VA
22042, USA
e-mail: Robin.West@inova.org

J. Ferguson
Department of Orthopaedic Surgery, Medstar
Georgetown University Hospital, 3800 Reservoir Rd.,
NW, Washington, DC 20009, USA

A. Butler
Georgetown University School of Medicine,
3900 Reservoir Rd., NW, Washington,
DC 20009, USA

The first clinical description of CECS was by Mavor in 1956, when a patient with bilateral leg pain with exercise presented after a recent intensification in his training regimen. The patient underwent bilateral lower extremity fasciotomies and, after a short period of convalescence, had a complete resolution of symptoms and returned to a more intense training regimen [1]. In the Proceedings of the Royal Society of Medicine in 1954, Freedman offers an earlier account of possible CECS from an Antarctic expedition. He presents the case of Dr. Edward Wilson, a surgeon and zoologist who was a member of the unfortunate Terra Nova Expedition to the South Pole in 1912. Dr. Wilson's journal entries describe a worsening swelling, erythema, and edema within the anterior compartment of his left leg after a rigorous march over the ice. Freedman attributes the symptoms in Wilson's journal to "ischemic necrosis of the anterior crural muscles due to exertion," a diagnosis he claims to have seen in his practice [2]. Throughout the next several decades, this diagnosis gained significant awareness as treatment was shown to be effective in selected cases.

French et al. were the first to document correlation between elevated intracompartmental pressures and clinical symptoms of chronic exertional compartment syndrome [3]. In 1962, the authors described the cases of two young, active patients whose participation in sport was limited due to anterior tibial pain associated with physical training. Initially suspected to be an unusual presentation of

© Springer International Publishing Switzerland 2016
T.L. Miller (ed.), *Endurance Sports Medicine*, DOI 10.1007/978-3-319-32982-6_9

intermittent claudication, these patients were found to have no evidence of vascular disease and upon provocation via exercise that reproduced symptoms were noted to have firm and swollen anterior compartments in both legs. With Mavor's work as the only cited exception, the authors commented on a lack of formal literature on such clinical presentations at the time of their writing. However, they did note that conversations with colleagues yielded an understanding that such presentations are not at all uncommon in a young, active, and otherwise healthy patient population. After measurement of tissue pressure in the anterior compartments of their subjects via needle manometry before and after exercise revealed levels significantly higher than in normal controls, the authors performed bilateral fasciectomies which resulted in a complete resolution of symptoms and full return to activity.

Epidemiology

As previously stated, CECS is a syndrome of athletes. It is most often seen in distance runners but can affect anyone who participates in endurance-style training with a focus on lower extremity training. In fact, military recruits are a unique population in which CECS has been well documented and studied due to their intensive marching and running regimens [4–6]. It has been estimated that 95 % of all cases of CECS occur in the leg [5]. Second only to medial tibial stress syndrome, the incidence is not well defined due to the difficulty in diagnosis and delay in presentation. It has been estimated to be between 14 and 27 % in patients with undiagnosed leg pain [7]. For those diagnosed with CECS, 87 % are athletes and 53–69 % are runners [8, 9]. It equally affects men and women athletes in their 20s and 30s and is linked to an increase in training regimen. Unlike traumatic compartment syndrome, CECS is more often than not bilateral, with reported rates of bilateral symptoms ranging from 63 to 95 % in the literature [10–16]. CECS is further distinguished from acute compartment syndrome in that it increases in severity over time if the inciting activity is continued and will typically remit with rest. However, it will return with similar character and intensity should activity be reinstated [10, 17–19]. The anterior compartment is most commonly affected, involved in 40–60 % of cases [8, 11]. The deep posterior compartment is the second most commonly affected (32–60 %), followed by the lateral compartment (12–35 %), and rarely the superficial posterior [8, 9, 18]. Roughly one-third have single-compartment involvement, and another third have two-compartment disease [11].

Anatomy/Physiology

A simple review of the anatomy of the lower leg reveals that there are four soft tissue compartments containing all of the muscular and neurovascular structures. These are arranged around the tibia and fibula, with the interosseous membrane and fascia forming the borders of the compartments. The four compartments are the anterior, lateral, superficial posterior, and deep posterior and will be described in detail in the following paragraphs. Figures 9.1, 9.2, and 9.3 are cross section magnetic resonance images of the proximal, mid, and distal tibia, respectively.

The anterior compartment contains the primary dorsiflexors of the ankle and extensors of the toes. These include the tibialis anterior, the extensor hallucis longus, the extensor digitorum longus, and the peroneus tertius. It also contains the deep peroneal nerve, which supplies the muscles of this compartment and transmits sensory information from the skin of the first dorsal web space. The anterior tibial artery and anterior tibial vein can be found along with the deep peroneal nerve for the majority of the length of the compartment, just anterior to the interosseous membrane and between the tibialis anterior and extensor digitorum longus. The artery arises from the popliteal artery and supplies the entire compartment along its path. It provides several branches along the length of the compartment, crosses the ankle anteriorly, and finally terminates as the dorsalis pedis over the dorsum of the foot.

The lateral compartment contains the evertors of the ankle, namely, the peroneus longus and

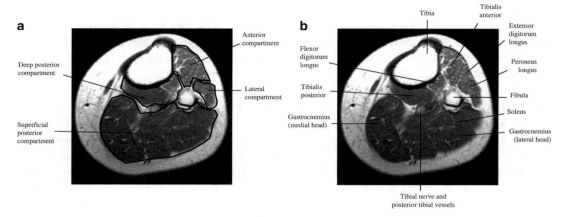

Fig. 9.1 (**a**) Axial MRI cut of proximal tibia outlining the compartments of the leg. (**b**) Axial MRI cut identifying structures of the proximal tibia

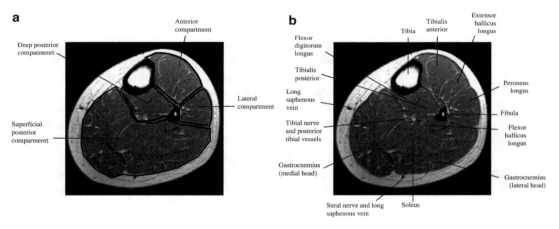

Fig. 9.2 (**a**) Axial MRI cut of mid-tibia outlining the compartments of the leg. (**b**) Axial MRI cut identifying structures of the mid-tibia

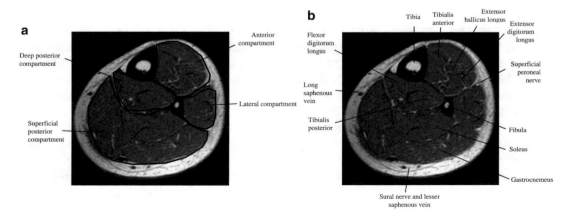

Fig. 9.3 (**a**) Axial MRI cut of distal tibia outlining the compartments of the leg. (**b**) Axial MRI cut identifying structures of the distal tibia

peroneus brevis. The superficial peroneal nerve splits off the common peroneal nerve just inferior to the fibular head. It has a relatively short course within the lateral compartment where it innervates the peroneal muscles, before piercing the fascia between the peroneus longus and extensor digitorum longus. It terminates as the medial and intermedial dorsal cutaneous branches, supplying the skin overlying the lateral aspect of the leg and the majority of the dorsum of the foot.

The superficial posterior compartment is comprised of the gastrocnemius and soleus muscles which insert together into the calcaneal tuberosity and are the primary plantarflexors of the foot. The sural nerve, a purely sensory nerve supplying the posterolateral portion of the leg and lateral foot, also runs in this compartment. There are no vessels within the superficial posterior compartment.

Within the deep posterior compartment lie the flexor hallucis longus, flexor digitorum longus, and tibialis posterior. These muscles flex the great toe and the lateral toes and invert the foot, respectively. The tibial nerve is the continuation of the sciatic nerve after giving off the common peroneal nerve. The tibial nerve runs under the arch of the soleus and within this compartment, supplying all muscles of both the superficial and deep posterior compartments. It terminates in branches that supply muscles on the plantar aspect of the foot, as well as the majority of the sensation to the plantar surface.

Compartment syndrome is a diagnosis that is commonly thought of in the setting of trauma. Typically seen after a tibial fracture (in 70 % of cases) or crush injury to the lower leg, increased pressure within one or more compartments of the leg can lead to painful ischemia. As seen above, the leg contains many structures in a relatively small, defined space. In extreme cases, elevated pressure can progress to the point of compressing the soft tissue structures. Depending on which compartment(s) are affected, arteries and/or nerves may be compressed, as the fascia of the lower leg has less compliance than these soft tissues. The result is nerve compression and a loss of perfusion distally. Compartment syndrome due to a traumatic injury is often rapidly progressive and is an orthopedic emergency with indications for immediate surgical intervention.

CECS, in contrast, is not a surgical emergency but can be a debilitating phenomenon for those that it affects. It is defined as pain in the lower leg that occurs with activity and resolves with rest. The pain is typically in the anterior compartment and occurs in a predictable fashion, such as after a certain distance of running. It then resolves after termination of activity, again in a predictable fashion. This classic presentation supports the theory that the pain is due to reversible tissue ischemia that results from decreased perfusion caused by elevated compartment pressure, just as in traumatic compartment syndrome. However, the inciting factor is not bleeding from fracture or muscle damage, but instead it is a result of muscle hypertrophy and increased fluid content within a defined osseofascial compartment [8].

While the exact physiologic mechanism of CECS is not a matter of scientific fact, the leading hypothesis is that of pain caused by ischemia. During exercise, normal muscle physiology leads to an increase in blood flow as oxygen demand increases. In fact, intracompartmental pressure has been found to increase 3–4 times during exercise in normal controls [20]. This leads to an increase in total volume within compartments, by as much as 20 % [21]. In athletes with low physiologic volume reserve or in those who have developed significant hypertrophy of muscles as a result of increased or prolonged training, this increase in volume is not tolerated well. However, when the exercise is discontinued, the oxygen demand of the muscles decreases. This allows for a decrease in circulatory volume and thus a drop in the compartmental pressure. The ischemia resolves as well, and thus the pain stimulus is removed, which results in the resolution of the patient's complaints.

The borders of the compartment—fascia, bones, and the interosseous membrane between the tibia and fibula—all have less elasticity than the soft tissues within. These relatively rigid borders provide a physiologic limit to the degree of perfusion and volumetric expansion that a given compartment can tolerate. Once the metabolic demands of the muscles exceed the rate of perfusion, tissue ischemia begins to occur. With ischemia, there is a shift to anaerobic respiration and elevated levels of lactate, as well as a local release of kinins. This is theorized to be the direct cause of pain within that compartment [8]. If exercise is terminated, the perfusion demands decrease, and the volume within the compartment begins to decrease. Once perfusion returns to the levels of demand, tissue ischemia resolves and normal physiology resumes.

Other factors that are theorized to contribute to the onset of symptoms are the muscle bulk itself, thickening of the fascia, vascular congestion, direct irritation of fascia or periosteal nerves, and connective tissue stiffness [22]. The ongoing debate as to the cause of pain has been supported by the findings that imaging evidence of tissue ischemia cannot be consistently reproduced at intracompartmental pressures that are typically noted in the symptomatic patient suffering from CECS of the leg [23–25]. Overtraining and rapidly increasing an exercise regimen are clear risk factors. The use of anabolic steroids or creatine may also increase the risk of CECS by raising the water content of muscle [8]. The quality and thickness of the fascia has been investigated and has not been shown to be significantly different between patients with known CECS and asymptomatic controls [26].

Diagnosis

When a patient presents with complaints of leg pain with exercise, a thorough history should first be obtained. Type of activity and onset of symptoms should be detailed, as well as when the symptoms resolve. The astute clinician can often delineate CECS from other diagnoses based on these factors, and the work-up that follows will help to confirm suspicions. As the participation rates, and subsequently injury rates, for recreational running have increased dramatically in recent decades, the patient with such a presentation has become increasingly common [27].

The pain of CECS typically begins within the first 30 min of exercise and is described as a dull ache or cramping in the affected compartment.

It may radiate to the ankle or foot on the affected side, with anterior or lateral compartment pain radiating to the dorsum of the foot and posterior compartment pain radiating more to the medial aspect of the foot. Paresthesias and, in extreme cases, even weakness may develop.

Once a history has been obtained that is suspicious for CECS, a thorough exam should be performed. In the initial outpatient setting, the exam is typically normal as the patient at rest is asymptomatic. The full work-up of CECS requires an exercise challenge and full recovery period, with close monitoring throughout. The exercise challenge should be adequate to re-create the patient's symptoms based on information obtained in the history. This is commonly performed using a treadmill, as it allows for a controlled environment and interval measurement of compartment pressures. Evaluation of the patient should be performed before, during, and after the designated exercise period. This evaluation should consist of the same physical exam performed for acute compartment syndrome seen in the trauma setting: each compartment's tension and compressibility should be assessed, any subjective or objective paresthesias should be noted, and pulses should be checked bilaterally, regardless of whether the complaints are bilateral.

Though history and physical exam findings are often used to make a diagnosis, the gold standard for diagnosis is intracompartmental pressure (ICP) monitoring [28]. Again, this should be performed before, during, and after the exercise challenge. The technique for measurement most commonly described in the literature is that of the slit catheter [20]. Other techniques include microcapillary infusion, wick catheterization, and needle manometry. Specifically, the most widely used device is the Stryker Intracompartmental Pressure Monitoring System (Kalamazoo, MI) due to its low cost relative to other systems and similar reliability [5]. The system uses a slit catheter that can be inserted directly into the leg and is able to directly measure the pressure within the specific compartment. There is some debate as to whether the clinician should measure all four compartments or just the affected compartment [28–30]. In one study, the authors measured only the affected compartment, and 21.5 % of patients failed to improve after fasciotomy. The other compartments were tested postoperatively and found to be elevated at a diagnostic level. Further surgery was declined [29]. Other authors specifically advocate for not measuring asymptomatic compartment, citing a lack of reproducibility in protocol and variability to the measurement within a given compartment [21, 28]. For this reason, strict needle placement and orientation should be used to maximize accuracy and reproducibility throughout the examination period, as changes in the pressure within a compartment are diagnostic.

Despite the fact that there is no universally accepted protocol for diagnosing CECS via ICP, many clinicians use the description by Pedowitz et al. as a guideline for needle manometry [14]. The appropriate leg position for measurement is with the leg in 0–20° of ankle plantar flexion and between 10 and 30° of knee flexion [22, 31]. The anterior compartment should be measured midway between the tibial crest and the intermuscular septum or alternatively at a point 2 cm lateral to the tibial crest. The lateral compartment should be measured midway between the anterior and posterior intermuscular septa. The superficial posterior compartment can be measured either posteromedially or posterolaterally, and both heads of the gastrocnemius can be assessed. The deep posterior compartment should be tested from a medial approach, inserting the needle just posterior to the tibia to avoid the posterior tibial artery and tibial nerve. The distance from the tibial tubercle should be held constant between measurements to reduce variability. One author describes 10 cm from the tibial tuberosity as an appropriate distance, while another uses 3 cm [31, 32]. There is no consistent site used in the literature.

While there is no consensus on exact values that should be used to diagnose CECS via needle manometry, most authors use some version of the guidelines set forth by Pedowitz [33–35]. Essentially, any one of the following parameters are diagnostic: pre-exercise pressure ≥ 15 mmHg, 1-min post-exercise ≥ 30 mmHg, and 5-min post-exercise ≥ 20 mmHg [14]. Additionally, elevation in any compartment of ≥ 10 mmHg from pre- to post-exercise may be considered diagnostic [30].

Despite intracompartmental pressure monitoring being the gold standard for diagnosis, it should not be used in isolation to make a determination about surgery. The confidence intervals for measurements between patients and controls frequently overlap, which brings the validity of the test into question [35]. However, based on the results of a large systematic review, Aweid et al. recommend for ICP measurements to be made 1-min post-exercise challenge to maximize the diagnostic accuracy. This is founded in their discovery of a lack of overlap between the ranges of mean ICP levels in patients with CECS and asymptomatic controls that have been reported in the literature. Despite these recommendations, the authors do note the lack of quality data available in the current literature to establish standardized ICP measurements for the diagnosis of CECS [20]. This suggests that pressure monitoring should be used to aid the clinician in confirming a diagnosis of CECS that is suspected clinically, and after other possible diagnoses have been ruled out [33].

Conversely, if compartment pressures are below diagnostic levels, patients may still benefit from surgical treatment. Verleisdonk et al. performed fasciotomies in 18 patients in whom CECS was suspected clinically, but ICP measurements were within the normal range. Twelve of the 18 showed significant improvement, but the remainder had no change in pain. Using a dynamic ICP measurement technique to enable the assessment of ICP in real time as exercise is performed, Roscoe et al. produced the greatest positive likelihood ratio using a diagnostic cutoff value of 105 mmHg measured, while the most intense phase of an exercise challenge was being performed by the patient, corresponding to a sensitivity of 65 % and specificity of 95 % [31]. While considerably higher than the pressures described in the Pedowitz criteria, Aweid et al. noted a range of intra-exercise intracompartmental pressure in CECS patients of 42–150 mmHg in their review of the literature [20].

Although imaging is not the modality of choice for diagnosing CECS, obtaining plain film radiographs or more advanced imaging to rule out stress fracture or other pathology should be included in the initial work-up. The radiographs of a patient with CECS will be normal, whereas other diagnoses may have positive findings (see below). Magnetic resonance imaging (MRI) is not required to make a diagnosis, but T2 sequences may show increased signal intensity within the affected compartment [22, 36, 37]. Ringler et al. describe using an intra-MRI active dorsiflexion exercise protocol and found T2 signal intensity to correlate well to clinical diagnoses and intracompartmental measurements for patients with suspected CECS [38]. Near-infrared spectroscopy has also been shown to correlate well to clinical diagnoses and intracompartmental measurements for patients with suspected CECS [4]. The advantage of these techniques includes the lack of invasive procedure, while limitations may include cost and coordination with exercise challenge protocols. Other imaging modalities such as diffusion tensor imaging and SPET have not demonstrated diagnostic utility [25, 36].

Differential Diagnosis

During the work-up, there are several common diagnoses in the differential that should be considered in conjunction with CECS. These include medial tibial stress syndrome, stress fracture, nerve entrapment syndromes, claudication, and fascial defects.

In contrast to CECS, medial tibial stress syndrome, commonly referred to as "shin splints," may present as pain with activity that may either improve or worsen with ongoing exertion. It has been found to have a higher incidence than CECS [39]. This lower incidence, along with the absence of clear evidence of CECS on resting physical exam, may be partly to blame for the relative frequency with which the diagnosis of CECS is missed [40]. The patient will often describe pain along the posteromedial aspect of the tibia from the midpoint distally toward the ankle. It will typically improve somewhat after cessation of activity, but not to the point of resolution. The differential should include deep posterior CECS,

but during the exam, there will be point tenderness over the posteromedial tibia and fascia of the soleus. Additionally, further diagnostic work-up should show normal compartment pressures, and bone scintigraphy may reveal linear uptake within the tibia [22, 33, 39, 41].

If the patient has pain with minimal activity or general weight bearing, there should be a high index of suspicion for tibial stress fracture [39]. Patients will describe a localized area of pain over the distal leg, which is usually relieved by rest. The history may include a change in training regimen, and symptoms may interfere with activities of daily living, not just exercise. Exam will reveal point tenderness, even at rest. Percussion over the area will usually cause a sharp increase in pain. Initially, radiographs will be negative, but as the pathology persists, the "dreaded black line" may appear, or there may be evidence of callous formation. If radiographs are normal but there is a high clinical suspicion, an MRI can confirm the diagnosis [22, 39, 41].

Nerve entrapment syndromes are less common sources of leg pain. Pain should be present within a specific nerve distribution, which should cross the compartment borders and therefore can be well delineated with a careful exam. Additionally, nerve entrapment may progress to paresthesias and even weakness in more severe cases. Loss of sensation or weakness in a muscle group that correlates to the anatomic distribution will reveal the nerve affected. Electromyography and nerve conduction studies can confirm the diagnosis [22, 41].

Popliteal artery entrapment syndrome is likely due to a congenital anomaly resulting in an abnormal course of the popliteal artery within the fossa. Pain is typically posterior and presents in males under the age of 30, typically occurring after periods of intense exertion, such as high-level athletics. It is thought to be a result of entrapment of the popliteal artery over the medial head of the gastrocnemius muscle in the fossa, so symptoms should be worse with passive dorsiflexion or active plantar flexion. Though the exact cause of pain is undetermined, ischemia as well as direct neurovascular compression has been described [42]. Exam is often normal at rest, although ipsilateral changes in the pulses of the ankle with motions described above is pathognomonic for disease. This is rare, as bilateral involvement is common [41]. Imaging via MRI or MRA will often aid in diagnosis, with arteriography serving as the gold standard to confirm the diagnosis. A Doppler ultrasound with the ankle in the provocative positions of dorsiflexion and plantar flexion can also be used to make the diagnosis.

Intermittent claudication, while a common cause of bilateral leg pain with activity, is rare in a young, healthy population. The physiology of the pain is similar to CECS—inadequate perfusion and resultant ischemia. However, the cause of the perfusion deficit is due to vascular disease, such as atherosclerosis, and not attributable to elevated pressure within the compartment. Exam should focus on the vascular status of the individual, including pulses, skin changes, and Doppler studies or angiogram.

Finally, the diagnosis of fascial defects is one that may overlap with CECS [33]. They are often asymptomatic, but may cause localized muscle ischemia or even nerve entrapment if the defect is near the superficial peroneal nerve. Much like in CECS, elevated volume within the compartment during exercise will exacerbate symptoms. However, the cause of pain would be related to the herniation of the affected structure through the fascia. Physical exam may actually demonstrate the fascial defects in thinner individuals, and the pain should be more localized than in the case of CECS. Compartment pressures should be tested to definitively rule out CECS, and MRI may be considered to rule out other causes of pain [22].

Treatment

CECS is a limiting diagnosis in terms of the patient's ability to perform the desired activity, but it is not a surgical emergency. If the individual is willing to modify his lifestyle and decrease the intensity or duration of the inciting activity, then conservative management may be possible. Nonsteroidal anti-inflammatory drugs (NSAIDs),

icing, orthotics, stretching regimens, and even massage therapy have been employed [21, 43]. There has been some suggestion that altering the running and gait biomechanics of symptomatic athletes, namely, to bias more of a forefoot or midfoot strike rather than a heel strike pattern, may in fact reduce symptoms [44, 45]. In general, conservative management is often ineffective, as most patients wish to return to their previous level of activity or sports participation [9]. Regardless, a trial of conservative management should be employed for up to 3 months in the event that a surgery could be avoided.

If conservative management fails, then there is an indication for surgical intervention to relieve the pressure from the affected compartment. The treatment for acute compartment syndrome in the trauma setting involves long incisions and total release of all four compartments, with delayed closure once the swelling has subsided. For CECS, the fascia can be released with a less invasive approach, and skin incisions should always be closed primarily since there should not be an issue with tissue tension at rest. Success seems to be dependent on the compartment affected, with the anterior and lateral compartments demonstrating higher rates of improvement [46]. Releases of the anterior and lateral compartments have a reported 65–100 % success rate after surgical release, while the deep posterior compartment improves in only 50–75 % [5, 18, 21]. Overall, the results of a systematic review indicated that surgical release has an 81–100 % success rate in patients who have first failed a traditional course of conservative management [20].

There are a variety of approaches described in the literature for performing a fasciotomy in the lower leg, including one- and two-incision open techniques, endoscopic assisted (also via one or two incisions), and, in recurrent cases, fasciectomy [18]. While clinical evidence to support one technique over another is lacking in terms of outcomes, recovery, or complications, some authors have demonstrated a slightly higher success rate with two-incision vs. one-incision techniques [8, 47]. The typical incisions for performing fasciotomies are anterolateral for anterior and lateral compartment releases and posteromedial for superficial and deep posterior compartments. The anterolateral incision is centered over the anterior intermuscular septum, approximately midway between the crest of the tibia and the fibula. The posteromedial incision is made approximately 1 cm posterior to the medial border of the tibia. After incision, soft tissue is dissected down to fascia, and the fascia is released under direct visualization throughout its entire length using Metzenbaum scissors. The fascia is left open and the subcutaneous tissue and skin is then closed primarily. Many authors recommend the use of a drain placed intraoperatively to prevent hematoma formation in an area already susceptible to compressive symptoms [29, 48].

Two-Incision Technique

Rorabeck initially outlined a two-incision technique beginning with two 4-cm incisions separated by 15 cm, located at the midpoint between the tibial crest and fibula (Figs. 9.4 and 9.5). Soft tissue is dissected down to fascia, and the skin is undermined in both directions. The superficial peroneal nerve (Fig. 9.6) and anterior intermuscular septum are identified through the lower incision. The skin flap between incisions should be sufficiently mobilized from the subcutaneous tissue in order to visualize the entire length of the fascia with proper retraction. Depending on which compartment is to be released (anterior

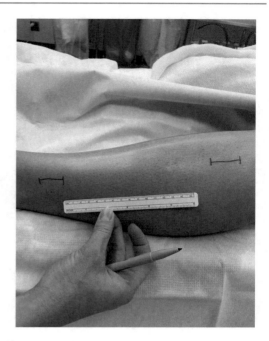

Fig. 9.5 Plan for anterior compartment two-incision skin incisions, with incisions approximately 15–20 cm apart

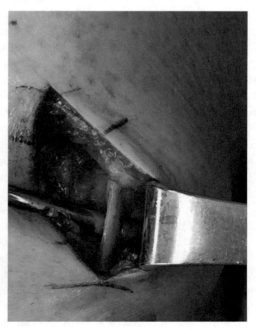

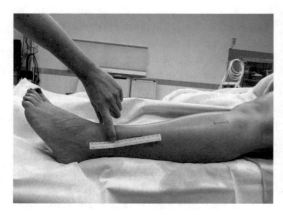

Fig. 9.4 Plan for anterior compartment two-incision skin incisions, with incisions 3–4 cm in length

Fig. 9.6 Identification and protection of the superficial peroneal nerve

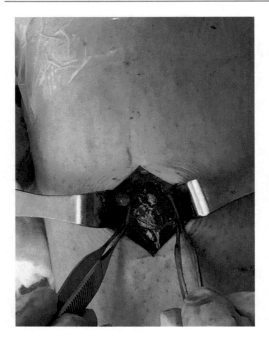

Fig. 9.7 Fascia of the anterior compartment incised

versus lateral), the skin is retracted anteriorly or posteriorly, respectively. The fascia is then incised (Fig. 9.7) approximately 1 cm anteriorly from the intermuscular septum for the anterior compartment and 1 cm posterior to the septum for the lateral compartment. It is then carried proximally and distally using Metzenbaum scissors under direct visualization [46].

Mouhsine describes making two 2-cm incisions over the anterior compartment 15 cm apart. He also recommends undermining but also uses a finger to bluntly dissect the subcutaneous tissue down to fascia as well as connecting the incisions. His other modification to Rorabeck's description is to perform blunt dissection of the fascia with a gloved finger if direct visualization cannot be attained over its entire length [18].

In the case of posterior compartment involvement, the two incisions are made 1 cm posterior to the medial tibial border. The saphenous nerve and vein should be dissected out and visualized through the proximal incision and then retracted anteriorly. The subcutaneous tissue should be dissected down to the muscle, and the soleus bridge is identified. After releasing the soleus,

the fascia of the deep posterior compartment is identified. It is incised over the flexor digitorum longus over its entire length [46].

Lohrer described a minimally invasive technique using a gynecologic speculum to dilate the subcutaneous approach and releasing the fascia under visualization via an endoscope. They advocate for endoscopic release for the anterior and lateral compartments. Due to their reported risk of hemorrhage from perforating vessels, they do not recommend its use for the deep posterior compartment [48]. Wittstein et al. also employ an endoscopic approach but use a transverse incision proximally and a balloon dissector to delineate the fascia from the overlying soft tissue. They cite an enhanced cosmetic effect while maintaining adequate visualization of the fascia and structures at risk [49]. Sebik et al. similarly describe the benefits of endoscopic technique, citing the theoretical avoidance of excessive scar tissue that may lead to symptom recurrence or risk of wound breakdown or infection that is relatively more characteristic of open incisions [50].

When fascial herniations are present in conjunction with CECS, they should be incorporated into the incision, regardless of the approach. The use of a tourniquet is not recommended due to risk of hemorrhage and improved hemostasis prior to closure when not using one [18, 29, 48].

During release of the lateral compartment, there is a risk of injury to the superficial peroneal nerve as it exits the compartment by piercing the fascia at the junction of the middle and distal thirds of the leg, roughly 10 cm superior to the lateral malleolus [18]. When releasing the posterior compartments, the saphenous nerve and veins course from posterior to anterior along the medial aspect of the lower leg.

Outcomes

The literature on CECS is limited and plagued by a lack of strong studies due to low numbers and a lack of randomization. The lack of agreed-upon surgical indications also contributes to the difficulty in interpreting the data. Despite this fact, there is still a strong body of evidence that surgical release is beneficial in helping athletes return to activity.

Parker et al. reported on 73 patients who underwent fasciotomies after failed conservative management for CECS. They found that anterior-only release had higher patient satisfaction rates for return to sports in 3 months. Those that had combined anterior and lateral releases did not do as well, and some never returned to the same level of participation. Based on this data, they do not recommend releasing the lateral compartment prophylactically but rather only when there are symptoms specific to that compartment. These authors also discovered that treatment success rates were significantly higher in patients under the age of 23 than in their older counterparts [21].

There seems to be an even lower rate of success with release of the deep posterior compartment. Van Zoest et al. evaluated 46 patients with unilateral symptoms of deep posterior CECS [51]. Of the 27 who had diagnosis confirmed with intracompartmental pressure monitoring and underwent subsequent release, only 19 % had a good to excellent result. Forty-eight percent deemed surgical treatment a failure. The failure in treatment is a question of whether all four compartments should be released or whether CECS was the true cause of pain preoperatively. Winkes et al. performed a systematic review of studies specifically evaluating release of the deep posterior compartment [9]. They cite a largely diverse ICP cutoff, lack of standardization of diagnosis and operative intervention, and lack of high-power studies as possible sources of lower success rates for deep posterior release.

Complications

As with any surgical intervention, fasciotomies for CECS are not without the occasional complication. The overall complication rate is somewhere between 4.5 and 13 % [18]. Complication rates have been noted to be lower when the anterior compartment alone is released relative to when multi-compartment releases are performed [21]. While superficial peroneal nerve damage is the most devastating, superficial infection, adhesions, scarring, and hematomas have also been reported [48, 52]. Lack of relief or recurrence of symptoms is typically due to insufficient release and should be viewed as a complication as well. Waterman et al. report age, bilateral symptoms, perioperative incidents, and activity limitations as risk factors for surgical failure in a large cohort of military service members who underwent fasciotomy to treat CECS [53]. Occasionally recurrence is due to fascial healing through fibrosis [5], and a revision fasciectomy surgery should be performed to prevent healing postoperatively. Other potential causes of surgical failure that have been postulated are improper diagnosis or inadequate fascial release of all affected compartments or residual nerve entrapment [6].

Recovery/Return to Sport

Success in treatment is outlined as minimal to no pain and with full return to sport [21]. A conservative time frame to offer to patients for returning to full activity after surgical treatment is approximately 3 months. The initial postoperative care is focused on range of motion and soft tissue healing. A splint is commonly employed for comfort measures and may consist of a simple short-leg posterior slab. If used, this should be discontinued quickly to prevent stiffness. The patient is made weight bearing as tolerated and can expect to be full weight bearing at about a week. Low-impact activity and ambulation distance should gradually increase over the course of the next 3–5 weeks, until unrestricted activity to tolerance is allowed at the 6-week mark [8, 9].

Summary

In any young and active patient presenting with pain in the lower leg, chronic exertional compartment syndrome should be included in the differential diagnosis. If clinical history features pain that is reproducibly associated with exercise, and physical exam at the time of initial presentation is normal, the suspicion for CECS should be raised significantly. While details of technique and diagnostic value are debated in the literature, intracompartmental pressure measurement, and more recently some imaging studies, may aid the clinician in making the final diagnosis. As conservative management of this condition has historically been less effective than surgical treatment, many patients are eventually offered fasciotomy. With proper diagnosis, treatment, recovery, and rehabilitation, surgical release can reliably offer patients a return to full activity.

References

1. Mavor G. The anterior tibial syndrome. J Bone Joint Surg. 1956;38:513–7.
2. Freedman B. Dr. Edward Wilson of the Antarctic; a biographical sketch, followed by an inquiry into the nature of his last illness. Proc R Soc Med. 1954;47(3):183–9.
3. French E, Price W. Anterior tibial pain. Br Med J. 1962;2(5315):1290–6.
4. van den Brand JG, Verleisdonk EJ, van der Werken C. Near infrared spectroscopy in the diagnosis of chronic exertional compartment syndrome. Am J Sports Med. 2004;32(2):452–6.
5. Verleisdonk EJ, Schmitz RF, van der Werken C. Long-term results of fasciotomy of the anterior compartment in patients with exercise-induced pain in the lower leg. Int J Sports Med. 2004;25(3):224–9.
6. Waterman BR, Laughlin M, Kilcoyne K, Cameron KL, Owens BD. Surgical treatment of chronic exertional compartment syndrome of the leg: failure rates and postoperative disability in an active patient population. J Bone Joint Surg Am. 2013;95(7):592–6.
7. Styf J. Diagnosis of exercise-induced pain in the anterior aspect of the lower leg. Am J Sports Med. 1988;16(2):165–9.
8. Rajasekaran S, Kvinlaug K, Finnoff JT. Exertional leg pain in the athlete. PM & R. 2012;4(12):985–1000.
9. Winkes M, Hoogeveen A, Scheltinga M. Is surgery effective for deep posterior compartment syndrome of the leg? A systematic review. Br J Sports Med. 2014;48:1592–8.
10. Blackman PG. A review of chronic exertional compartment syndrome in the lower leg. Med Sci Sports Exerc. 2000;32 Suppl 3:S4–10.
11. Davis DE, Raikin S, Garras DN, Vitanzo P, Labrador H, Espandar R. Characteristics of patients with chronic exertional compartment syndrome. Foot Ankle Int. 2013;34(10):1349–54.
12. Detmer DE, Sharpe K, Sufit RL, Girdley FM. Chronic compartment syndrome: diagnosis, management, and outcomes. Am J Sports Med. 1985;13(3):162–70.
13. Gerow G, Matthews B, Jahn W, Gerow R. Compartment syndrome and shin splints of the lower leg. J Manipulative Physiol Ther. 1993;16(4):245–52.
14. Pedowitz RA, Hargens AR, Mubarak SJ, Gershuni DH. Modified criteria for the objective diagnosis of chronic compartment syndrome of the leg. Am J Sports Med. 1990;18(1):35–40.
15. Reneman RS. The anterior and the lateral compartmental syndrome of the leg due to intensive use of muscles. Clin Orthop Relat Res. 1975;113:69–80.
16. Touliopolous S, Hershman EB. Lower leg pain. Diagnosis and treatment of compartment syndromes and other pain syndromes of the leg. Sports Med. 1999;27(3):193–204.
17. Edwards P, Myerson MS. Exertional compartment syndrome of the leg: steps for expedient return to activity. Phys Sportsmed. 1996;24(4):31–46.
18. Mouhsine E, Garofalo R, Moretti B, Gremion G, Akiki A. Two minimal incision fasciotomy for chronic exertional compartment syndrome of the lower leg. Knee Surg Sports Traumatol Arthrosc. 2006;14(2):193–7.
19. Wilder RP, Magrum E. Exertional compartment syndrome. Clin Sports Med. 2010;29(3):429–35.
20. Aweid O, Del Buono A, Malliaras P, Iqbal H, Morrissey D, Maffulli N, et al. Systematic review and recommendations for intracompartmental pressure monitoring in diagnosing chronic exertional compartment syndrome of the leg. Clin J Sport Med. 2012;22(4):356–70.
21. Packer JD, Day MS, Nguyen JT, Hobart SJ, Hannafin JA, Metzl JD. Functional outcomes and patient satisfaction after fasciotomy for chronic exertional compartment syndrome. Am J Sports Med. 2013;41(2):430–6.
22. Bong MR, Polatsch DB, Jazrawi LM, Rokito AS. Chronic exertional compartment syndrome: diagnosis and management. Bull Hosp Joint Dis. 2005;62(3–4):77–84.
23. Amendola A, Rorabeck CH, Vellett D, Vezina W, Rutt B, Nott L. The use of magnetic resonance imaging in exertional compartment syndromes. Am J Sports Med. 1990;18(1):29–34.
24. Balduini FC, Shenton DW, O'Connor KH, Heppenstall RB. Chronic exertional compartment syndrome: correlation of compartment pressure and muscle ischemia utilizing 31P-NMR spectroscopy. Clin Sports Med. 1993;12(1):151–65.
25. Trease L, van Every B, Bennell K, Brukner P, Rynderman J, Baldey A, et al. A prospective blinded evaluation of exercise thallium-201 SPET in patients with suspected chronic exertional compartment syndrome of the leg. Eur J Nucl Med. 2001;28(6):688–95.
26. Dahl M, Hansen P, Stal P, Edmundsson D, Magnusson SP. Stiffness and thickness of fascia do not explain chronic exertional compartment syndrome. Clin Orthop Relat Res. 2011;469(12):3495–500.
27. Fields KB. Running injuries—changing trends and demographics. Curr Sports Med Rep. 2011;10(5):299–303.

28. Hislop M, Batt ME. Chronic exertional compartment syndrome testing: a minimalist approach. Br J Sports Med. 2011;45(12):954–5.
29. Cook S, Bruce G. Fasciotomy for chronic compartment syndrome in the lower limb. ANZ J Surg. 2002;72(10):720–3.
30. Hutchinson M. Chronic exertional compartment syndrome. Br J Sports Med. 2011;45(12):952–3.
31. Roscoe D, Roberts AJ, Hulse D. Intramuscular compartment pressure measurement in chronic exertional compartment syndrome: new and improved diagnostic criteria. Am J Sports Med. 2015;43(2):392–8.
32. Rajasekaran S, Beavis C, Aly AR, Leswick D. The utility of ultrasound in detecting anterior compartment thickness changes in chronic exertional compartment syndrome: a pilot study. Clin J Sport Med. 2013;23(4):305–11.
33. George CA, Hutchinson MR. Chronic exertional compartment syndrome. Clin Sports Med. 2012;31(2):307–19.
34. Hislop M, Tierney P. Intracompartmental pressure testing: results of an international survey of current clinical practice, highlighting the need for standardised protocols. Br J Sports Med. 2011;45(12):956–8.
35. Roberts A, Franklyn-Miller A. The validity of the diagnostic criteria used in chronic exertional compartment syndrome: a systematic review. Scand J Med Sci Sports. 2012;22(5):585–95.
36. Sigmund EE, Sui D, Ukpebor O, Baete S, Fieremans E, Babb JS, et al. Stimulated echo diffusion tensor imaging and SPAIR T2-weighted imaging in chronic exertional compartment syndrome of the lower leg muscles. J Magn Reson Imaging. 2013;38(5):1073–82.
37. Yilmaz TF, Toprak H, Bilsel K, Ozdemir H, Aralasmak A, Alkan A. MRI findings in crural compartment syndrome: a case series. Emerg Radiol. 2014;21(1):93–7.
38. Ringler MD, Litwiller DV, Felmlee JP, Shahid KR, Finnoff JT, Carter RE, et al. MRI accurately detects chronic exertional compartment syndrome: a validation study. Skeletal Radiol. 2013;42(3):385–92.
39. Ali T, Mohammed F, Mencia M, Maharaj D, Hoford R. Surgical management of exertional anterior compartment syndrome of the leg. West Indian Med J. 2013;62(6):529–32.
40. Paik RS, Pepple DA, Hutchinson MR. Chronic exertional compartment syndrome. BMJ. 2013;346:f33.
41. Edwards Jr PH, Wright ML, Hartman JF. A practical approach for the differential diagnosis of chronic leg pain in the athlete. Am J Sports Med. 2005;33(8):1241–9.
42. Turnipseed WD. Popliteal entrapment in runners. Clin Sports Med. 2012;31(2):321–8.
43. Blackman PG, Simmons LR, Crossley KM. Treatment of chronic exertional anterior compartment syndrome with massage: a pilot study. Clin J Sport Med. 1998;8(1):14–7.
44. Diebal AR, Gregory R, Alitz C, Gerber JP. Forefoot running improves pain and disability associated with chronic exertional compartment syndrome. Am J Sports Med. 2012;40(5):1060–7.
45. Franklyn-Miller A, Roberts A, Hulse D, Foster J. Biomechanical overload syndrome: defining a new diagnosis. Br J Sports Med. 2014;48(6):415–6.
46. Rorabeck CH. A practical approach to compartmental syndrome. Part III. Management. Instr Course Lect. 1983;32:102–13.
47. Slimmon D, Bennell K, Brukner P, Crossley K, Bell SN. Long-term outcome of fasciotomy with partial fasciectomy for chronic exertional compartment syndrome of the lower leg. Am J Sports Med. 2002;30(4):581–8.
48. Lohrer H, Nauck T. Endoscopically assisted release for exertional compartment syndromes of the lower leg. Arch Orthop Trauma Surg. 2007;127(9):827–34.
49. Wittstein J, Moorman 3rd CT, Levin LS. Endoscopic compartment release for chronic exertional compartment syndrome: surgical technique and results. Am J Sports Med. 2010;38(8):1661–6.
50. Sebik A, Dogan A. A technique for arthroscopic fasciotomy for the chronic exertional tibialis anterior compartment syndrome. Knee Surg Sports Traumatol Arthrosc. 2008;16(5):531–4.
51. van Zoest WJ, Hoogeveen AR, Scheltinga MR, Sala HA, van Mourik JB, Brink PR. Chronic deep posterior compartment syndrome of the leg in athletes: postoperative results of fasciotomy. Int J Sports Med. 2008;29(5):419–23.
52. Edmundsson D, Toolanen G, Sojka P. Chronic compartment syndrome also affects nonathletic subjects: a prospective study of 63 cases with exercise-induced lower leg pain. Acta Orthop. 2007;78(1):136–42.
53. Waterman BR, Liu J, Newcomb R, Schoenfeld AJ, Orr JD, Belmont Jr PJ. Risk factors for chronic exertional compartment syndrome in a physically active military population. Am J Sports Med. 2013;41(11):2545–9.

Shoulder Injuries and Conditions in Swimmers

10

Tyler R. Johnston and Geoffrey D. Abrams

Background

Shoulder pain is the most common musculoskeletal complaint among swimmers, with an incidence of up to 91% and more than 20% of swimmers reporting a history of shoulder pain which affects performance [1–7]. These injury rates stem from the fact that swimming is uniquely positioned as an almost exclusively upper extremity endurance sport, with elite swimmers logging one million or more arm cycles per year per limb [5].

The development of shoulder pain in competitive swimmers was initially recognized by Kennedy at the 1972 Summer Olympic Games [8]. This condition, termed "swimmer's shoulder," initially presents as pain after practice or competition. Without proper treatment or rest, shoulder discomfort progresses to occur during swimming activities and eventually leads to decreased performance or an inability to compete. The development of "swimmer's shoulder" is directly proportional to the age of the athlete, years of practice, and the level of competition [3].

T.R. Johnston • G.D. Abrams (✉)
Department of Orthopedic Surgery, Stanford University, 450 Broadway St., #6342, Redwood City, CA 94063, USA
e-mail: gabrams@stanford.edu

Epidemiology

McMaster et al. performed one of the largest studies examining shoulder pain in competitive swimmers [4]. Administering surveys to nearly 1300 swimmers in the United States with an average age of 19 years, they found that 71% of males and 75% of females reported shoulder pain at some time during their careers. The prevalence of shoulder pain at the time of survey was 17% in males and 35% for females.

Another large study of 137 competitive swimmers ranging in age from 14 to 23 years reported a history of shoulder pain in 52% of elite (top-level) swimmers and 57% of championship-level swimmers [5]. In contrast to the McMaster et al. findings, a higher percentage of males reported a history of shoulder pain versus females (46% versus 40%); however, when broken down by gender and level of competition, elite-level females had the greatest incidence of self-reported shoulder dysfunction.

The most common area of localized shoulder pain in competitive swimmers is anterosuperior (44%), followed by diffuse (26%), anteroinferior (14%), posterosuperior (10%), and least commonly posteroinferior (4%) [9]. Additionally, in the freestyle stroke, where 50–80% of practice time is spent, swimmers most frequently identify the first half of pull-through as the most painful phase (70%), followed by 18% in the early recovery phase [7, 9, 10].

© Springer International Publishing Switzerland 2016
T.L. Miller (ed.), *Endurance Sports Medicine*, DOI 10.1007/978-3-319-32982-6_10

Pathophysiology

Currently, the term "swimmer's shoulder" does not relate to one specific diagnosis. Instead, it encompasses a variety of interrelated and overlapping disorders of the rotator cuff, capsulolabral structures including the biceps, and periscapular muscles, which end in the final common pathway of shoulder pain.

Pain development and aggravation has been associated with multiple factors including increased training and competition time, increased stretching, the use of hand paddles, and increased weight training and resistance activities [4, 7, 11–14]. Subtle faulty stroke technique and training errors without appropriately balanced land-based exercises compound baseline risks, leading to muscle imbalances, changes in shoulder mobility, and alterations in scapulothoracic motion and rotator cuff mechanics [1, 2].

Some authors believe that rotator cuff-related pain, from a variety of inciting factors, is the most common finding in the pathologic swimmer's shoulder [2, 8, 15]. Kennedy and Hawkins proposed that avascular zones within the supraspinatus and long head of the biceps tendon were the cause of shoulder pain in swimmers [8]. More recently, others have proposed a role for muscular imbalance within the periscapular muscles as well as glenohumeral instability [2, 16, 17].

In short, inciting factors for rotator cuff-related pain in the swimmer's shoulder can be broken down into intrinsic and extrinsic factors. Intrinsic factors are related to tendon injury originating from inside the tendon, possibly from molecular inflammation from direct tendon overload, which leads to degeneration of the collagen fibrils and subsequent tendinopathy. Extrinsic factors, such as muscle imbalances, scapular dyskinesis, and alterations in range of motion and stability, relate to pathology originating outside the rotator cuff tendons yet exert significant downstream effects (Table 10.1).

Table 10.1 Extrinsic causes of rotator cuff-related pain in the swimmer's shoulder

Overuse/muscular overload	Coracoacromial arch configuration
Hypovascularity	Muscle imbalance
Scapular dyskinesis	Joint laxity

Training Factors

Training duration and intensity is clearly a factor in the development of "swimmer's shoulder." While no correlation has been shown between stroke distance, stroke specialty, and rate of shoulder pain development [14, 18, 19], greater than 50% of swimmers reported provocation with increased intensity and/or distance [20]. High training volume has been repeatedly implicated as a risk factor for shoulder pain development, with Sein et al. demonstrating a significant correlation between weekly mileage and number of hours per week of swimming with MRI evidence of supraspinatus tendinopathy [7]. Additionally, the relationship between pain development and the use of hand paddles, resistance activities, and increased training intensity and/or distance has been described [4, 5, 13, 20].

Technique errors can also be a contributing factor to the development of shoulder injury and "swimmer's shoulder." Stroke technique errors have been noted to be present in a high proportion of elite collegiate swimmers, with 61% demonstrating dropped elbow during pull-through and 53% during recovery phase, among other errors [21]. This improper stroke technique has been shown to lead to altered biomechanics, and this has been associated with development of shoulder pain in swimmers [22].

Scapular Dyskinesis

The combination of unique biomechanical demands and fatigue associated with swimming as an upper extremity endurance sport predisposes the swimming athlete's shoulder to altered kinematics. Scapular dyskinesis is an important common pathway for many "swimmer's shoulder" pathologies. This pathway has been previously recognized for its role in overuse pain syndromes in throwing and other overhead athletes—the so-called SICK (Scapular malposition, Inferior medial border prominence, Coracoid pain and malposition, and dysKinesis of scapular movement) scapula [23]. Characterized as an "overuse muscular fatigue syndrome," in symptomatic shoulders, the scapula is placed in a more

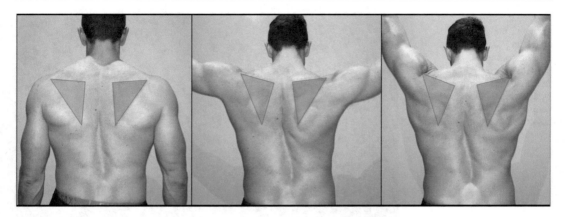

Fig. 10.1 Posterior view of a patient with scapular dyskinesis. Note the more abducted, protracted, and laterally displaced position of the involved scapula (*red*) versus the asymptomatic left (*green*) shoulder

abducted, protracted, and laterally displaced position, increasing risk for impingement (Fig. 10.1). This abnormal positioning is particularly relevant during the recovery phase of swimming strokes, where a combination of body roll and ability to repeatedly retract the scapula typically protects at-risk structures including subacromial bursa, supraspinatus tendon, and posterosuperior labrum [2]. It is no surprise that multiple studies have identified a high percentage of scapulothoracic musculature dysfunction or asynchrony in swimmers, particularly protraction and winging, and have shown a significant correlation with symptomatic shoulders [1, 6].

Using topographic analysis, Warner et al. demonstrated a significant correlation of axioscapular muscle dysfunction with glenohumeral instability (64%) and impingement syndrome (100%) in swimmers, whereas this finding was not significant in control patients [24]. This has been corroborated in a meta-analysis which demonstrated abnormal scapular position and motion in subjects with shoulder impingement or rotator cuff tendinopathy [25]. Furthermore, exaggerated thoracic kyphosis, present in a significant portion of swimming athletes, has been shown to be an aggravating factor in scapular dyskinesis development [2, 25]. While it remains to be conclusively demonstrated where scapular dyskinesis falls exactly in the sequential cause-effect pathway of development of shoulder pain, this likely depends on the underlying pathology. Regardless, abnormal scapular motion must be addressed during treatment algorithms.

Shoulder Instability and Range of Motion Deficits

Ninety percent of forward propulsion force in swimming is generated by the upper extremity, as it must "pull" the rest of the swimmer's body over the shoulder [9]. Akin to the development of pathological changes in overhead throwing athletes, some posit that repetitive, high-energy overhead stresses at the shoulder result in progressive attenuation of the shoulder's static stabilizers (capsulo-ligamentous structures), leading to increased laxity as well as potential instability and impingement symptoms if dynamic stabilizers are unable to compensate [26].

Others believe that the pathological changes within the shoulders of overhead athletes result from a stress-induced contraction of the postero-inferior glenohumeral ligament and subsequent loss of internal rotation [27]. This can then lead to a posterosuperior translation of the humeral head upon the glenoid and lead to a variety of pathologies within the shoulder including internal and external impingement, labral tears, and rotator cuff strain (Fig. 10.2). This has been termed glenohumeral internal rotation deficit (GIRD).

One investigation examined shoulder range of motion in a small group of competitive swimmers [28]. These groups were dichotomized based on shoulder symptoms, with the control group of swimmers having no present or past shoulder pain. Although not significant, they found a trend toward decreased internal rotation in swimmers with painful shoulders. Beach et al. described an

Fig. 10.2 Arthroscopic image of the shoulder from the posterior portal demonstrating a posterosuperior labral tear associated with undersurface of the rotator cuff inflammation in an overhead athlete

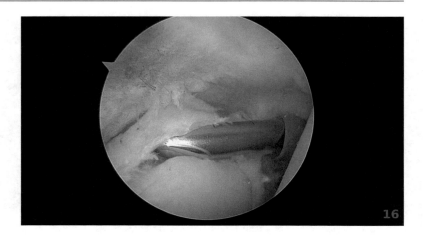

average 40° internal rotation deficit and 10° increased external rotation range of motion in 32 collegiate and club swimmers versus normative data [10]. In another study, Contreras-Fernandez et al. evaluated shoulder internal and external range of motion in competitive swimmers as well as a control group. They reported an average internal rotation deficit of 10° and average external rotation deficit of 20° in swimmers versus those healthy controls [29]. Others have reported increased external rotation and abduction range of motion in swimmers versus controls [1, 6].

Multiple studies have taken this association a step further and reported a direct correlation between increased range of motion and development of shoulder pain in swimmers [4, 7, 14, 30]. Interestingly, in a 12-month prospective cohort study, Walker et al. demonstrated that competitive swimmers with either high or low external rotation range of motion were at significantly higher risk of developing significant interfering shoulder pain (>8× more likely) and/or a significant shoulder injury (>32× more likely) versus those with mid-range external rotation [31].

Along with increased external and abduction range of motion, increased glenohumeral joint laxity has also been described in swimmers with painful shoulders, as clinically measured by anterior-posterior drawer, sulcus sign, and apprehension signs [28, 30]. Sein et al. also noted a statistically significant association between extreme shoulder pain and increased laxity, measured using a combination of mechanical testing with a validated "laxometer" and clinical sulcus sign [7]. Furthermore, in their comparison of elite versus recreational swimmers, Zemek and Magee demonstrated that elite swimmers have significantly greater glenohumeral joint laxity on three out of five clinical laxity tests, as well as increased generalized hypermobility versus their recreational counterparts [32].

It must be remembered, however, that increased shoulder range of motion is adaptive in swimmers and affords the benefits of (1) reducing drag with the arms and body positioned to minimize forward axial surface area and (2) increasing stroke length, which has been shown to be correlated with increased swimming speed [33–35]. In swimming, the distinction between adaptive changes leading to shoulder laxity and pathological changes leading to instability is more difficult to detect as there is no dominant side from which to obtain a direct comparison (such as in baseball).

Muscle Imbalance

Some investigations have documented differences in muscle strength ratios between swimmers and nonswimmers. Specifically, swimmers have been shown to have increased adduction-to-abduction strength ratios (2.05 in swimmers versus 1.53 in nonswimmers) and internal rotation-to-external rotation strength ratios (1.89 in swimmers versus 1.35 in nonswimmers) [10, 36]. While this strength pattern reflects adaptive changes in the swimmer's shoulder muscles which are beneficial in generating increased forward speed through the water, it may also contribute to the development of shoulder pathology. As stability of the shoulder ultimately depends on the interplay of static and dynamic stabilizers, the effects of muscle imbalance are left to be compensated for by the remaining dynamic stabilizers (the rotator cuff and parascapular musculature). The compensatory capacity of these structures is finite, and once the ability to compensate is overcome, instability can occur, leading to inflammation, pain, and altered stroke mechanics, further perpetuating the problem [35].

Muscle Fatigue

When considering both glenohumeral instability and scapular dyskinesis contributions to shoulder pain in swimmers, the effects of muscle fatigue due to repetitive motion and high training volume cannot be overlooked. In a study of 78 previously pain-free competitive swimmers, Madsen et al. demonstrated a significantly increasing prevalence of scapular dyskinesis over the course of a single 100-min training session, with a final cumulative prevalence of 82 % versus 0 % at the beginning of the training session [37]. This finding underscores prevalence of scapular dyskinesis even in asymptomatic athletes and identifies the significant contribution of muscle fatigue with endurance-based training. Both the serratus anterior and subscapularis have been shown to be continuously active throughout freestyle and butterfly strokes, making them susceptible to fatigue [9]. In their cinematographic and electromyographic analysis of painful and pain-free shoulders in swimmers, Pink et al. demonstrated significantly decreased electromyographic activity in the serratus anterior in painful shoulders in both freestyle and butterfly strokes, especially during the pull-through power-generating phase of stroke [22, 38]. They suggest that these muscles experience increased fatigue in swimmers with painful shoulders, contributing to the production of an unstable scapula [9].

In the freestyle stroke specifically, it was observed that rhomboid activity antagonistically increased in a compensatory manner, while decreased activity of subscapularis during recovery was noted to be associated with a general increase in infraspinatus muscle activity [38]. This investigation concluded that while normal muscle activation patterns were lost during painful strokes on account of fatigue, antagonistic muscles were recruited to compensate and prevent impingement. For both freestyle and butterfly strokes, painful shoulders correlated with muscle activation patterns leading to a wider hand entry point, thought to occur in order to decrease shoulder impingement. On the other hand, with painful freestyle or butterfly strokes, there was no significant alteration in pectoralis major or latissimus dorsi activity [22, 38]. These studies emphasize and underscore the central importance of parascapular and rotator cuff balance and healthy activation patterns. Furthermore, muscle fatigue clearly plays an important role in the development of abnormal kinematics during the swimming stroke and likely works synergistically with scapular dyskinesis and underlying laxity to produce common symptomatic phenotypes of shoulder pathology.

Intrinsic Tendon Degeneration

Intrinsic tendon degeneration, encompassing tendinopathy, tendinosis, and tendinitis, has also been implicated as a mechanism in the development of the swimmer's shoulder, primarily in relation to the rotator cuff and specifically the supraspinatus tendon [7]. Overall, this process of tendon degeneration is macroscopically characterized by a healthy, white, firm, fibroelastic tendon giving way to a gray, soft, and fragile tissue [39]. Histopathologically this correlates to mucoid degeneration and fibrocartilage metaplasia of healthy elongated tenocytes, with normal parallel-organized collagen fibers replaced by disoriented and frayed fibers [40, 41]. This process coincides with upregulated apoptosis pathways associated with oxidative stress, all of which can be induced in vitro and ex vivo in human and animal tendon model systems through high dose cyclic strain [42]. This degenerative process is characteristically devoid of inflammatory cells but instead features a characteristic extracellular matrix degeneration facilitated by metalloproteinase enzymes [42].

This distinctive progression has been demonstrated in vivo in a rat supraspinatus tendon overuse model [43]. After 16 weeks of increased daily running stress, rat tendons were significantly thickened and had accumulated water and ground substance while collagen fibers were disorganized. This resulted in significantly reduced modulus of elasticity and maximum stress of failure [43]. A similar pathway has been investigated specifically in the supraspinatus tendon in swimmers. One investigation examined the supraspinatus tendons of 52 young elite swimmers using MRI [7]. They found that a majority of subjects (69%) had evidence of supraspinatus tendinopathy based on MRI signal, which correlated strongly with shoulder pain, increased tendon thickness, and number of hours of swimming per week as well as weekly mileage [7]. They concluded that swim-volume-induced supraspinatus tendinopathy is a primary contributor to shoulder pain in elite swimmers.

Diagnosis, Evaluation, and Management

It should be emphasized that the earlier in pathologic progression a problem is identified, the more specific a diagnosis and appropriate a treatment can be. If athletes wait to report pain, there is increased likelihood that inciting symptoms can be masked by generalized inflammation and global pain, resulting in an imprecise diagnosis and lengthened treatment. Specifically, Pink and Tibone recommend teaching and emphasizing the difference between "pain and soreness" as a means to minimize damage associated with an injury and ultimately hasten return to play [9].

Following identification of a symptomatic shoulder in the swimming athlete, a treatment plan should first consist of a review of any recent training regimen changes. This will aid in identifying new sources of overuse at the shoulder. Whether it

be increased training time, distance, or strengthening and stretching protocols, these should be reviewed and revised to help the athlete return to pre-injury state. Treatment should progress in a thoughtful, stepwise manner based on severity of symptoms, beginning with active rest, reducing aggravating activity or training intensity, and icing, in concert with stroke analysis and exercises directed toward any identified dysfunction [2]. Importantly, if kickboard-based activities are to be used for active rest, this must include modification of arm position to limit placing the board out in front of the swimmer as this places the shoulder in maximal forward flexion and internal rotation, a setup to aggravate impingement symptoms [9]. In the case that symptoms persist or increase to a level of daily pain independent of swimming, treatment should be escalated to include complete rest from swimming activities for 2-week intervals as well as anti-inflammatory use and consideration of corticosteroid injection as appropriate [2]. Finally, if symptoms persist despite rest and treatment for greater than 3 months, typically advanced imaging should be pursued, and consideration may be given to surgical intervention, as discussed below.

Given their common contribution to shoulder pain in swimmers, the following specific sources of pain should be actively considered and addressed early on: impaired posture, core strength, scapular dyskinesis, tight posterior capsule, impaired rotator cuff strength, and glenohumeral instability [29].

Core Strength, Impaired Posture, and Scapular Dyskinesis

Reduced core strength and endurance and abnormal scapular posture have been associated with symptomatic shoulders in swimmers as well as overhead athletes, which is logical given the fact that the abdominal and lumbar musculature and shoulder girdle positioning form the foundation of the upper extremity kinetic chain [11, 25, 44]. Accordingly, these deficiencies should be addressed with a multipronged approach involving joint and soft-tissue mobilization and flexibility training focused on pectoralis minor, scalene, and

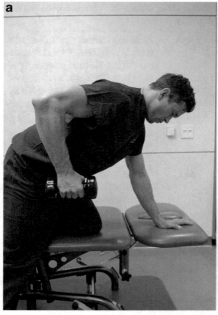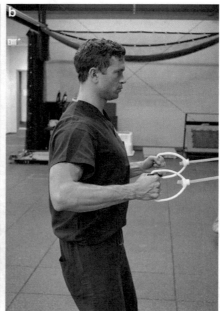

Fig. 10.3 (**a**, **b**) Performance of the (**a**) "lawn mower" and (**b**) low-row exercises to strengthen the periscapular musculature (middle and lower trapezius, serratus ante- rior, and rhomboid muscles) in swimmers diagnosed with scapular dyskinesis as a contributing factor to "swimmer's shoulder"

levator scapulae muscles [29]. This should be combined with well-proven scapular stabilizing exercises to strengthen middle and lower trapezius, serratus anterior, and rhomboid muscles, including low rows, "lawn mower", hands up/"robbery" exercises, shrugs, and push-ups with plus (Fig. 10.3a, b) [9, 25, 45]. Instruction should focus on improving neuromuscular control, training scapular retraction prior to and during humeral motion, as well as scapular stabilization in the protracted position [29]. Lynch et al. demonstrated the efficacy of an 8-week postural correction intervention in division I collegiate athletes to improve head position and rounded shoulder posture and reported a trend of associated decreased pain and shoulder dysfunction [46].

Tight Posterior Capsule

Posterior capsule tightness is associated with anterior shoulder laxity as well as glenohumeral internal rotation deficit (GIRD). While swimmers often regularly participate in shoulder stretches, the posterior capsule is traditionally

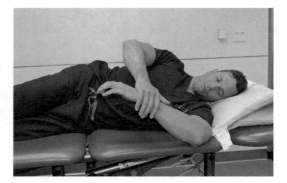

Fig. 10.4 Demonstration of the "sleeper stretch" to address a tight posterior shoulder capsule in those with shoulder internal range of motion deficits

neglected. If such deficits are identified, they must be addressed through capsular mobilizations with posterior-directed forces at the humerus to stretch the posterior capsule, as well as self-stretching techniques, including the so-called sleeper stretch (Fig. 10.4) [29, 35]. Such techniques have been shown to be therapeutic and protective against future injuries in overhead athletes including baseball pitchers and tennis players [23, 27].

Rotator Cuff Strength

If rotator cuff weakness is identified, strengthening exercises may include isometric, concentric, eccentric, and plyometric options. Importantly, cuff exercises should be integrated into the rehab protocol only after an appropriate base of healthy scapula kinematics, including elevation and retraction, has been established. Closed-chain exercises such as humeral head depressions and rotations on a ball, "wall washes," and punches are useful to promote and train sound scapular and cuff activation patterns, in concert with isolated external and internal rotator exercises [23, 29].

Glenohumeral Instability

While laxity is common in the swimming population, it should be treated if the swimmer progresses to instability (defined as laxity in the setting of concomitant shoulder dysfunction). A first step is to minimize exercises that have laxity-potentiating effects, including stretching and overhead resistance-based activities. Rehabilitation then focuses on optimizing dynamic scapular positioning by addressing scapular dyskinesia and strengthening scapular stabilizers and strengthening dynamic glenohumeral stabilizers (rotator cuff) with progressive resistance [29, 47]. Burkhead and Rockwood reported an 83 % efficacy with good or excellent results of such a program when treating atraumatic instability in patients at a minimum of 2 years of follow-up [48].

Shoulder-Specific Conditions

Subacromial Impingement

Subacromial impingement is defined by tendon injury from compression against the coracoacromial arch. Impingement pain is most frequently reported during initial catch and recovery phases of stroke [49]. This can be further characterized as primary (due to bony structural anatomy) ver-

Table 10.2 Types of swimmer's shoulder, adapted from Bak [2]

Type A	Isolated external impingement with subacromial bursitis and rotator cuff pathology. Normal acromial pathology with possible thickening of the coracoacromial ligament. No hyperlaxity or instability. Frequent scapular dyskinesis
Type B	Isolated internal impingement with labral degeneration and partial, articular-sided rotator cuff lesions. No instability. Frequent scapular dyskinesis
Type C	Complex impingement with both external and internal impingement contributions, commonly with minor instability. Frequent scapular dyskinesis
Type D	Isolated minor instability, commonly with bilateral shoulder laxity and scapular dyskinesis. Rare pain
Type E	Other pathologies including AC joint arthrosis, SLAP tears, biceps pathology, etc. Scapular dyskinesis may be present

SLAP superior labral anterior posterior

sus secondary impingement, where abnormal motion of the scapula and/or humerus contributes to the pathology (Table 10.2) [50].

The exam should consist of inspection of the swimmer while standing, with the scapulae visible. The examiner should inquire regarding presence of a painful arc and assess for scapular dyskinesis in forward flexion and abduction planes. Scapular assistance and scapular retraction tests are useful to ascertain if these maneuvers can relieve pain and improve scapular motion [51, 52]. Active range of motion should be assessed in this position while isolating humeral motion from scapular contributions. Impingement signs should be evaluated using the Neer and Hawkins tests [2].

A complete plain radiograph shoulder series may be valuable to identify a primary (bony) cause of impingement and may also reveal calcification in the supraspinatus tendon or subacromial bursa as indicators of pathology. MRI may lend diagnostic value to rule out concomitant rotator cuff or labral pathology.

In a great majority of cases, there will be no evidence of primary impingement. In fact, some now believe that the incidence of primary shoulder impingement is extremity low and question its existence altogether. Given the well-described pathomechanics of muscle imbalance at the glenohumeral and scapulothoracic joints, a conservative physical therapy treatment begins with rest and is designed to correct scapular dyskinesis and optimize stroke mechanics to limit impingement. This includes avoiding or limiting the stroke characteristics with the highest risk of impingement: (a) large amounts of humerus internal rotation during pull-through, (b) late initiation of humeral external rotation during recovery, and (c) small scapular tilt angle [49]. Physical therapy should also include correction of any noted scapular dyskinesia or otherwise abnormal stroke biomechanics, focusing on normal strength and endurance of cuff and scapular stabilizers, as well as improving flexibility of the anterior capsule, pectoralis minor, and rotator cuff [35]. Furthermore, given that a significant correlation has been demonstrated between shoulder dysfunction and core instability in overhead athletes, physical therapy should incorporate core training as an integral part of rehabilitation [44]. Per physician discretion, this may also be combined with use of corticosteroid injection to the subacromial bursa to calm local inflammation and facilitate therapy.

Following an exhaustive trial of conservative management, arthroscopic decompression is the final treatment option. While surgical treatments have demonstrated greater than 70 % reduction in pain and improved function in long-term follow-up in the general population [53], postsurgical outcomes are modest and unpredictable based on the limited available swim-specific literature. Specifically, the average time to return to swimming training following arthroscopy has been reported between 2.9 and 4 months [54, 55]. While sample size was notably small, a retrospective review reported only a 56 % rate of return to swimming in 18 athletes who underwent arthroscopy for a variety of pathologies, including impingement [54]. In a later series by Butler et al., all cases of diagnosed impingement referred to orthopedic subspecialist were successfully treated with a combination of physical therapy with or without subacromial steroid injection, and none underwent surgical decompression [55].

Internal Impingement

Internal impingement refers to a constellation of pathology originating from contact between the posterosuperior aspect of the glenoid, labrum, and rotator cuff (Fig. 10.2). This injury pattern originates from abnormal shoulder mechanics, most notably from a tight posteroinferior capsule, and can result in posterosuperior labral injuries and articular-sided rotator cuff tears. Accordingly, pain is commonly localized to the posterior aspect of the shoulder and may be temporally associated with the recovery phase of stroke [2, 56].

In addition to previously described evaluation of scapular dyskinesis and active range of motion at the shoulder, shoulder instability should also be evaluated as a potential contributing factor. Instability exam should include sulcus and anterior-posterior drawer tests, apprehension-relocation tests, load-and-shift test, and generalized hyperlaxity evaluation [2]. The posterior impingement test, performed while supine by placing the shoulder at 90° abduction followed by maximal external rotation of arm, should reproduce posterior shoulder pain, with the sensitivity of this test reported to be >75 % for detecting posterior labrum and rotator cuff tears [56].

Plain radiographs are usually unremarkable. MRI can be useful to evaluate the nature of the soft-tissue injury including rotator cuff tears and labral pathology, with a reported >95 % sensitivity and specificity [56]. MRIs of clinically diagnosed and arthroscopically confirmed shoulders with internal impingement demonstrate the constellation of findings of undersurface tears of supraspinatus and/or infraspinatus tendons, cystic changes in posterosuperior humeral head, and abnormalities of the posterosuperior labrum versus controls [57].

Initial treatment consists of active rest versus complete activity cessation, which may be required for a prolonged period. Patients will likely benefit from physical therapy, with a focus on posterior capsular stretching and improving potential internal rotation deficits. If an internal rotation deficit is identified (i.e., GIRD), this should be addressed with a posterior shoulder stretching regimen including sleeper stretches, which has been shown to be therapeutic and protective against future injuries in overhead athletes [23, 27]. Furthermore, physical therapy should include exercises and strengthening to correct scapular dyskinesis (particularly protraction) that additionally contribute to internal impingement. While there has been a great deal of debate in the literature regarding the true importance of anterior instability in association with internal impingement, it is recommended that this also be evaluated and addressed when appropriate with strengthening of dynamic shoulder stabilizers to improve glenohumeral stability [58].

Surgical treatment may be considered after a thorough and exhaustive nonoperative trial, with the primary operative options being debridement of partial-thickness rotator cuff pathology as well as fixation of labral tears. Data on the efficacy of these interventions are unfortunately limited to nonswimming athletes. Sonnery-Cottet et al. reported a 79% return to tennis following arthroscopic debridement but with a significant portion of patients reporting some persistent pain [59]. Some have argued that subtle or unrecognized anterior laxity may also be a cause of failure of debridement alone in these cases and accordingly have recommended this be assessed and addressed surgically, but data is limited [56].

Multidirectional Instability

Multidirectional instability is defined as instability in two or more directions. Accordingly associated pain may be from a variety of different sources as the humeral head loses its ability to center itself on the glenoid secondary to loss of dynamic stabilizer function. The pain profile can include anterosuperior impingement-area pain, posterosuperior pain, as well as fatigue/pain in parascapular musculature [60].

Exam/Imaging

As previously described, examination should include evaluation of range of motion and laxity measures, including generalized hyperlaxity evaluation (Beighton criteria), load-and-shift test, and particularly the sulcus sign [60, 61].

The Gagey hyperabduction test has also been shown to effectively assess laxity of the inferior glenohumeral ligament in shoulders with instability versus controls [62]. Importantly, a demonstration of increased laxity is not diagnostic of multidirectional instability, and furthermore, unidirectional anteroinferior instability is possible in the patient with multidirectional hyperlaxity. Additionally, scapular dyskinesis is common in this population and must be evaluated.

Diagnosis is primarily clinical. Plain radiographs do not typically lend significant diagnostic value as bony injury is uncommon, but glenoid dysplasia or hypoplasia may be identifiable. MRI may be useful to detect labral or glenohumeral ligament tears or other associated soft-tissue injuries [47].

Treatment

The mainstay of treatment for multidirectional instability of the shoulder remains rehabilitation with regimens focused on treatment of scapulothoracic dyskinesia and improving the strength and endurance of dynamic glenohumeral stabilizers, including the scapular stabilizers and rotator cuff. This results in improved humeral head centering [47, 60]. Therapeutic regimens have been shown to be effective in the literature, with 83% of treated patients with traumatic or atraumatic instability obtaining good or excellent results with a specific strengthening regimen [48].

It is recommended that surgical treatment only be considered in patients who continue to experience debilitating symptoms following at least 6 months of directed therapy. Open inferior capsular shift has been shown to yield consistent results at 2-year follow-up [63] with arthroscopic capsular plication and rotator interval closure also demonstrating some utility in the treatment of multidirectional instability [47].

References

1. Bak K, Fauno P. Clinical findings in competitive swimmers with shoulder pain. Am J Sports Med. 1997;25(2):254–60.

2. Bak K. The practical management of swimmer's painful shoulder: etiology, diagnosis, and treatment. Clin J Sport Med. 2010;20(5):386–90.

3. Kennedy J, Hawkins R, Krissoff W. Orthopaedic manifestations of swimming. Am J Sports Med. 1978;6(6):309–22.

4. McMaster W, Troup J. A survey of interfering shoulder pain in United States competitive swimmers. Am J Sports Med. 1993;21(1):67–70.

5. Richardson A, Jobe F, Collins H. The shoulder in competitive swimming. Am J Sports Med. 1980; 8(3):159–63.

6. Rupp S, Berninger K, Hopf T. Shoulder problems in high level swimmer-impingement, anterior instability, muscular imbalance? Int J Sports Med. 1995;16(8): 557–62.

7. Sein M, Walton J, Linklater J, Appleyard R, Kirkbride B, Kuah D, et al. Shoulder pain in elite swimmers: primarily due to swim-volume-induced supraspinatus tendinopathy. Br J Sports Med. 2010;44:105–13.

8. Kennedy J, Hawkins R. Swimmers shoulder. Phys Sportsmed. 1974;2:34–8.

9. Pink M, Tibone J. The painful shoulder in the swimming athlete. Orthop Clin North Am. 2000; 31(2):247–61.

10. Beach M, Whitney S, Dickoff-Hoffman S. Relationship of shoulder flexibility, strength, and endurance to shoulder pain in competitive swimmers. J Orthop Sports Phys Ther. 1992;16:262–8.

11. Tate A, Turner G, Knab S, Jorgensen C, Strittmatter A, Michene L. Risk factors associated with shoulder pain and disability across the lifespan of competitive swimmers. J Athl Train. 2012;47(2):149–58.

12. Greipp J. Swimmer's shoulder: the influence of flexibility and weight training. Phys Sportsmed. 1985;13: 92–105.

13. McMaster W, Troup J, Arrendondo S. The incidence of shoulder problems in developing elite swimmers. J Swim Res. 1989;5:11–6.

14. Hill L, Collins M, Posthumus M. Risk factors for shoulder pain and injury in swimmers: a critical systematic review. Phys Sportsmed. 2015;43(4):412–20.

15. Hawkins R, Kennedy J. Impingement syndrome in athletes. Am J Sports Med. 1980;8:151–8.

16. Schmitt L, Snyder-Mackler L. Role of scapular stabilizers in etiology and treatment of impingement syndrome. J Orthop Sports Phys Ther. 1999;29(1):31–8.

17. Su K, Johnson M, Gracely E, Karduna A. Scapular rotation in swimmers with and without impingement syndrome: practice effects. Med Sci Sports Exerc. 2004;36(7):1117–23.

18. Wymore L, Reeve R, Chaput C. No correlation between stroke specialty and rate of shoulder pain in NCAA men swimmers. Int J Shoulder Surg. 2012;6(3):71–5.

19. Wolf B, Ebinger A, Lawler M, Britton C. Injury patterns in Division I collegiate swimming. Am J Sports Med. 2009;37(10):2037–42.

20. Stocker D, Pink M, Jobe F. Comparison of shoulder injury in collegiate- and master's-level swimmers. Clin J Sport Med. 1995;5(1):4–8.

21. Virag B, Hibberd E, Oyama S, Padua D, Myers J. Prevalence of freestyle biomechanical errors in elite competitive swimmers. Sports Health. 2014;6(3): 218–24.

22. Scovazzo M, Browne A, Pink M, Jobe F, Kerrigan J. The painful shoulder during freestyle swimming. Am J Sports Med. 1991;19:577–82.

23. Burkhart S, Morgan C, Kibler B. The disabled throwing shoulder: spectrum of pathology. Part III: The SICK scapula, scapular dyskinesis, the kinetic chain, and rehabilitation. Arthroscopy. 2003;19(6):641–61.

24. Warner J, Micheli L, Arslanian L, Kennedy J, Kennedy R. Scapulothoracic motion in normal shoulders and shoulders with glenohumeral instability and impingement syndrome. Clin Orthop Relat Res. 1992;285:191–9.

25. Ludewig P, Reynolds J. The association of scapular kinematics and glenohumeral joint pathologies. J Orthop Sports Phys Ther. 2009;39(2):90–104.

26. Kvitne R, Jobe F. The diagnosis and treatment of anterior instability in the throwing athlete. Clin Orthop Relat Res. 1993;291:107–23.

27. Burkhart S, Morgan C, Kibler B. The disabled throwing shoulder: spectrum of pathology. Part I: Pathoanatomy and biomechanics. Arthroscopy. 2003; 19(4):404–20.

28. Bak K, Magnusson S. Shoulder strength and range of motion in symptomatic and pain-free elite swimmers. Am J Sports Med. 1997;25(4):454–9.

29. Contreras-Fernandez J, Verdugo R, Feito M, Rex F. Shoulder pain in swimmers. In: Ghosh S, editor. Pain in perspective. Rijeka: InTech; 2012.

30. McMaster W, Roberts A, Stoddard T. Correlation between shoulder laxity and interfering pain in competitive swimmers. Am J Sports Med. 1998; 26(1):83–6.

31. Walker H, Gabbe B, Wajswelner H, Blanch P, Bennell K. Shoulder pain in swimmers: a 12-month prospective cohort study of incidence and risk factors. Phys Ther Sport. 2012;13(4):243–9.

32. Zemek M, Magee D. Comparison of glenohumeral joint laxity in elite and recreational swimmers. Clin J Sport Med. 1996;6(1):40–7.

33. Troup J. The physiology and biomechanics of competitive swimming. Clin Sports Med. 1999;18(2): 267–85.

34. Chengalur S, Brown P. An analysis of male and female Olympic swimmers in the 200-meter events. Can J Sport Sci. 1992;17(2):104–9.

35. Weldon E, Richardson A. Upper extremity overuse injuries in swimming. Clin Sports Med. 2001;20(3): 423–38.

36. McMaster W. Assessment of the rotator cuff and a remedial exercise program for the aquatic athlete. In: Miyashita J, Mutoh M, Richardson A, editors. Medicine and science in aquatic sports. Basel: Karger; 1994. p. 213–7.

37. Madsen P, Bak K, Jensen S, Welter U. Training induces scapular dyskinesis in pain-free competitive swimmers: a reliability and observational study. Clin J Sport Med. 2011;21:109–13.

38. Pink M, Jobe F, Perry J, Browne A, Scovazzo M, Kerrigan J. The painful shoulder during the butterfly stroke. An electromyographic and cinematographic analysis of twelve muscles. Clin Orthop Relat Res. 1993;288:60–72.

39. Khan K, Cook J, Bonar F, Harcourt P, Astrom M. Histopathology of common tendinopathies. Update and implications for clinical management. Sports Med. 1999;27(6):393–408.

40. Fukuda H, Hamada K, Yamanaka K. Pathology and pathogenesis of bursal sided rotator cuff tears viewed from en bloc histologic sections. Clin Orthop. 1990; 254:214–21.

41. Hashimoto T, Nobuhara K, Hamada T. Pathologic evidence of degeneration as a primary cause of rotator cuff tear. Clin Orthop Relat Res. 2003;415: 111–20.

42. Xu Y, Murrell G. The basic science of tendinopathy. Clin Orthop Relat Res. 2008;466:1528–38.

43. Soslowsky L, Thomopoulos S, Tun S, Flanagan C, Keefer C, Mastaw J, et al. Overuse activity injures the supraspinatus tendon in an animal model: a biomechanical study. J Shoulder Elbow Surg. 2000;9:79–84.

44. Radwan A, Francis J, Green A, Kahl E, Maciurzynski D, Quartulli A, et al. Is there a relation between shoulder dysfunction and core instability? Int J Sports Phys Ther. 2014;9(1):8–13.

45. Kibler W, Sciascia A, Uhl T, Tambay N, Cunningham T. Electromyographic analysis of specific exercises for scapular control in early phases of shoulder rehabilitation. Am J Sports Med. 2008;36:1789–98.

46. Lynch S, Thigpen C, Mihalik J, Prentice W, Padua D. The effects of an exercise intervention on forward head and rounded shoulder postures in elite swimmers. Br J Sports Med. 2010;44(5):376–81.

47. Gaskill T, Taylor D, Millett P. Management of multidirectional instability of the shoulder. J Am Acad Orthop Surg. 2011;19:758–67.

48. Burkhead W, Rockwood CJ. Treatment of instability of the shoulder with an exercise program. J Bone Joint Surg Am. 1992;74:890–6.

49. Yanai T, Hay J. Shoulder impingement in front-crawl swimming: II. Analysis of stroke technique. Med Sci Sports Exerc. 2000;32(1):30–40.

50. Page P. Shoulder muscle imbalance and subacromial impingement syndrome in overhead athletes. Int J Sports Phys Ther. 2011;6(1):51–8.

51. Kibler W, Sciascia A, Dome D. Evaluation of apparent and absolute supraspinatus strength in patients with shoulder injury using the scapular retraction test. Am J Sports Med. 2006;34(10):1643–7.

52. Uhl T, Kibler W, Gecewich B, Tripp B. Evaluation of clinical assessment methods for scapular dyskinesis. Arthroscopy. 2009;25:1240–8.

53. Hartwig C, Burkhard R. Operative release of the impingement syndrome. Indication, technique, results. Arch Orthop Trauma Surg. 1996;115(5):249–54.

54. Brushøj C, Bak K, Johannsen H, Faunø P. Swimmer's painful shoulder arthroscopic findings and return rate to sports. Scand J Med Sci Sports. 2007;17:373–7.

55. Butler D, Funk L, Mackenzie T, Herrington L. Sorting swimmers shoulders: an observational study on swimmers that presented to a shoulder surgeon. Int J Shoulder Surg. 2015;9(3):90–3.

56. Drakos M, Rudzki J, Allen A, Potter H, Altcheck D. Internal impingement of the shoulder in the overhead athlete. J Bone Joint Surg Am. 2009;91:2719–28.

57. Giaroli E, Major N, Higgins L. MRI of internal impingement of the shoulder. Am J Roentgenol. 2005;185(4):925–9.

58. Wilk K, Meister K, Andrews J. Current concepts in the rehabilitation of the overhead throwing athlete. Am J Sports Med. 2002;30(1):136–51.

59. Sonnery-Cottet B, Edwards T, Noel E, Walch G. Results of arthroscopic treatment of posterosuperior glenoid impingement in tennis players. Am J Sports Med. 2002;30:227–32.

60. Ren H, Bicknell R. From the unstable painful shoulder to multidirectional instability in the young athlete. Clin Sports Med. 2013;32(4):815–23.

61. Beighton P, Horan F. Orthopedic aspects of the Ehlers-Danlos syndrome. J Bone Joint Surg (Br). 1969;51:444–53.

62. Gagey O, Gagey N. The hyperabduction test. J Bone Joint Surg (Br). 2001;83:69–74.

63. Pollock R, Owens J, Flatow E, Bigliani L. Operative results of the inferior capsular shift procedure for multidirectional instability of the shoulder. J Bone Joint Surg Am. 2000;82:919–28.

Common Injuries and Conditions in Rowers

11

Clinton Hartz and Abigail Lang

Introduction

Rowing is a popular endurance sport that requires coordination, technique, and strength. Rowing is a low-impact sport, but the repetitive motions of the rowing stroke can predispose rowers to injury. Additionally, injury can result as additional stress or strain is placed on the body due to improper form or technique. Overall, most rowing injuries occur as a result of chronic overuse.

Brief History

Rowing has a long history dating back to ancient times. Originally used in war times and for transportation, rowing began as a competitive sport in the eighteenth century. Rowing was one of the original scheduled events in the first modern Summer Olympic Games in 1896. More recently, the popularity of rowing has grown since the introduction of Title IX in 1972 with the rise in numbers of women's collegiate varsity rowing programs.

Basic Technique and Biomechanics

According to the 2015 US Rowing Rules of Racing, rowing is defined as "[the] propulsion of a displacement boat through water by the muscular force of one or more rowers … in which oars are levers … and in which the rowers are sitting with their backs to the direction of forward movement of the boat" [1]. Boat types can include different numbers of rowers (most often one, two, four, or eight rowers), with or without coxswains. Rowers can also be classified by weight, and there are separate competitions for lightweight rowers. Boats may also have either sweeping or sculling oars; sweep rowers only control one oar, while scullers control two oars.

Proper technique and fluid motion in the rowing stroke are important to both prevent injury and maximize efficiency in rowing. The stroke propels the boat by the rower exerting a force through his or her oar acting as a lever to pull the boat forward through the water. The stroke has both an active drive and subsequent recovery phase. The typical phases of the rowing stroke include [2, 3]:

Catch—The catch is the initial motion of the stroke in which the oars are placed in the water. The knees and hips are flexed. The back is also flexed, and the rower appears "curled." The arms and shoulders are extended fully in this phase as the rower prepares to initiate the active drive (Fig. 11.1).

11

C. Hartz (✉) • A. Lang
Division of Sports Medicine, Department of Family Medicine, Ohio State University, Columbus, OH 43210, USA
e-mail: clinton.hartz@osumc.edu

© Springer International Publishing Switzerland 2016
T.L. Miller (ed.), *Endurance Sports Medicine*, DOI 10.1007/978-3-319-32982-6_11

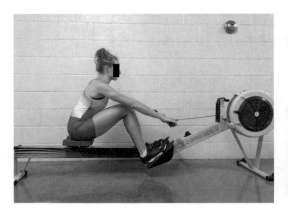

Fig. 11.1 The catch phase

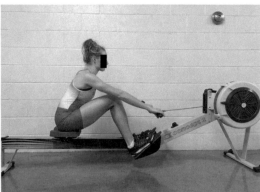

Fig. 11.3 The recovery phase

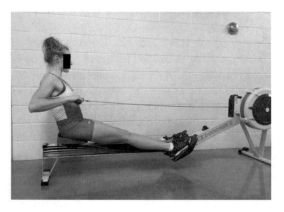

Fig. 11.2 The drive, finish, and rerelease phases

Drive—During the drive, the rower extends his or her legs to create power and push with plantar flexion of the feet. The drive continues with knee, then hip, and then back extension. As the legs extend, the upper body starts to utilize force to pull the oar through the water. The arms flex at the elbow and the shoulders are adducted and extended. At the end of the drive, the arms pull through to complete the motion (Fig. 11.2).

Finish/release—During the end of the drive, known as the finish and release, the rower takes his or her oar out of the water (the extraction). The rower at this point has maximally extended his or her legs with the torso leaning backwards (Fig. 11.2).

Recovery—During recovery, the rower prepares to start the active phase of the stroke. The torso

and lower legs flex, and the arms are once again extended to prepare for the catch. The oar handles are also rotated to prepare for the catch and the placement of the oars in the water again for the next drive (Fig. 11.3).

Mechanisms of Injury and Initial Assessment

Understanding the basics of the biomechanics of rowing and the demands on the rower's body allows for the endurance medicine physician to anticipate and predict common injury patterns to allow for the prompt treatment and rehabilitation of the athlete. Many muscle groups are used throughout the rowing stroke. Strong core muscles along with back flexors and extensors are essential to stabilize the body of the rower to help with a smooth and fluid motion of the stroke.

The repetitive motion of the rowing stroke predisposes athletes to overuse injuries. Epidemiological studies show that the majority of rowing injuries occur as a result of chronic overuse with a smaller minority of injuries occurring from an acute traumatic event [4]. Increases in training length, adjustments in positioning, and differences in technique can also contribute to the development of injuries.

The initial approach to evaluation of injuries should include a thorough history, including the mechanism of the injury, the athlete's training regimen, recent changes in position or form, previous injuries, and additional relevant past medical history. The physical exam should include assessment of the acute injury as well as making note of any observations of areas of muscle hypertrophy, atrophy, or weakness.

Treatment and rehabilitation plans should be tailored to the individual rower's complaint and level of training. Most common rowing injuries can be managed conservatively with a gradual return to previous level of competition.

Common Injuries and Treatment

Lower Back

Low back injuries are very common in rowing, and the incidence of injuries is increasing [5–8]. Many mechanisms have been proposed to account for the nature of lower back injuries in rowing. A common theory is that lumbar hyperflexion, which often occurs in rowing, increases stress on spinal structures. For example, excessive lumbar flexion caused by fatigue of the erector spinae muscles of the back increases pressure on the spine [9]. Other risk factors for development of back pain include increasing the frequency and amount of time spent in training sessions [10, 11]. Most low back injuries in rowing are chronic in nature, and non-specific lower back pain accounts for the majority of cases. Other common injuries and their management are described in more detail below.

Spondylolysis

Spondylolysis signifies the presence of a lesion or stress fracture in the pars interarticularis, most often in the lumbar spine. In rowing, spondylolysis is often nontraumatic, and the stress fracture in the pars occurs as a result of repetitive stress and pressure on the vertebrae associated with physical activity.

The initial presentation of spondylolysis is most commonly lower back pain without radicular symptoms; this can be exacerbated by back extension. Imaging usually starts with plain films making sure to get oblique views to assess the lumbar spine. Additionally, a CT or bone scan is also used to image early lesions when there is high clinical suspicion of spondylolysis: the MRI is being used more frequently for the diagnosis of spondylolysis.

Treatment includes rest and rehabilitation; however, there is still debate as to whether to place athletes in a brace or not. Physical therapy is needed to strengthen the core and back muscles to stabilize the spine and stretch out hamstrings. Bracing may also be used to stabilize the spine and minimize pain, but controversy still exists on the appropriate treatment. Surgical laminectomy or spinal fusion is rarely needed and is reserved for cases of failed nonsurgical management or worsening spondylolisthesis described below.

Spondylolisthesis

Spondylolisthesis can occur in the presence bilateral stress fractures in the pars interarticularis that can develop into an anterior slippage on its subadjacent vertebra. This can result in a mild to severe slippage, resulting in mild low back to severe pain with radicular symptoms and/or bowel or bladder dysfunction [12]. The Meyerding Grading System is used for classifying spondylolisthesis. The slips are graded on the basis of the percentage that one vertebral body has shifted forward over the vertebral body below on a I–V scale [13]. Low-grade spondylolisthesis can usually be treated conservatively with relative rest, anti-inflammatories, physical therapy, and a return to activity within 3–6 months [13]. However, there is some controversy regarding routine management for spondylosis and low-grade spondylolisthesis on whether to use lumbosacral orthosis and cessation of sports with rehabilitation [14]. While duration of rest and the use of an orthosis are controversial, there is wide agreement in the literature that a period of rest is essential and rowers need to be pain-free before returning to their sport [14, 15]. However, there are no high-level evidence studies with specific recommendations on rehab, bracing, or surgery [14].

Disk Injuries/Herniation

Increased pressure on intervertebral disks while rowing can increase risk for a disk herniation. This is usually the result of improper support or weak spinal musculature that can lead to increased forces on the spine. These motions and the necessity of repetitive back flexion and extension in rowing can add additional pressure on the spine that further increases the risk of disk herniation.

The initial exam of a case of suspected disk herniation should start with a comprehensive neurological examination of lower extremities. Range of motion on physical exam is often decreased due to either pain or muscle spasms; other potential findings include positive straight leg raise, decreased patellar and Achilles reflexes on affected side, or radicular symptoms. An MRI is the imaging modality of choice to identify disk pathology.

Initial treatment in most cases is conservative, while the use of anti-inflammatories, analgesics, and muscle relaxants may help relieve discomfort initially. Physical therapy is also a good initial treatment option to work on core strengthening. At times a prolonged period of rest requiring the discontinuation of rowing for a period of time is often necessary to prevent reinjury. Neurologic signs also known as "red flags," i.e., bowl or bladder issues or failure of nonsurgical management, can be indications for surgery.

Sacroiliac Joint Dysfunction (SIJD)

Sacroiliac (SI) joint dysfunction results from irritation of the sacroiliac ligaments. Pain is often localized in the buttocks, pelvis, and groin [16, 17]. On physical exam there is at time pain on palpation over the affected SI joint and pain with flexion and extension, with a positive flexion abduction and external rotation (FABER) testing. First-line therapy should again be conservative with anti-inflammatories, analgesic medications, and relative rest. Physical therapy and posture correction can also help to alleviate pain. If these modalities are not improving symptoms an intra-articular steroid injection may also be used for pain relief [17]. Surgery is reserved for failure of conservative treatment.

Knee

Knee injuries are also common in rowing. There is a significant force placed through the patellofemoral joint during the drive phase with repetitive flexion and extension of the knees throughout the rowing stroke. Potentially leading to two of the most common knee injuries encountered in rowers are the iliotibial band friction syndrome and the patellofemoral syndrome.

Iliotibial Band Friction Syndrome

The iliotibial band (ITB) friction syndrome is a type of overuse tendonitis. The iliotibial band becomes compressed against the lateral femoral condyle (Gerdy's tubercle), which leads to inflammation and pain. The physical exam typically shows lateral knee pain, the IT band is often tight, and Ober's test may be positive [7]. Conservative treatment consisting of rest, anti-inflammatories, ice, and stretching often is enough to alleviate pain. When prolonged conservative management is not working, a corticosteroid injection, preferably under ultrasound guidance, can be done under IT band at Gerdy's tubercle.

Patellofemoral Syndrome

Patellofemoral syndrome usually presents with anterior knee pain. Patellofemoral syndrome, or chondromalacia patella, occurs as a result of increased stress of the cartilage underneath the patella. This is mostly the result of abnormal tracking of the patella contributing to increased friction and deterioration of the underlying cartilage. It has been proposed that the fixed foot position of rowers may contribute to an increased incidence of abnormal patellar tracking which could contribute to the prevalence of patellofemoral syndrome in rowers [6]. As the cartilage behind the patella wears down, an inflammatory response can begin which can lead to pain.

The initial presentation of rowers with patellofemoral syndrome includes retropatellar pain. Pain is worse with actions that load the patellofemoral joint, such as climbing stairs and squatting. Additionally, on physical exam, there can be a grinding or clicking sound may be felt or heard with knee flexion and extension. Similarly, tight quadriceps, hip flexors, and IT bands may also be noted [7].

Treatment consists initially of physical therapy to strengthen the quadriceps muscle to help stabilize the patella and prevent abnormal tracking with or without anti-inflammatories, icing, and analgesics which can also be utilized to minimize pain. The use of kinesio taping can also be used to stabilize the patella to prevent excessive abnormal tracking, but studies are lacking on efficacy.

Rib

Rib pain is another relatively common injury in rowers, including stress responses, fractures, inflammation, and somatic dysfunction.

Rib Stress Fractures

Rib stress fractures are relatively unique to rowing. It has been reported that up to 8–16 % of high-level rowers will have a rib stress fracture over a career [18]. Additionally, rib stress fractures have been shown to be more common in elite rowers, as evidenced by an increased incidence of injuries in international-level rowers as compared to national rowers [19]. Decreased joint mobility, malalignment, and decreased bone mineral density also have been shown to be factors associated with the development of rib stress fractures [18].

Rib stress fractures can present with non-specific pain or as areas of point tenderness along the ribs. Severe pain that increases with movement or deep inspiration can occur as well [7]. The fifth to ninth ribs are most often involved and locate in the posterior lateral position, and this may be due to extra load placed on the outside chest wall while rowing [6]. Physical exam may reveal areas of point tenderness, callus formation, a rib spring, and/or pain during movements similar to those required in the rowing stroke [7].

The diagnosis of a rib stress fracture is often clinical, but if imaging is needed, often a bone scan, CT scan, or MRI is utilized, as plain radiographs are often negative in the acute setting. Treatment of rib stress fractures consists of rest and rehab to work on core, upper back and improve rib cage flexibility. Athletes continue any activity gradually as long as they remain pain-free. If there is a history of nutritional deficiency or multiple stress fractures, calcium and vitamin D supplementation is also often recommended.

Costochondritis

Costochondritis is another common rib injury in rowers. Athletes often complain of pain and soreness located at the costochondral joints, pain with deep inspiration, and musculoskeletal chest pain. Inflammation is localized to the costochondral cartilage of the rib cage and swelling is not often present [20]. The mechanism is thought to be due to increased tension or strain on these areas contributing to the inflammation and pain associated with the condition [7]. Costochondritis is treated conservatively with anti-inflammatory medications and activity modification and is usually self-limited.

Wrist and Forearm

Wrist and forearm injuries, like intersection syndrome, De Quervain's tenosynovitis, medial and lateral epicondylosis, are other common injuries in rowing. These injuries are usually overuse syndromes and are the most common injuries observed. These are often the result of poor form and technique that can precipitate these injuries [7]. Conservative treatment is the main form of management for most of the wrist and forearm injuries. The use of physical therapy to work on upper back and core, in addition to icing, anti-inflammatories, and analgesics, are standard initial therapy choices. Most wrist and forearm injuries improve with adequate rest, bracing as needed, and time off from the sport. If conservative treatment measures fail, ultrasound-guided steroid injections can be trialed. Surgery is only rarely used if more conservative treatment measures fail.

Intersection Syndrome ("Oarsmen's Wrist")

Intersection syndrome, or "oarsmen's wrist," is characterized by distal forearm pain. Occasionally crepitation and swelling can be seen. Pain and swelling is noted on the radial side of the forearm approximately four to eight centimeters proximal to the radial styloid; intersection syndrome is defined by this area of pain to distinguish the diagnosis from De Quervain's tenosynovitis [21]. Inflammation and pain develop in this area because it is at this spot where the first extensor compartment tendons cross over the second compartment extensor tendons, more specifically where the tendons of the abductor pollicis longus and extensor pollicis brevis cross over the compartment containing the extensor carpi radialis longus and brevis. Movements with repetitive flexion and extension of wrist, such as those involved with the positioning of the oars in rowing, increase the risk for developing the syndrome. Management and treatment again relies on conservative measures, including rest, ice, anti-inflammatories, analgesics, and splinting; if not improving with conservative treatment, an ultrasound-guided injection can be considered.

Tenosynovitis

Tenosynovitis, or inflammation of a tendon sheath, is another common overuse injury in rowing. The most common form is De Quervain's tenosynovitis which consists of pain secondary to inflammation of the sheath surrounding the tendons of the extensor pollicis brevis and abductor pollicis longus that make up the first dorsal/extensor compartment of the forearm. On physical exam a positive Finkelstein's test (resisted abduction of the thumb) that reproduces pain along the distal radius is used to diagnose De Quervain's tenosynovitis. Another common tenosynovitis seen in rowing is extensor tenosynovitis or "sculler's thumb." This extensor tenosynovitis is thought to be common in rowing due to the "feathering" motion in which rowers remove the blade from the water and rotate the oar before replacing it in the water during the finish and recovery phases of the rowing stroke [7]. Wrist extensor tenosynovitis is thought to be due to compression of the radial extensor tendons underneath the abductor pollicis longus and extensor pollicis brevis muscles [7, 22].

The management of tenosynovitis, regardless of location, begins with conservative measures used to treat other overuse syndromes. Splinting, anti-inflammatories, and rest are common initial treatments.

Exertional Compartment Syndrome

Another more serious injury called chronic exertional compartment syndrome of the forearm has been seen on occasion in rowers. Athletes usually present with pain, tingling, tightness, or cramping induced during exercise and training, and the pain typically resolves with rest. The pain is associated with increased pressure in muscular compartments, with potential to cause chronic pain and nerve damage if not treated. The measurement of compartment pressures before and after exercise is used to diagnose chronic exertional compartment syndrome. Conservative treatment with rest is often the initial step in management. Indications for surgical fasciotomy include unequivocal clinical findings, pressure within 15–20 mmHg, rising tissue pressure, significant tissue injury, and 6 h of total limb ischemia [23]. Injuries are at high risk of compartment syndrome if conservative treatment does not resolve the symptoms [24, 25].

Dermatology and Skin Conditions

Due to contact with the oars and boat, rowers often develop blisters and abrasions as a result of friction. These injuries are usually self-limited and heal with time.

Blisters

Blisters often develop on the palms of rowers. The development of blisters often occurs after a period of rest or cross-training, when the rower is not used to the friction caused by the grip on the oars. As the rower gets back into routine training, blistering often decreases as the skin heals. Modifying the rower's grip or taping the areas predisposed to blistering can also help. Open blisters increase the risk of infection including osteomyelitis (Fig. 11.4), making proper hygiene and covering of wounds imperative.

Abrasions

Like blisters, abrasions are most often minor injuries that heal with time and adjustment to the demands of rowing. Sculler's knuckles occur

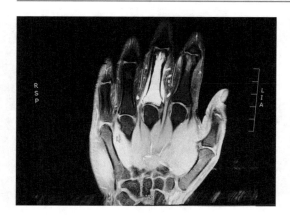

Fig. 11.4 Osteomyelitis in rower after open blister

during training when rowers are sculling and controlling two oars—the hands cross over each other and can result in scraping and scarring of the knuckles. Slide blisters or "slide bites" often occur on the back of rower's calves as a result of contact with the sliding mechanism of the rowing seat. Wearing protective sleeves on the lower legs can help prevent this irritation. Rower's rump is another skin irritation that develops due to prolonged rowing on unpadded seats. Topical corticosteroids and adding padding to the seat can help treat rower's rump.

Conclusion

Most common injuries in rowing occur as a result of overuse. Understanding the basic motions of the rowing stroke can help the sports medicine physician anticipate common injuries and assist in developing appropriate treatment plans. Common injuries include non-specific lower back pain, rib stress fractures, blisters and abrasions, extensor tenosynovitis of the wrist, and patellofemoral pain syndromes. Avoidance of rapid increases in training can help prevent injuries. Proper posture and technique can also minimize additional stress and strain on rower's body.

References

1. The rules of rowing. 2015. http://www.usrowing.org/docs/default-source/governance/ConsolidatedROR_REF_LOC_2015_Final_Edited_Version.pdf?sfvrsn=0.
2. Nilsen T. Basic rowing technique. Zürich: FISA Development Programme; 1987.
3. Mazzone T. Sports performance series: kinesiology of the rowing stroke. Natl Strength Cond Assoc J. 1988;10(2):4–13.
4. Smoljanovic T, Bojanic I, Hannafin JA, Hren D, Delimar D, Pecina M. Traumatic and overuse injuries among international elite junior rowers. Am J Sports Med. 2009;37:1193–9.
5. Hickey GJ, Fricker PA, McDonald WA. Injuries to elite rowers over a 10-yr period. Med Sci Sports Exerc. 1997;29(12):1567–72.
6. McNally E, Wilson D, Seiler S. Rowing injuries. Semin Musculoskelet Radiol. 2005;9(4):379–96.
7. Rumball et al. Rowing Injuries. Sports Med 2005; 35(6):537–555.
8. Smoljanovic T, Bohacek I, Hannafin JA, Terborg O, Hren D, Pecina M, et al. Acute and chronic injuries among senior international rowers: a cross-sectional study. Int Orthop. 2015;39(8):1623–30.
9. Caldwell JS, McNair PJ, Williams M. The effects of repetitive motion on lumbar flexion and erector spinae muscle activity in rowers. Clin Biomech. 2003;18(8):704–11.
10. Teitz CC, O'Kane J, Lind BK, Hannafin JA. Back pain in intercollegiate rowers. Am J Sports Med. 2002; 30(5):674–9.
11. Reid DA, McNair PJ. Factors contributing to low back pain in rowers. Br J Sports Med. 2000;34:321–2.
12. Sys J, Michielsen J, Bracke P, Martens M, Verstreken J. Nonoperative treatment of active spondylolysis in elite athletes with normal X-ray findings: literature review and results of conservative treatment. Eur Spine J. 2001;10(6):498–504.
13. Lasanianos NG, Triantafyllopoulos GK, Pneumaticos SG. Spondylolisthesis Grades. In: Trauma and orthopaedic classifications. London: Springer; 2015. p. 239–42.
14. Bouras T, Korovessis P. Management of spondylolysis and low-grade spondylolisthesis in fine athletes. A comprehensive review. Eur J Orthop Surg Traumatol. 2015;25 Suppl 1:S167–75.
15. Standaert CJ, Herring SA. Expert opinion and controversies in sports and musculoskeletal medicine: the diagnosis and treatment of spondylolysis in adolescent athletes. Arch Phys Med Rehabil. 2007;88:537–40.

16. Timm KE. Sacroiliac joint dysfunction in elite rowers. J Orthop Sports Phys Ther. 1999;29(5):288–93.

17. Vanelderen P, Szadek K, Cohen SP, De Witte J, Lataster A, Patijn J, et al. Sacroiliac joint pain. Pain Pract. 2010;10(5):470–8.

18. McDonnell KL, Hume PA, Nolte V. Rib stress fractures among rowers: definition, epidemiology, mechanisms, risk factors and effectiveness of injury prevention strategies. Sports Med. 2011;41:883–901.

19. Verrall G, Darcey A. Lower back injuries in rowing national level compared to international level rowers. Asian J Sports Med. 2014;5(4), e24293.

20. Grindstaff TL, Beazell JR, Saliba EN, Ingersoll CD. Treatment of a female collegiate rower with costochondritis: a case report. J Man Manip Ther. 2010; 18(2):64–8.

21. Hanlon DP, Luellen JR. Intersection syndrome: a case report and review of the literature. J Emerg Med. 1999;17(6):969–71.

22. Williams J. Surgical management of traumatic non-infection tenosynovitis of the wrist extensors. J Bone Joint Surg (Br). 1977;59:408.

23. Lagerstrom CF, Reed 2nd RL, Rowlands BJ, Fischer RP. Early fasciotomy for acute clinically evident posttraumatic compartment syndrome. Am J Surg. 1989;158:36–9.

24. Hutchinson MR, Ireland ML. Common compartment syndromes in athletes. Treatment and rehabilitation. Sports Med. 1994;17(3):200–8.

25. Rowdon G. Chronic exertional compartment syndrome. Medscape; 2015 (Published Online).

Common Injuries and Conditions in Crossfit Participation

12

Brian D. Giordano and Benjamin M. Weisenthal

Introduction

Crossfit is a conditioning program known for its focus on successive ballistic motions that build strength and endurance. Crossfit workout sessions use a wide variety of exercises, ranging from running and rowing, to Olympic lifting (snatch, clean, and jerk), powerlifting (squat, dead lift, bench), and gymnastic movements (pull-ups, toes to bar, muscle ups, ring dips, rope climbs, push-ups, pistols, handstand push-ups). These exercises are combined into high-intensity workouts that are performed in rapid succession, with limited to no recovery time. It has been adopted in both military and civilian populations with widespread anecdotal reports of impressive sustained fitness gains. These findings parallel existing literature demonstrating that high-intensity, single modal exercise is an effective and efficient means of enhancing physical performance without a large time investment [1–3]. The rising popularity of Crossfit is not surprising given the positive affective response that exercise participants have exhibited with interval training

and the social support associated with joining a Crossfit gym [4, 5].

Crossfit endorses a business model unlike that of other commercial gyms. Gyms are required to pay an initial and annual fee to use the Crossfit name. The requirement to open a gym or be a trainer is to have a Level 1 Crossfit certification, which can be obtained in a weekend at a seminar. Crossfit headquarters allow its credentialed owners to develop on their own within the parameters of the business model. They believe that the market will select for the best gyms and those that do not provide adequate services will fail. Therefore, there can be a wide variation in quality between Crossfit gyms based on the experience of the owner and coaches.

Injury rates among Crossfit participants have been investigated in several observational studies. Hak and colleagues collected 132 responses from Crossfit participants and established an injury rate of 3.1 per 1000 h trained, with 9 of the 186 injuries requiring surgical intervention. Weisenthal and colleagues collected 386 responses with an injury rate of 2.4 per 1000 h trained. This is comparable to long-distance running, training periods for triathletes, weight lifting, powerlifting, and gymnastics [6, 7]. However, the reported rate is lower than that associated with competitive contact sports such as rugby [8]. Although the reported injury rates have been routinely low, as popularity, access, and involvement in Crossfit increase, physicians will likely begin to encounter injuries due to

B.D. Giordano (✉)
Orthopaedics and Rehabilitation, University of Rochester Strong Memorial, 601 Elmwood Avenue, Rochester, NY 14642, USA
e-mail: brian_giordano@urmc.rochester.edu

B.M. Weisenthal
Orthopedics, Vanderbilt University Medical Center, 1215, 21st Ave., S#4200, Nashville, TN 37232, USA

© Springer International Publishing Switzerland 2016
T.L. Miller (ed.), *Endurance Sports Medicine*, DOI 10.1007/978-3-319-32982-6_12

147

Crossfit in their clinic [9]. As such, it is important that physicians are aware of the movements and potential risk they pose for injury in Crossfit workouts.

Injuries in Crossfit can occur via several common training faults. Poor form is a commonly cited cause of concern [8]. This results primarily from two situations: inadequate initial education on the movement or deterioration of good form due to fatigue. Overtraining is another cause of injury, with overuse-related tendonitis occurring primarily in the shoulder and knee [10]. This can result from programming that focuses on one area of the body and does not adequately distribute the stress of exercising [11]. As well, athletes who have a clinically silent preexisting tendonitis are likely to unmask this injury over the course of the strenuous nature of Crossfit workouts. In addition, injuries can occur as a direct consequence of the riskier activities in Crossfit. Examples of these are an athlete falling from the bar during toes to bar, a barbell dropping on the back following a missed snatch, or hyperextending the elbow in a wide overhead grip (such as the snatch or overhead squat). Lastly, there has been a report of rhabdomyolysis following a Crossfit workout [12]. Mainstream media have expressed significant interest in the sport of Crossfit, its philosophies, and some of the more dramatic injuries that have been documented.

When a physician evaluates a Crossfit athlete, it is important to define a general training fault, the specific movement that caused or exacerbates their pain, and several aspects of their training and athletic history. In order to learn exactly what the athlete is doing, the physician has to understand the mechanisms and language of the exercises. The majority of injuries in Crossfit are acute, mild, and most likely will not require surgery [6, 8]. In these cases, athletes are often aware of a specific movement that caused their pain and can even pinpoint a specific time. This helps to define the general mechanism of injury and the potential etiology. It is important to determine whether this occurred as the result of inadequate education on the movement prior to initiating the workout or was a result of breakdown in form due to fatigue. If the athlete reports a more insidious onset, then their training frequency, type, previous athletic interests, and prior injuries should be explored in more detail. In both cases, this information will help to determine the proper treatment for the athlete's injury and identify any faults that may exist in their training program to prevent further injuries.

In this chapter, we explore the important philosophies, training methods, and themes of Crossfit that will help the treating physician evaluate injuries that occur among these athletes. We will review the exercises associated with injury in each subset of movements within Crossfit. Since there are limited studies examining injuries incurred specifically during Crossfit, we will review existing literature related to sports or activities that utilize each separate subset of movements. Lastly, we will discuss specific concerns related to Crossfit athletes with regard to the combination of these distinct movements.

Weight lifting

Weight lifting in Crossfit is divided into two primary categories: Olympic lifting and powerlifting. The classic powerlifting exercises are the dead lift, back squat, and bench press. Olympic lifting exercises include the snatch, clean, and jerk. In competitive weight lifting, the goal of each of these is to lift as much weight as possible in a single attempt. In Crossfit, the incorporation of these movements is intended to achieve two separate objectives: (1) to improve strength, by using a high weight for low repetitions, and (2) to facilitate and optimize metabolic conditioning, when a low weight is used for many repetitions. In the dead lift, the athlete begins in a hip width stance with the barbell positioned over the midfoot and extends the hip and knees until the weight is at waist level with the back in full extension. In the back squat, the athlete begins with a loaded barbell across the upper back and shoulders and then flexes at the hip and knees until the thighs are below parallel with the floor and then presses the weight back up [11]. In both of these exercises, the extensors of the spine, hip, knee, and ankle keep the body from collapsing under the load.

For the bench press, the athlete is supine with the barbell over their chest with the arms extended, and the bar is lifted off a rack and brought to the chest and pushed back up again. In this exercise, the shoulder muscles (pectoralis major and minor, deltoids, core muscles, and anterior rotator cuff) provide the primary support for the motion of the barbell. In the snatch, an athlete initiates the lift with the barbell on the ground. Using a wide grip, the athlete lifts the bar rapidly up and over his or her head in one smooth motion. In the clean, the athlete starts with the barbell on the ground with a grip similar to the dead lift and then lifts the bar quickly onto the front of his or her shoulders in one motion. Finally, in the jerk, the barbell is initially rested on the shoulders, and the athlete then explosively pushes the bar upward, using a small dip to initiate the motion. As the bar is raised, the arms are extended, and the bar is caught with the arms extended over the athlete's head (Fig. 12.1) [10, 13].

Crossfit athletes frequently report that injuries incurred are acute in onset, with the majority experiencing no history of discomfort in that body region prior to the injury. Most of these injuries are fairly mild, with sprain/strain being relatively common [6]. Studies examining weight lifters corroborate this finding, with muscular strains and ligamentous sprains accounting for 40–60 % of the acute injuries. Training timed missed is usually less than 1 day in about 90.5 % of the injuries [11, 14]. More emergent acute injuries, such as tendon ruptures, joint dislocations, and muscular tears, are uncommon in Crossfit athletes and in weight lifters [6, 11]. Chronic injuries tend to be due to repetitive stress with insufficient recovery time. In weight lifting, this occurs in entry-level athletes who increase their training too quickly or in high-level athletes focused on performance [11]. With the intense nature of Crossfit, and the use of high repetitions at lower weight, combined with gymnastic movements, chronic injuries of attrition are far more likely. Tendonitis/tendinopathy is the most common chronic injury accounting for 12–25 % of all strength-training injuries. Most commonly, overuse tendonitis afflicts the shoulder and knee. Stress fractures occurring at sites of repetitive loads are less common, but more worrisome, as they can destabilize with improper attention and potentially lead to overt fractures in rare cases (Fig. 12.2).

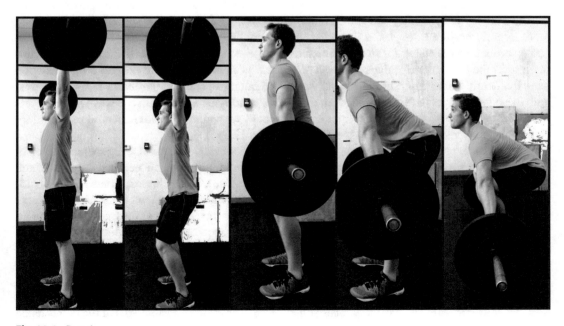

Fig. 12.1 Snatch

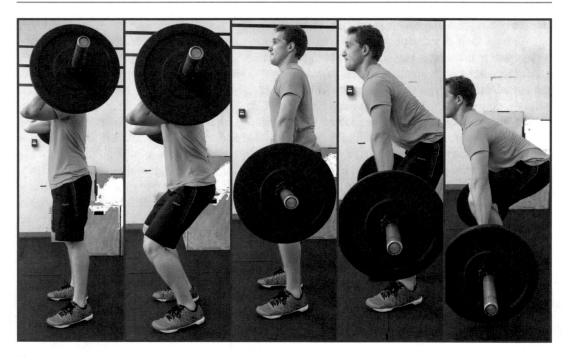

Fig. 12.2 Clean

The lumbar spine is particularly at risk due to repetitive loaded flexion and extension and potential development of spondylolysis [11]. In Crossfit, the push press and jerk are often used in the metabolic conditioning portions of the class. As the athletes fatigue, they tend to assume a more lordotic posture through the lumbar spine and place themselves at risk for stress reaction or fracture in the pars interarticularis. Crossfit athletes frequently report injuring their lower back with these movements [6, 8]. A Swedish study of elite level Olympic and powerlifters demonstrated an injury rate of 2.6 injuries per 1000 h, with the lumbar spine reportedly as the common injury location [10]. Most occurrences of low back pain in athletes are self-limited sprains or strains [11, 14]. However, when an athlete succumbs to fatigue due to repetitive lifting, as commonly seen in Crossfit workouts, there is less knee and hip range of motion and a greater spine peak flexion, which may place increased pressure on the intervertebral disks [15]. In addition, squatting and dead lifting can increase both compressive and shear force across the lumbar spine [16].Therefore, persistent pain should prompt

concern for disk herniation or exacerbation of preexisting degenerative lumbar disk disease [17]. Furthermore, lumbar hyperextension during bench and overhead press represents a failure of form and is commonly seen in Crossfit in the setting of fatigue as a strategic adaptation to accomplish the lifting task [13]. In the pathologic state, this maladaptation can result in clinically significant spondylolytic stress reaction or fracture [17]. In addition to stress fractures, an underlying spondylolisthesis or spondylolysis could put an individual at increased risk of injury (Fig. 12.3) [13].

Crossfit athletes report a higher prevalence of shoulder injuries when compared to elite and competitive Olympic weight lifters [8, 10, 11, 13, 16]. Crossfit workouts tend to use lighter weights for higher repetitions and incorporate gymnastics into their workouts, both of which increase stress on the shoulder girdle. A cross-sectional study of weight lifters demonstrated considerable soft tissue damage involving the rotator cuff, biceps tendon, and capsular and ligamentous insertions [13]. The authors postulated that the demands on the shoulder and motions involved (extreme

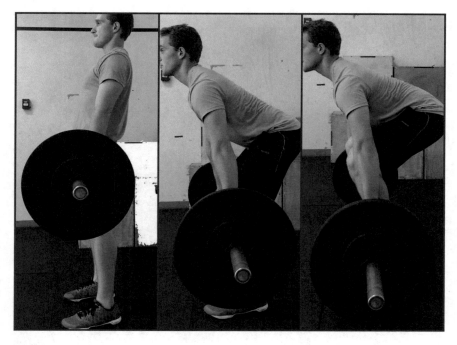

Fig. 12.3 Dead lift

overhead position, as in the overhead press or jerk) increased the risk of injury to the rotator cuff, acromioclavicular joint, and glenohumeral capsule. In addition, an athlete occasionally must drop a missed snatch behind themselves, which can result in extreme external rotation and extension of the shoulders [14]. In addition, osteolysis of the distal clavicle has been reported to occur in powerlifters, and presumably Crossfit athletes would be subject to similar risks, although peak loads are somewhat smaller [10, 11].

Knee injuries are more commonly reported in Olympic weight lifting versus powerlifting [11, 16]. In Olympic lifting, there is more emphasis on an upright position in the squat and the ability to squat deeper than parallel, requiring deep loaded knee flexion. This position enables the athlete to more effectively catch a heavy clean or snatch. However, it causes increased anterior displacement of the center of gravity, augmenting patellofemoral joint reactive forces, which can potentially result in patellofemoral pain and patellar tendonitis [13]. For an athlete with persistent pain, chronic inflammatory problems from persistent tendinitis is the likely diagnosis

[14]. Traumatic cruciate and collateral ligament injuries, common in cutting and pivoting sports, are rare in the sport of weight lifting (Figs. 12.4 and 12.5).

Other rare injuries can occur during weight lifting, which are not directly related to repetitive stresses on the body. Dropping weights is a rare but potentially catastrophic event. In a Crossfit competition in California in 2014, an athlete missed a heavy snatch and the barbell came into contact with his lower thoracic spine causing a traumatic spinal cord injury, resulting in paraplegia. Unfortunately, this pattern of injury has been previously reported during weight lifting [11, 13]. Elbow dislocations can occur in the snatch, due to the wide grip and aggressive rotation or over rotation of the shoulders [11]. Compartment syndrome, primarily of the forearm, has been described as a consequence of aggressively gripping a barbell during a workout [10]. Callous tears are very common in Crossfit and weight lifting. Rectal prolapse has occurred among powerlifters due to the heavy loads incurred during their lifts, but this has not been reported in any Crossfit athletes [11].

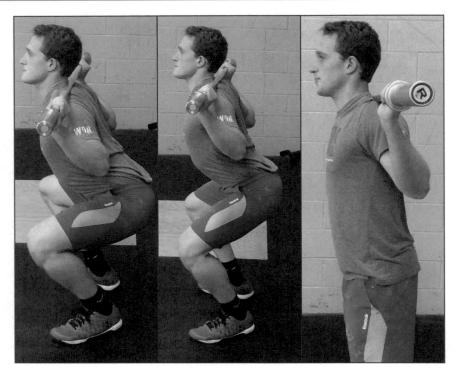

Fig. 12.4 Squat

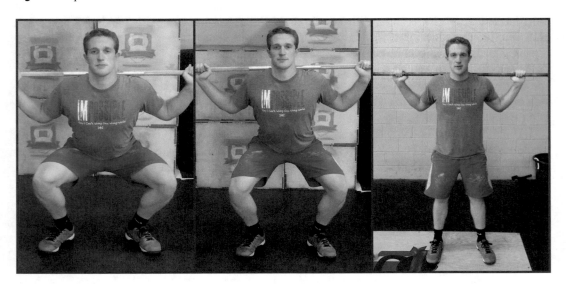

Fig. 12.5 Squat

Endurance

Running and indoor rowing on the ergometer are the two most common endurance exercises in Crossfit. Typical distances used in metabolic condition portions of classes range from 150 to 2000 m in rowing and 200–1600 m in running. These distances are performed several times in a workout and are combined with gymnastic and weight-lifting movements. Crossfit Endurance is a program within Crossfit that focuses almost entirely on high-intensity interval distances of these two monostructural exercises. It is commonly used as a supplement to the traditional Crossfit classes in the athletes who wish to improve their cardiovascular workload. Crossfit athletes are less likely to be injured in either of these two movements compared with typical endurance athletes, as their mileage is far less. The risk to Crossfit athletes, however, is when stresses from these exercises are combined with weight lifting and gymnastics, and when fatigue becomes a factor, overall potential for injury increases.

Indoor rowing on the ergometer is used in metabolic conditioning portions of the Crossfit classes. In colder climates, it is used more frequently in the winter, when running is no longer an attractive option. As many rowing injuries are overuse injuries due to changes in training volume, this is concerning [18]. In rowers, the knee and back are the two most commonly injured body areas, both of which are at risk in a number of other movements in Crossfit [19, 20]. In rowing, there is constant flexion and extension of the knee under loaded conditions. Patellofemoral chrondromalacia patella and iliotibial band syndrome are common sequelae of this mechanism. In rowing, the lower back functions as a braced cantilever during each stroke, which enables the transfer of power from the legs to the flywheel. As the erector spina muscles fatigue, there is increased lumbar flexion. The spine is well suited to handle compression; however, the shear load created by the lumbar flexion makes the intervertebral disks susceptible to injury. Disk herniation on MRI was demonstrated by 95.2 % of male rowers and 78.9 % of females; however, only 27 % of females and 15 % of males had neurologic signs or symptoms. In addition to discogenic pain, strains, sprains, spondylosis, and facet joint arthropathy are potential sequel of the long-term repetitive stresses of rowing [21]. Stress fractures of the ribs are a concern for rowers; however, the mileage of Crossfit rowers is significantly less, and therefore they are at a reduced risk for this to occur.

Running does not usually cause injuries in the Crossfit athlete unless preexisting pathology is present and is exacerbated by the demands of the exercises. The predominant site of injury related to running is the knee. Other areas of injury in running that overlap with Crossfit exercises are the Achilles tendon/calf and hip/pelvis [22, 23]. Common overuse injuries of the knee include patellofemoral pain syndrome, iliotibial band syndrome, and medial tibial stress syndrome. When running is combined with a heavy squat routine or intense Olympic weight lifting, then patellofemoral pain may manifest. Achilles tendinopathy is a common cause of calf pain in runners [24]. This is worrisome, as high repetition box jumps are often used in the conditioning portion of Crossfit, and this motion places strain on the gastrocsoleus and Achilles complex. There have been anecdotal reports of Achilles tendon ruptures with high repetition box jumps. Muscle strains and tendonitis are the most common etiologies of hip pain due to running. Bursitis, exacerbation of hip osteoarthritis, stress fractures, snapping hip syndrome, and acetabular labral tears are all potential etiologies [25].

Gymnastics

Gymnastics movements are a common component of Crossfit workouts and are the most frequently reported cause of shoulder injuries [6]. While gymnastics encompasses a wide range of activities, there are some movements that are used more frequently and put the participant at greater risk for injury. These include pull-ups, toes to bar, handstand push-ups, ring dips, muscle ups, push-ups, and pistols (one-legged squats). Large numbers of pull-ups are often incorporated into Crossfit workouts. The muscles used for a strict pull-up fatigue quickly. Therefore, athletes compensate with a "kipping" motion, meaning they use momentum from the lower body to generate an explosive force to complete the repetition [8]. A similar-type kipping motion is used in toes to bar, where an athlete generates a force in their lower body in order to touch their feet to the bar. Handstand push-ups can be programmed in large numbers. In this exercise, athletes assume a handstand position against a wall with their arms extended and then flex at the elbow until their head reaches the ground and then press back

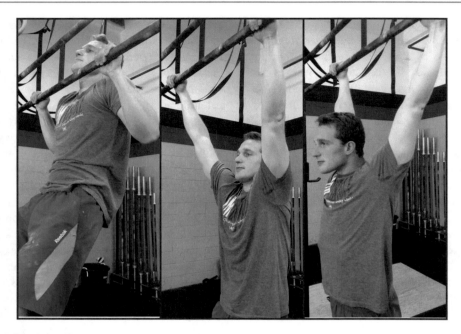

Fig. 12.6 Kipping pull-up

up again. Muscle ups require an athlete to hang from the rings and pull him or herself into a ring-dip position, with the arm flexed to 90°, and then push him or herself up until the arms are fully extended (Figs. 12.6 and 12.7).

Studies of male gymnasts correspond with data from Crossfit, demonstrating that the shoulder is the most commonly injured joint in these movements [6, 26]. Kipping, both in the pull-up and toes to bar, places the shoulder in a position of hyperflexion, internal rotation, and abduction at the bottom of the hang [8]. Handstand push-ups place the shoulder in a position of extreme loaded hyperflexion, which imparts stress upon the rotator cuff and shoulder capsule. Both the push-up and burpee tax the anterior shoulder musculature, as in the bench press. Lastly, in ring dips and muscle ups, the athlete is required to press up and to stabilize the rings. This means that they can fall forward, which may lead to anterior translation of the humerus and an increased risk of shoulder dislocation (Fig. 12.8).

The wrist and lower back are sites of frequent injury in gymnastics. The wrist is the most commonly injured area in female gymnasts and the second most commonly injured area in male gymnasts

[26]. This is most likely due to movements such as the handstand, which subjects the wrist to a combination of axial compression in extreme hyperextension [27]. Injuries to the spine/trunk compromise 13.7–24 % of gymnastic injuries, with the lumbar spine representing the most frequently injured region [26, 28]. The handstand position, as seen in the press and jerk, can cause an athlete to assume a hyperlordotic posture through the lumbar spine. This can result in stress fractures of the pars interarticularis and eventually spondylolysis. In addition, pistols (one-legged squats) are commonly programmed into lower extremity Crossfit workouts, which place strain on the lower back. Athletes are encouraged to squat below parallel on one leg. It is difficult to maintain balance with an upright chest in this position, so athletes compensate with lumbar flexion and anterior drift of the knee. This puts increased shear force on the vertebral bodies. Lastly, athletes often perform many handstand push-ups in a row without a break. This may lead to fatigue of periscapular musculature and inability to resist gravity in the eccentric portion of the motion. As a result, athletes may place a considerable axial load on the head and cervical spine as they impact the ground (Fig. 12.9).

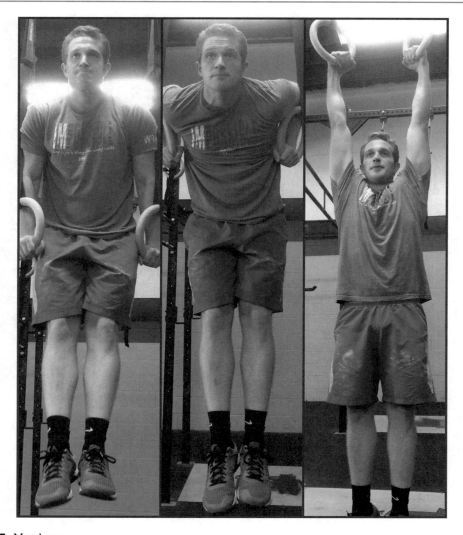

Fig. 12.7 Muscle up

Other

There are several exercises and injuries related to Crossfit that do not fit into a general category. Box jumps, often conducted at a height of 20 or 24 inches, have anecdotally been associated with Achilles tendon rupture, although the exact mechanism is unclear. This could be the result of an acutely overloaded tendon or an overuse condition [29]. Kettlebells are frequently used in Crossfit workouts. There have been reports of extensor pollicis brevis tendon damage presenting

as de Quervain's disease with kettlebell training [30]. Occasionally, athletes fall off the bar in toes to bar. This poses a significant risk, as it usually occurs when the athlete is raising his or her feet toward bar and, therefore, is unable to slow the descent. Lastly, rope climbs, usually to 15 feet, are incorporated into Crossfit workouts. If an athlete fatigues, or does not appreciate the appropriate means of descent, they can fall from that distance.

Another concern with Crossfit athletes is the development of rhabdomyolysis. Suspicion should be raised in an individual who presents

Fig. 12.8 Ring dip

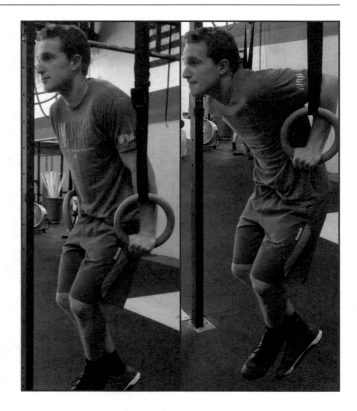

Fig. 12.9 Handstand push-up

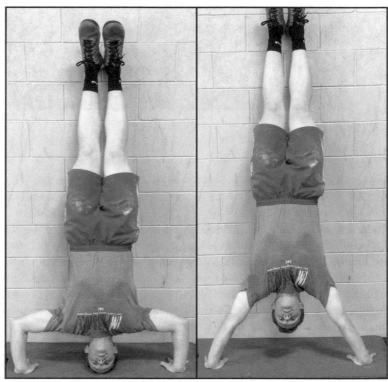

with muscle stiffness in the days following a period of exercise, as well as swelling, and pain out of proportion to the expected fatigue post exercise. It is confirmed clinically by myoglobinuria and an elevated serum creatinine phosphokinase. It should be readily identified and treated to prevent acute renal failure [31]. While this is a concern for Crossfit athletes, it has been reported very infrequently in single cases [12]. Larger-scale studies of Crossfit athletes have reported no reports of rhabdomyolysis [8].

Conclusion

Crossfit is an extreme conditioning program that utilizes successive ballistic motions to build strength and endurance. Injuries related to Crossfit present the treating physician with certain challenges. Despite significant overlap between body areas stressed by the demands of Crossfit exercises, injury rates are relatively low and in concordance with established injury rates for the various components of the workout (i.e., weight lifting, running, gymnastics, etc.). Nevertheless, Crossfit owners continue to pursue training strategies that optimize safety in their gyms. This contention is further supported by evidence that suggests that the degree trainer involvement directly correlates with injury rate [6].

Crossfit is a rapidly growing sport. While its injury rate is comparable to most adult fitness activities such as gym/fitness club training, running, and triathlon training, physicians are likely to interact more frequently with Crossfit participants as the sport grows in popularity [6–8]. It is important to recognize that quality control may vary from gym to gym and depends heavily on the coach operating and maintaining the gym. Therefore, the risk of injury is dependent upon factors related to the quality of the gym and the athlete-dependent factors. Both of these issues should be addressed to treat the current injury and to prevent further injuries. The key to defining the etiology of a Crossfit injury is to understand the different exercises and their related mechanisms. By doing so, a physician can adequately counsel the athlete on their course of

recovery. By recognizing larger faults in their training, such as poor form or programming, the physician can help the athlete decide if exercise modification or even participation at a different gym may help them achieve their athletic training objectives and promote optimal wellness.

References

1. Boutcher SH. High-intensity intermittent exercise and fat loss. J Obes. 2011;2011, 868305.
2. Gremeaux V, Drigny J, Nigam A, Juneau M, Guilbeault V, Latour E, et al. Long-term lifestyle intervention with optimized high-intensity interval training improves body composition, cardiometabolic risk, and exercise parameters in patients with abdominal obesity. Am J Phys Med Rehabil. 2012;91(11):941–50.
3. Smith MM, Sommer AJ, Starkoff BE, Devor ST. Crossfit-based high intensity power training improves maximal aerobic fitness and body composition. J Strength Cond Res. 2013;27(11):3159–72.
4. Jung ME, Bourne JE, Little JP. Where does HIT fit? An examination of the affective response to high-intensity intervals in comparison to continuous moderate- and continuous vigorous-intensity exercise in the exercise intensity-affect continuum. PLoS One. 2014;9(12), e114541.
5. Heinrich KM, Patel PM, O'Neal JL, Heinrich BS. High-intensity compared to moderate-intensity training for exercise initiation, enjoyment, adherence, and intentions: an intervention study. BMC Public Health. 2014;14. 789-2458-14-789.
6. Weisenthal B, Beck C, Maloney M, DeHaven K, Giordano B. Injury rate and patterns among crossfit athletes. Orthop J Sports Med. 2014;2(4):1–7.
7. Giordano B, Weisenthal B. Prevalence and incidence rates are not the same. Orthop J Sports Med. 2014;2(7):1–2.
8. Hak PT, Hodzovic E, Hickey B. The nature and prevalence of injury during crossfit training. J Strength Cond Res. 2013. [Epub ahead of print].
9. Bergeron MF, Nindl BC, Deuster PA, Baumgartner N, Kane SF, Kraemer WJ, et al. Consortium for health and military performance and American College of Sports Medicine consensus paper on extreme conditioning programs in military personnel. Curr Sports Med Rep. 2011;10(6):383.
10. Raske A, Norlin R. Injury incidence and prevalence among elite weight and power lifters. Am J Sports Med. 2002;30(2):248–56.
11. Lavallee ME, Balam T. An overview of strength training injuries: acute and chronic. Curr Sports Med Rep. 2010;9(5):307–13.
12. Larsen C, Jensen MP. Rhabdomyolysis in a well-trained woman after unusually intense exercise. Ugeskr Laeger. 2014;176(25), V01140001.

13. Basford JR. Weightlifting, weight training and injuries. Orthopedics. 1985;8(8):1051–6.
14. Calhoon G, Fry AC. Injury rates and profiles of elite competitive weightlifters. J Athl Train. 1999;34(3):232–8.
15. Sparto PJ, Parnianpour M, Reinsel TE, Simon S. The effect of fatigue on multijoint kinematics, coordination, and postural stability during a repetitive lifting test. J Orthop Sports Phys Ther. 1997;25(1):3–12.
16. Keogh J, Hume PA, Pearson S. Retrospective injury epidemiology of one hundred one competitive Oceania power lifters: the effects of age, body mass, competitive standard, and gender. J Strength Cond Res. 2006;20(3):672–81.
17. Bono CM. Low-back pain in athletes. J Bone Joint Surg Am. 2004;86-A(2):382–96.
18. Newlands C, Reid D, Parmar P. The prevalence, incidence and severity of low back pain among international-level rowers. Br J Sports Med. 2015;49(14):951–6.
19. Menzer H, Gill GK, Paterson A. Thoracic spine sports-related injuries. Curr Sports Med Rep. 2015;14(1):34–40.
20. Boykin RE, McFeely ED, Ackerman KE, Yen YM, Nasreddine A, Kocher MS. Labral injuries of the hip in rowers. Clin Orthop Relat Res. 2013;471(8):2517–22.
21. Hosea TM, Hannafin JA. Rowing injuries. Sports Health. 2012;4(3):236–45.
22. van Gent RN, Siem D, van Middelkoop M, van Os AG, Bierma-Zeinstra SM, Koes BW. Incidence and determinants of lower extremity running injuries in long distance runners: a systematic review. Br J Sports Med. 2007;41(8):469–80. Discussion 480.
23. Taunton JE, Ryan MB, Clement DB, McKenzie DC, Lloyd-Smith DR, Zumbo BD. A prospective study of running injuries: the Vancouver Sun Run "In Training" clinics. Br J Sports Med. 2003;37(3): 239–44.
24. Cosca DD, Navazio F. Common problems in endurance athletes. Am Fam Physician. 2007;76(2): 237–44.
25. Paluska SA. An overview of hip injuries in running. Sports Med. 2005;35(11):991–1014.
26. Caine DJ, Nassar L. Gymnastics injuries. Med Sport Sci. 2005;48:18–58.
27. Barton N. Sports injuries of the hand and wrist. Br J Sports Med. 1997;31(3):191–6.
28. Kolt GS, Kirkby RJ. Epidemiology of injury in elite and subelite female gymnasts: a comparison of retrospective and prospective findings. Br J Sports Med. 1999;33(5):312–8.
29. Thomopoulos S, Parks WC, Rifkin DB, Derwin KA. Mechanisms of tendon injury and repair. J Orthop Res. 2015;33(6):832–9.
30. Karthik K, Carter-Esdale CW, Vijayanathan S, Kochhar T. Extensor Pollicis Brevis tendon damage presenting as de Quervain's disease following kettlebell training. BMC Sports Sci Med Rehabil. 2013;5. 13-1847-5-13.
31. Lee G. Exercise-induced rhabdomyolysis. R I Med J. 2014;97(11):22–4.

Hip Injuries in the Endurance Athlete

13

Joshua D. Harris

Introduction

Endurance athletes require extended periods of functional repetitive hip motion, articular congruity, and balanced musculotendinous coordination in order to successfully perform their sport [1]. Over 80 % of athletic hip and pelvis injuries are due to overuse [2]. The majority of endurance athletes with groin, hip, or pelvis pain have intra-articular diagnoses [3]. Recurrent episodes of high-intensity or extended duration sport without sufficient recovery may lead to overuse injury. These injuries may involve isolated single osseous or soft-tissue structures or a combination of multiple separate musculoskeletal entities. Overuse hip injuries in endurance athletes may occur in the setting of normal or abnormal anatomy and mechanics (e.g., femoroacetabular impingement [FAI]) [1]. As the quantity and quality of athletic hip preservation literature evolve and improve, normal anatomy and abnormal pathology are better understood, classified, and managed. Anatomic evaluation of athletic hip complaints has led to the utilization of the "layer concept," categorizing diagnoses into different layers: I (osteochondral), II (inert), III (contractile), and IV (neuromechanical) [4]. This has permitted not only better assessment and treatment of hip injuries but also implementation of effective prevention programs [5].

Anatomy

The hip is a deep, diarthrodial synovial ball-and-socket joint. The highly congruous spherical femoral head and acetabulum afford a highly stable, yet multiaxial, joint. Recent recognition of variable degrees of severity of nonarthritic hip pathoanatomy relative to FAI, dysplasia, and labral pathology has greatly improved the understanding of "normal hip anatomy." The hip articulation, in conjunction with the pelvic ring, forms the basis of the osteochondral layer, Layer I [4]. Layers II (inert) and III (contractile) comprise the stabilizing soft tissues enveloping the joint, working in synchronicity to prevent instability during normal physiologic motion. Layer II includes the static stabilizers (labrum, capsule, iliofemoral, pubofemoral, and ischiofemoral ligaments and zona orbicularis). Layer III includes the dynamic musculotendinous stabilizers crossing the hip joint and lumbosacral and pelvic floor complexes. Layer IV, the neuromechanical layer, includes the nervous and vascular structures that coordinate the kinetic chain in and around the hip.

J.D. Harris (✉)
Houston Methodist Orthopedics and Sports Medicine,
6550 Fannin Street, Smith Tower, Suite 2500,
Houston, TX 77030, USA
e-mail: joshuaharrismd@gmail.com

© Springer International Publishing Switzerland 2016
T.L. Miller (ed.), *Endurance Sports Medicine*, DOI 10.1007/978-3-319-32982-6_13

Layer I

The osteochondral layer provides the basis for arthrokinetic motion via joint congruity. Hip motion is primarily rotational, around a center of rotation, rather than translational [6]. Sphericity of the articulation combined with the near-frictionless articular cartilage surface permits a lifetime of normal joint function in most individuals. Static and/or dynamic conditions of asphericity may lead to early chondrolabral damage and arthrosis. In the endurance athlete, with tens of thousands of repetitive functional hip joint movements per day, this situation has the potential to accelerate. The loss of femoral head-neck junction sphericity (cam FAI) (Fig. 13.1a), femoral head overcoverage (pincer FAI) (Fig. 13.1b) or undercoverage (dysplasia) (Fig. 13.1c), and extra-articular impingement (trochanteric-pelvic [Fig. 13.1d, e], ischiofemoral [Fig. 13.1f], and subspine impingement [Fig. 13.1g, h]) all may disrupt normal joint mechanics (translation in addition to rotation). Other osseous femoral (version, neck-shaft angle), acetabular (version, depth), and lumbopelvic (pelvic incidence, sagittal, and coronal plane balance) parameters play a significant role in the multifactorial evaluation of normal hip and pelvis anatomy [7].

Osseous architecture of the femoral head, neck, and peritrochanteric region demonstrates compact cortical and cancellous trabecular bone. Radiographically, the proximal femur can be characterized by trabecular group (compressive, tensile, and greater trochanteric) and type (primary, secondary) (Fig. 13.2a) [8]. During gait, a coronal plane rotatory equilibrium exists between vectors of body weight and abductor tension to maintain a level pelvis (Fig. 13.2b) (Table 13.1). These vectors are responsible for the designation of "compressive" and "tensile" sides of the femoral neck [8]. Proximal femoral abnormalities in bone mineral density may be responsible for femoral neck fractures, including both acute traumatic and chronic overuse stress fractures.

Altered bone mineral density has also been observed on both the proximal femoral head-neck junction and acetabulums of patients with cam FAI morphology [9, 10]. In FAI, elevated bone mineral density exponentially increases subchondral bone stiffness, altering the joint contact stresses with incongruent joint surfaces, potentially instigating and propagating the degenerative arthrosis paradigm [11]. In fact, bone mineral density has shown a significant positive correlation with alpha angle, with the magnitude of deformity even more correlative than symptom status [10].

In symptomatic patients that have failed nonsurgical treatments, arthroscopic hip preservation continues to rapidly grow internationally as a successful treatment of intra-articular hip pathologies, including those of Layer I. Arthroscopic "normal" anatomy of the proximal femur and acetabulum has been the subject of several high-quality anatomical investigations [12, 13]. The superior margin of the anterior labral sulcus ("psoas u") has been designated as the standard clockface reference, denoting 3:00 on the acetabular clockface [12]. As opposed to the center of the transverse acetabular ligament, previously used as the referenced arthroscopic landmark at 6:00 [14, 15], the anterior labral sulcus is consistently and reproducibly visualized during hip arthroscopy. Other consistently identifiable arthroscopic landmarks include the anterior inferior iliac spine (1:30–2:30), direct and indirect heads of rectus femoris (2:00–2:30 and 11:30–2:00, respectively), iliocapsularis (2:00–2:30), iliopsoas (3:00–3:30), and lateral ascending vessels (11:30–12:00 on femur) [12]. These intraoperative landmarks have been confirmed to be radiographically identifiable (anteroposterior [AP] and false profile) during surgical fluoroscopy and during preoperative planning [16].

Layer II

Layer II is comprised of the inert, noncontractile soft-tissue structures in and around the hip. This includes the fibrocartilaginous acetabular labrum, which provides a joint-stabilizing suction seal during physiologic motion [17]. This seal has been negated in subjects with FAI during flexed and rotated positions, including pivoting necessary for participation in endurance sports [18].

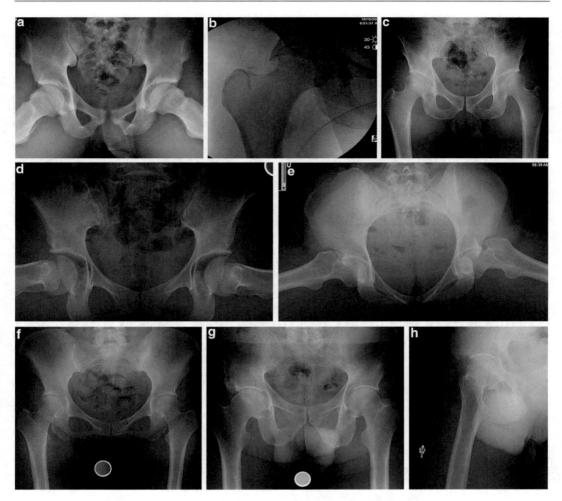

Fig. 13.1 (**a**) Dunn 45° plain radiograph of bilateral cam morphology in a 19-year-old collegiate runner, illustrating loss of anterolateral femoral head-neck offset, cortical sclerosis, and a significantly increased alpha angle. (**b**) Intraoperative anteroposterior (AP) fluoroscopy of far lateral and posterolateral pincer femoroacetabular impingement (FAI) overcoverage of the right hip of a 35-year-old female marathon runner. (**c**) Standing AP pelvis plain radiograph, illustrating bilateral acetabular dysplasia in a 25-year-old male triathlete. A reduced lateral center-edge angle, increased Tönnis angle, and increased femoral head extrusion index are observed. (**d**) AP "splits" plain radiograph of a 19-year-old collegiate cheerleader in 90° abduction and permissive limb external rotation, illustrating bilateral posterior trochanteric-pelvic impingement and a "vacuum" sign. (**e**) AP "splits" plain radiograph of a 19-year-old collegiate cheerleader (same as Fig. 13.1d) in 90° abduction and forced limb internal rotation, illustrating superior trochanteric-pelvic impingement. (**f**) AP pelvis plain radiograph of a 40-year-old female cyclist with increased femoral anteversion and suggestive of bilateral ischiofemoral impingement. (**g**) AP pelvis plain radiograph of a 45-year-old male half-marathon runner with a type III anterior inferior iliac spine (AIIS) and subspine impingement in his right hip. He reported a history of "groin strain" as a teenage playing football. (**h**) False-profile plain radiograph of a 45-year-old male half-marathon runner (same as Fig. 13.1g) with a type III AIIS and subspine impingement in his right hip

The labrum plays a significant role in pain generation inside the hip joint, secondary to the presence of free sensory nerve fibers and mechanoreceptors, with the highest relative concentration in the anterior zone, where most labral pathology is located [19–21]. The distribution of free nerve endings is greatest at the labral base and decreases toward the periphery [22].

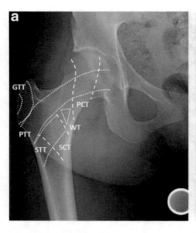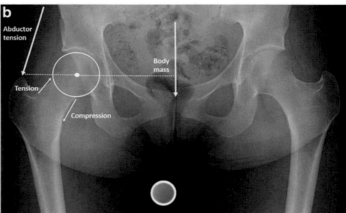

Fig. 13.2 (**a**) AP plain radiograph of an 18-year-old female collegiate cross-country runner with proximal femoral primary and secondary trabeculae outlined in the right hip. GTT (greater trochanteric trabeculae); PCT (primary compressive trabeculae); PTT (primary tensile trabeculae); SCT (secondary compressive trabeculae); STT (secondary tensile trabeculae); WT (Ward's triangle). Figure reprinted with permission from Elsevier Inc. (**b**) AP plain radiograph of an 18-year-old female collegiate cross-country runner (same as Fig. 13.2a) with balanced free-body diagram of force vectors outlined in the right hip. Hip center of rotation is marked with a *dot* and a *Möse circle* around the femoral head. The product of the force of the body weight and its associated moment arm equals the product of the abductor muscle force and its associated moment arm. For equilibrium, according to Newton's third law of motion, for every action (abductor muscle tension and body weight), there is an equal and opposite reaction (joint reaction force). Figure reprinted with permission from Elsevier Inc.

Table 13.1 Proximal femoral anatomy based on version, neck-shaft angle

		Anatomy	Coronal plane lever arm	Required abductor muscle force
Femoral version increased	Increased anteversion	Greater trochanter posterior, closer to hip center	Decreased	Increased
Femoral version decreased	Relative retroversion	Greater trochanter lateral, further from hip center	Increased	Decreased
Neck-shaft angle increased	Coxa valga	Greater trochanter above center of femoral head	Decreased	Increased
Neck-shaft angle decreased	Coxa vara	Greater trochanter below center of femoral head	Increased	Decreased

The hip capsule is composed of four discrete ligamentous structures: the iliofemoral (Y ligament of Bigelow), ischiofemoral, and pubofemoral ligaments and zona orbicularis. The iliofemoral ligament is the strongest of the four and is transversely cut during interportal capsulotomy (anterolateral to mid-anterior) in hip arthroscopy [23]. The latter permits excellent viewing of the central compartment: labrum, acetabular rim, articular cartilage of the acetabulum and femoral head, fovea, and ligamentum teres. A "T" capsulotomy, perpendicular to the interportal capsulotomy, permits excellent viewing of the peripheral compartment: proximal femoral head-neck junction, zona orbicularis, lateral and medial synovial folds, and lateral ascending vessels. Several biomechanical investigations have illustrated the importance of the iliofemoral ligament for retention of normal hip kinematics: Iliofemoral ligament sectioning (unrepaired capsulotomy) leads to increased external rotation, extension, and anterior and distal translation [24–27]. Clinically, during hip arthroscopy using a "T" capsulotomy, this translates to significantly better outcomes in patients who have a complete capsular repair (Fig. 13.3a–d) versus those who

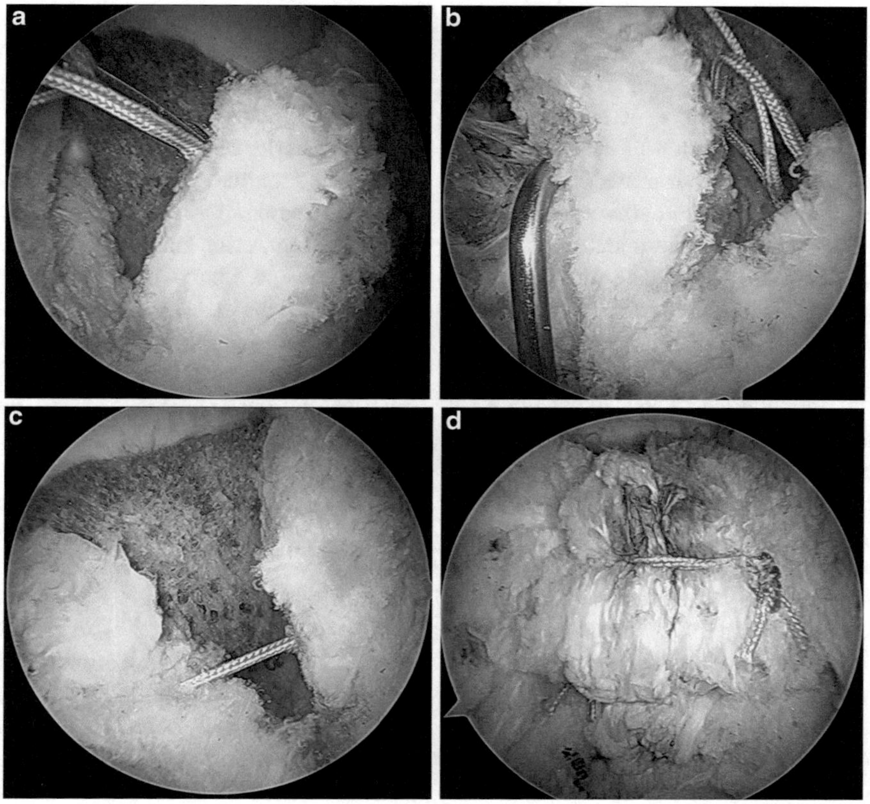

Fig. 13.3 (a) Right hip arthroscopy of a 20-year-old female collegiate gymnast. Viewing from modified mid-anterior portal and instrumenting from distal anterolateral accessory portal (DALA), a "T" capsulotomy has been made for improved peripheral compartment visualization of the cam morphology (following osteoplasty) and is now being repaired with a suture-penetrating and suture-passing device through the medial limb of the capsulotomy. Nonabsorbable, #2 suture is utilized. (b) Same patient as Fig. 13.3a, the suture is being retrieved after penetrating the lateral limb of the capsulotomy. (c) Same patient as Fig. 13.3a, each limb of the capsulotomy is approximated prior to standard arthroscopic knot-tying techniques. (d) Same patient as Fig. 13.3a, three high-strength nonabsorbable sutures have been utilized for "T" capsulotomy capsular plication of the iliofemoral ligament

have a partial repair (repaired "T" and unrepaired interportal capsulotomy) [28]. An unrepaired "T" capsulotomy may potentially leave the hip catastrophically unstable (dislocation) or prone to "microinstability" due to a disrupted "stability arc" [29–31]. The "stability arc" is a defined area of the anterior hip, defined by the medial and lateral limbs of the iliofemoral ligament as the static deep border and the iliocapsularis and rectus femoris as the dynamic superficial medial border and the gluteus minimus as the dynamic superficial lateral border [29]. In the setting of an unrepaired "T" capsulotomy, hip extension and external rotation dynamically pull the medial and lateral limbs of the iliofemoral ligament apart and evade the anterior stabilizing effect of the anterior capsule.

Layer III

Layer III consists of the dynamic musculotendinous units in and around the hip and pelvis. This includes the muscles whose action is to move the hip, the lumbopelvic-stabilizing girdle, and the pelvic floor. Several different extra-articular pathologies may be either the cause of the effect of intra-articular lesions, such as FAI or labral injury. In endurance athletes with FAI, increased stresses across the bony hemipelvis may result when athletes attempt to achieve supraphysiologic terminal range of motion via the hip required for participation in their sport [32]. These forces may be transmitted through the pubic symphysis (osteitis pubis), sacroiliac joint, and lumbosacral spine. Anatomical regions may help categorize these subsequent tendinopathies and/or enthesopathies: anterior enthesopathy (hip flexor strain, psoas impingement), medial enthesopathy (adductor and rectus tendinopathies—"athletic pubalgia," "core muscle injury," "sports hernia"), posterior enthesopathy (proximal hamstring syndrome, "piriformis syndrome," deep gluteal space syndrome), and lateral enthesopathy (peritrochanteric pain syndrome, gluteus medius tendinopathy, or tear).

The iliopsoas tendon may instigate an atypical direct anterior labral tear (3:00) (iliopsoas impingement) [33]. Further, the iliopsoas tendon has been shown to demonstrate an anterior stabilization role in the setting of hip arthroscopy. In three separate case reports with a post-arthroscopic dislocation, an iliopsoas tenotomy was performed [34, 35]. In addition, the effects of femoral version in the setting of iliopsoas tenotomy have been investigated. Significantly better outcomes have been observed in patients with femoral version less than 25° (versus greater than 25°) [36].

The posterior musculotendinous complex, primarily the proximal hamstring and gluteus maximus, is frequently involved in the endurance athlete. The inferior margin of the more superficial gluteus maximus is approximately 6 cm proximal to the deeper superior aspect of the proximal hamstring origin on the ischium [37]. The inferomedial origin, the conjoined semitendinosus/long-head biceps femoris tendons, is oval shaped and larger than the crescent-shaped semimembranosus footprint on the superolateral ischial tuberosity [37, 38]. The most lateral aspect of the tuberosity is approximately 1 cm from the sciatic nerve [37]. This explains the common posterior hip pain over the tuberosity and uncommon lower extremity radiculopathy in the sciatic nerve distribution. In runners, proximal hamstring (myotendinous junction and tuberosity origin) syndrome (Fig. 13.4a, b) is common in both short-distance sprinters and long-distance runners [39, 40]. In patients with FAI, compensatory posterior tilt of the pelvis (to avoid impingement)

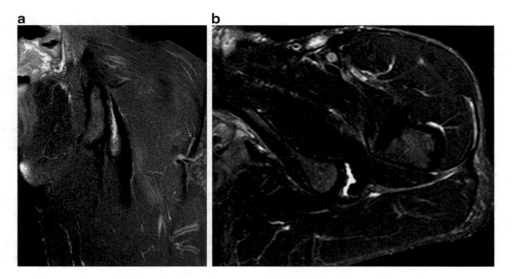

Fig. 13.4 (**a**) Coronal, T2-weighted MRI of a 38-year-old female ultramarathon runner with proximal hamstring syndrome demonstrating a partial-thickness, interstitial, insertional proximal hamstring tear with posterior hip and buttock pain at the ischial tuberosity. (**b**) Same patient as Fig. 13.4a, with an axial, T2-weighted MRI demonstrating partial-thickness proximal hamstring tear. Quadratus femoris is observed without any edema (ischiofemoral impingement). This MRI was performed 2 weeks following a 50-mile ultramarathon

leads to chronic hamstring shortening and eventual tendinopathy.

The medial hip and abdominopelvic musculo-tendinous complex are variable and highly intricate, leading to an often misunderstood, under-recognized, and undertreated entity termed core muscle injury or athletic pubalgia. Adductor-related pain, osteitis pubis, and core muscle injury are rarely seen in isolation and nearly always seen in combination with intra-articular diagnoses, especially FAI and labral injury [3]. Thus, a detailed understanding of the anatomy is paramount in timely identification and management. The anatomy centers around the pubis and pubic symphysis. The latter is a non-synovial joint stabilized by four ligaments and an intra-articular fibrocartilage disk [41]. The four ligaments conjoin the rectus abdominis, external and internal oblique, transversus abdominis, and gracilis and adductor aponeuroses. The most important ligament is the anteroinferiorly located arcuate ligament. The symphysis acts as the anterior pelvic fulcrum, around which the hip and pelvis muscle forces act. The rectus abdominis (creates a posterosuperior force) and adductor longus (creates an anteromedial force) unite anteriorly in a common sheath anterior to the pubis. This common aponeurosis joins the conjoint tendon (internal oblique and transversus abdominis), external oblique, pectineus (anterior), adductor brevis (posterior to adductor longus), adductor magnus (posterolateral), and gracilis (posteromedial). Core muscle injury ("sports hernia," "athletic pubalgia") occurs when any of these multiple structures is injured, resulting in increased stress and strain on the intact proximate structures, typically without a discrete recognizable hernia [42]. The superficial (external) inguinal ring is located just immediately lateral to the pubic aponeurosis (indirect hernia through the ring versus direct hernia through Hesselbach's triangle). This clearly complicates the diagnostic picture, given the close, complex, integrated anatomy and pathoanatomy in endurance athletes. The abnormal musculotendinous stress distribution may further potentiate symphyseal instability and then lead to a secondary musculotendinous injury (cyclical stress transmission).

Further, especially in endurance sports, imbalances or injuries to the core muscles result in increased fatigue, decreased endurance, and injury, exacerbating the stress transmission cycle [43]. Part of the innervation of the core muscles, the iliohypogastric, ilioinguinal, and genitofemoral nerves (part of Layer IV), may also be involved via entrapment, resulting in deep anterior and/or lateral hip pain.

Layer IV

Layer IV is comprised of the neurokinetic layer, thoracolumbosacral plexus, and lumbopelvic tissues, serving as the neural link to the hip and lower extremities. This essentially links the hip and pelvis to the remainder of the body. Any kink in the kinetic chain may result in dysfunction. Several studies have revealed either upstream or downstream effects of hip injury and other proximal or distal structures. In the endurance athlete, this has wide implications as to the determination of the cause or effect of hip injury. Elevated alpha angle has been associated with increased risk of anterior cruciate ligament (ACL) tear (27 times greater if alpha angle greater than 60°) [44]. In patients with chronic recurrent ankle sprains, significantly delayed gluteus maximus activation during prone hip extension has been identified [45]. It is unknown if whether the ankle is the instigator for the hip or vice versa. Similarly, patients with low back pain have consistently identified decreased hip range of motion (versus controls) [46–51]. Further, pelvic incidence (position-independent measure of lumbar lordosis and pelvis orientation) has been shown to be significantly lower in both cam and pincer FAI [7].

History

Endurance athletes presenting to the clinician should be thoroughly evaluated in a systematic fashion. The chief complaint is frequently helpful in determining the most important part of the history and physical examination: Is the source of pain coming from inside (intra-articular) or

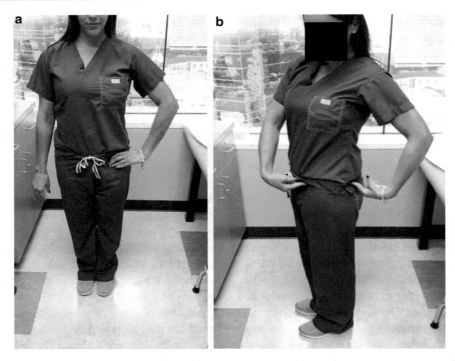

Fig. 13.5 (**a**) Left hip "C" sign, indicative of intra-articular source of hip pain. (**b**) Left hip "between the fingers" sign, indicative of intra-articular source of hip pain

outside (extra-articular) the hip joint? Although the typical patient complains of groin pain, illustrated by a "C" sign or a "between the fingers" sign (Fig. 13.5a, b), several different locations in and around the hip may be perceived for true intra-articular hip pain [47]. Patients may complain of pain in the groin (55–92 %), lateral hip (59–67 %), anterior thigh (35–52 %), buttock (29–71 %), low back (23 %), knee and below (22–47 %), or foot (2 %) [47].

The history of present illness should query several key aspects of the patient's reason for evaluation:

Onset (acute, chronic, traumatic, insidious), location (right, left, bilateral; deep, superficial; anterior, lateral, posterior), character (dull, sharp, burning, aching, throbbing), duration, frequency, exacerbating and relieving factors (sitting, standing, walking, running, jumping, laying down, twisting, pivoting, putting on socks and shoes, toilet, out of bed, coughing, sneezing, Valsalva), radiation of pain (below hip,

below knee, above to back), and associated symptoms (clicking, catching, popping, snapping, numbness, tingling, pins and needles, groin swelling or bulging/hernia).

Coxa saltans (snapping hip) is frequently due to one (or more) out of three potential causes:

1. external coxa saltans (snapping iliotibial band), frequently described by patients as "My hip is dislocating"; frequently this is visible (the snapping hip you can see);
2. internal coxa saltans (snapping iliopsoas), frequently described by patients as the snapping hip you can hear, but not see;
3. internal coxa saltans (labral tear), frequently described by patients as the snapping hip that they can feel, but you cannot see or hear

Prior treatments should be thoroughly assessed (physical therapy, oral medications, injections, surgeries). Prior injections should be specified (intra-articular, peritrochanteric, trigger point), especially regarding the use of ultrasound or fluoroscopic guidance and the response to injection. In hip osteoarthritis, intra-articular injection has been shown to be quite accurate in determining the source of pain [52, 53]. However, for other intra-articular nonarthritic diagnoses, such as FAI or labral injuries, the utility of injection is less well understood and less predictable [54]. A significant response to injection (greater than 50% pain relief) helps to rule in intra-articular pathology as the source of the patient's symptoms [54]. However, a positive response from injection is not a strong predictor of short-term functional outcomes following arthroscopic management of FAI and labral pathology [55]. Although the lack of a significant response (less than 50% pain relief) does not necessarily rule out intra-articular pathology [54], a negative response may be predictive of poor short-term surgical outcome [56]. The author gives all injection patients a pain diary following injection to document response to injection on a visual analog scale (0–10) at multiple time points (preinjection; 5, 30, 60 min; 2, 3, 6, 12, 24 h; 2, 3, 7, 14 days). This helps clearly delineate the response to the local anesthetic based on typical drug pharmacokinetics.

If prior surgery, the operative report and operative photographs should be scrutinized. Past medical and surgical history should be critically evaluated for other potential sources of groin, hip, or pelvic pain. This especially includes general surgical, urological, colorectal, and obstetric/gynecologic causes. Causes of potential unique sources of hip pathology should be elicited when indicated:

1. Femoral head avascular necrosis (chronic corticosteroid use, alcoholism, pancreatitis, sickle cell anemia, diabetes, scuba diving decompression illness [caisson disease], myeloproliferative disease, systemic lupus erythematosus, Gaucher's disease)
2. Inflammatory arthritides (rheumatoid arthritis, ankylosing spondylitis, psoriatic arthritis)
3. Legg-Calve-Perthes disease (4–14 years of age)
4. Slipped capital femoral epiphysis (8–16 years of age)

5. Transient osteoporosis of the hip (third trimester of pregnancy, middle-aged males)

For endurance athletes, a detailed athletic history is a key component of the evaluation, especially including existing risk factors:

1. History of prior overuse injury (including stress fracture)
2. Rapid increase in training intensity or mileage
3. Pain characterization during sport (progression with time to the point of stoppage or relieving with time)
4. Change in running shoes or equipment
5. Pain progression from after activity to with activity, to activities of daily living, to rest, and to female athlete triad (disordered eating, amenorrhea, low bone mineral density) or tetrad (triad plus endothelial injury) [57]

Physical Examination

The physical examination for endurance athletes with hip pain should be an extension of the focused history of present illness. Although comprehensive and systematic allowing for reproducibility and consistency, it should be adaptive as well, focused on the history elicited prior to the physical assessment. The first fundamental evaluation should be to determine if the source(s) of symptoms stems from inside or outside the joint. As with examination of any joint, visual inspection, palpation, motion, strength, and special testing is performed. Further, in order to understand if pathology is present in the involved hip or hemipelvis, the contralateral side should also be critically scrutinized. Extensions of the hip assessment should include a thoracolumbosacral spine evaluation, in addition to the distal limb. This includes coronal plane alignment, femoral version, tibial torsion, and pedal arch. Although the physical examination should focus on the presenting chief complaint, a comprehensive evaluation should also identify other abnormalities that may predispose the patient to other overuse injuries (i.e., injury prevention). Further, a caveat to the hip physical examination should be to avoid iatrogenic displacement of non-displaced femoral neck stress fractures with a hop test. If sufficient concern exists and radiographs are available, do not perform a hop test, as this dramatically alters the treatment and eventual outcome.

Inspection

Thorough inspection of the hip and pelvis requires a balance between sufficient exposure and modesty. The core, hip, pelvis, and entire lower extremity should be observed. In addition to the patient him/herself, shoe wear patterns should also be assessed. Prior surgical incisions, deformity, alignment, swelling, edema, ecchymosis, and erythema should be noted. Hip "snapping" may be observed in cases of external coxa saltans due to snapping iliotibial band. Gait evaluation by either observation in clinic or outside of clinic and on a treadmill or via digital video analysis gives a real-time evaluation of biomechanical factors that may predispose to stress injuries of the tibia. This includes scrutiny for potential abductor weakness or abductor fatigue via Trendelenburg sign.

Palpation

Palpation is a key component for evaluation of multiple causes of hip pain in the endurance athlete. Locations of tenderness suggestive of the source of pathology include:

1. Peritrochanteric (trochanteric bursitis, abductor tendinopathy or partial tear, snapping iliotibial band)
2. Proximal hamstring (proximal hamstring tendinopathy, partial tear, ischial bursitis)
3. Sacroiliac joint (sacroiliitis, referred from FAI)
4. Lumbosacral spine (degenerative disk disease, herniated nucleus pulposus, degenerative facet arthropathy, spondylolisthesis, sacral stress fracture [Fig. 13.6])
5. Groin (direct or indirect hernia, general surgical/urologic/obstetric/gynecologic causes, core muscle injury [athletic pubalgia])

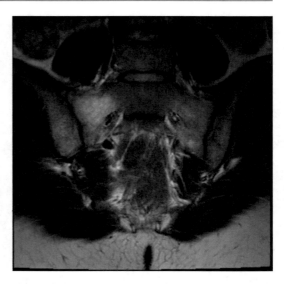

Fig. 13.6 Right-sided sacral ala stress fracture in a collegiate male cross-country runner

6. Adductor tendon (tendinopathy, tear, core muscle injury)
7. Pubis (pubic symphysis, pubic tubercle, pubic rami for core muscle injury or stress fracture [Fig. 13.7a, b])
8. Iliac crest (stress fracture, apophysitis [Fig. 13.8])

Motion, Strength, and Special Testing

Range of motion is an important component of the hip physical examination in endurance athletes. Although different clinicians may have their own specific routine for assuring completeness and minimizing patient movement between sitting, standing, supine, lateral, and prone, it is important to ensure that a complete exam is performed and documented for every patient. It is also often helpful to examine the "normal" hip before examination of the involved hip. It is important to assess for tightness or contracture in certain muscle groups, especially the iliopsoas, iliotibial band, common adductors, and hamstring complex. The Thomas test may be utilized to assess for hip flexor tightness [58]. The Ober test may elicit iliotibial band tightness and peritrochanteric pain syndrome [59]. For the hip, it is important to normalize the pelvic position

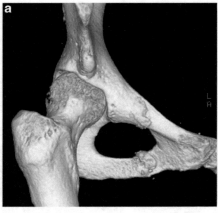

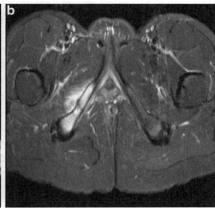

Fig. 13.7 (**a**) Three-dimensional CT scan of a 35-year-old female marathon runner with healing superior and inferior pubic rami stress fractures with visible fracture callus. (**b**) Same patient as Fig. 13.7a, axial T2-weighted pelvis MRI illustrating edema in the inferior right pubic ramus and extra-osseous soft-tissue edema, after acute injury-on-chronic groin pain

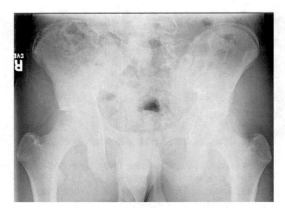

Fig. 13.8 AP pelvis plain radiograph of a 17-year-old male cross-country runner with right anterior iliac crest pain with running, illustrating an iliac crest apophysitis and stress fracture

by bringing the contralateral limb up to the chest to reduce lumbar lordosis, confounding and truly isolating the magnitude of hip flexion (Fig. 13.9a). Hip flexion, internal and external rotation (Fig. 13.9b, c, respectively), abduction (Fig. 13.9d), and extension (Fig. 13.9e) should be measured and compared to the contralateral limb. Measurements may be taken using visual inspection, goniometer, digital photography, motion analysis, or imaging-based techniques (plain radiographs, MRI, or CT scan). Strength testing may be performed using the MRC (Medical Research Council) manual muscle testing system [60]. Hip flexion, extension, abduction, adduction, and internal and external rotation should be tested. Muscle strains are the most common injury in and around the hip in endurance athletes [2]. The muscles that cross both the hip and knee (two joints—eccentric contraction; rectus femoris, sartorius, tensor fascia lata) are especially at risk [61]. Further, in distance runners, iliopsoas strains have been shown to be the most common cause of groin pain [62]. The iliopsoas test, provocation of pain with resisted hip flexion in an externally rotated position, may be performed to diagnose iliopsoas strain, iliopsoas impingement, or an iliopsoas labral tear [63]. The Ludloff test is performed by passively flexing the hip greater than 90°, while supine, isolating the iliopsoas, and a positive sign is reproduction of pain with resisted hip flexion in that flexed position [64].

Impingement testing is performed in endurance athletes to assess for FAI and labral pathology. The key with all impingement testing is to assure that, in a positive test, the reproduction of pain during the examination maneuver is the same pain location during provocative sport. Although sensitive (94–99 %), the anterior impingement (flexion-adduction-internal rotation) test demonstrates poor specificity (5–9 %) [65]. It is the most common screening examination maneuver to detect intra-articular pathology. The subspine impingement maneuver is performed with

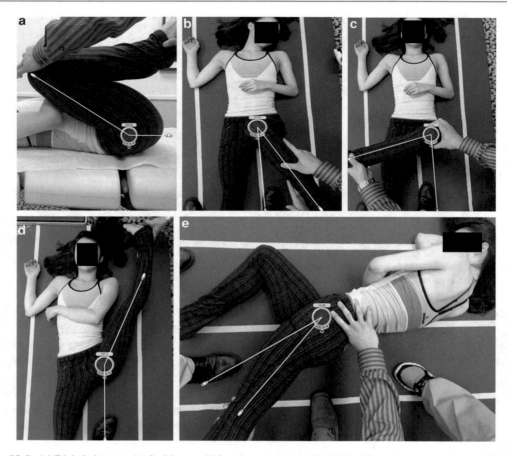

Fig. 13.9 (**a**) Digital photograph of a 22-year-old female professional ballet dancer, illustrating measurement of right hip flexion. (**b**) Same patient as Fig. 13.9a, illustrating measurement of left hip internal rotation. (**c**) Same patient as Fig. 13.9a, illustrating measurement of left hip external rotation. (**d**) Same patient as Fig. 13.9a, illustrating measurement of left hip abduction. (**e**) Same patient as Fig. 13.9a, illustrating measurement of left hip extension

straight hip flexion in the sagittal plane [66]. The lateral impingement test is performed to maximal coronal plane abduction and permissive limb external rotation [30]. Once maximal abduction is reached, the limb is then internally rotated (trochanteric-pelvic impingement test) [30]. Posterior impingement may be tested with hip extension and external rotation [30]. The posterior impingement test may be performed supine with the patient at the side edge of the table and the leg off the side of the table or with the patient at the end of the table and the leg far off the end. It is important to assess the posterior impingement test for two possible end points: pain or apprehension of hip instability. The FABER (flexion-abduction-external rotation)

distance test is another impingement maneuver performed in the supine position, with the affected hip flexed and externally rotated and the affected ankle on the contralateral knee, above the patella [67]. A distance greater than 3 cm (compared to the contralateral limb) is a positive test [67]. The Stinchfield test is a supine-resisted active straight-leg raise test with the knee extended and the hip flexed approximately 20° [68]. A positive Stinchfield is the most specific physical examination maneuver for intra-articular pathology [68].

In addition to the posterior impingement apprehension test, several other tests in the endurance athlete may indicate atraumatic microinstability:

1. In the external rotation recoil test, a positive finding is present when release of maximal passive lower extremity external rotation, while supine, fails to demonstrate normal spring-like recoil back to the pre-external rotation position [69, 70].
2. In the dial test, the lower extremity is maximally internally rotated, while supine, and the limb is then allowed to passively externally rotate (positive finding is indicated when greater than 45° of passive external rotation occurs and lacks a mechanical end point) [71].
3. In the traction test, a positive finding occurs upon the feeling of instability or looseness with limb distraction, while supine [30, 72, 73].

Imaging Evaluation

Imaging for hip pain in the endurance athlete should always begin with plain radiographs. The clinician should always remember to "treat the patient and not the X-ray." The reason for the latter is the prevalence of abnormal radiographic findings in asymptomatic subjects [74]. The prevalence of asymptomatic cam and pincer FAI was 37% and 67%, respectively. Cam morphology was significantly more common in athletes (55%) than nonathletes (23%). The prevalence of asymptomatic labral tear was 68%. Weight-bearing anteroposterior (AP) pelvis and a combination of ipsilateral lateral hip views (supine Dunn 45°, standing Dunn 45°, supine Dunn 90°, frog-leg lateral, Lauenstein lateral, cross-table lateral, false profile) should be obtained and scrutinized for adequacy. The standing AP pelvis should demonstrate symmetry of obturator foramina, collinearity of pubic symphysis and coccyx (approximately 2 cm proximal to most superior aspect of symphysis), and an elongated femoral neck (lower extremity internal rotation). On the standing AP pelvis, acetabular coverage (lateral center-edge angle, Tönnis angle, femoral head extrusion index) (pincer FAI versus dysplasia), neck-shaft angle (coxa vara, coxa valga), neck primary and secondary trabeculae (femoral neck stress fracture), alpha angle (far lateral cam FAI), and Tönnis grade of osteoarthritis should

be assessed. On the false-profile view, anterior inferior iliac spine (AIIS) morphology (types I, II, III) and anterior center-edge angle (anterior acetabular coverage) may be assessed. On the Dunn, frog-leg, cross-table, and Lauenstein lateral views and measurement of head-neck offset (millimeters), head-neck offset ratio (unitless), and alpha angle (degrees) permit a thorough two-dimensional characterization of femoral head-neck junction asphericity (a three-dimensional issue).

Femoral neck stress fractures are another common cause of hip pain in endurance athletes. Four different classifications exist to classify femoral neck stress fractures. Three of these systems may exclusively utilize plain radiographs. The most clinically relevant, easily applied, and generalizable, with the highest interobserver and intra-observer reliability, is the system created by Kaeding and Miller [75]. This system utilizes five grades, one through five. Grade 1 is a painless asymptomatic stress response visible on imaging. Grade 2 also illustrates a stress response without a fracture line. However, Grade 2 injuries are symptomatic. Grades 3 and 4 injuries both have a visible fracture line. Grade 3 injuries are non-displaced and Grade 4 are displaced. Grade 5 injuries are nonunions. The Devas classification divided fractures into compression and tension sides [76]. The Blickenstaff and Morris classification has three types: type 1 (callus, without fracture line), type 2 (non-displaced fracture line), and type 3 (displaced fracture) [77]. The Fullerton and Snowdy classification also has three types: tension side, non-displaced; compression side, non-displaced; displaced [78].

Magnetic resonance imaging (MRI) and computed tomography (CT) offer complimentary three-dimensional osseous and soft-tissue information in and around the hip and pelvis. Standard series should include a combination of T1-, T2-, and proton density-weighted coronal, axial, sagittal, axial oblique, and radial series [79]. The unique three-dimensional, nearly spherical, anatomy of the hip joint makes it highly difficult to view the thin (1–2 mm) opposing articular cartilage and labrum with standard planar series because of partial volume averaging in MRI. Radial sectioning, at 30° increments, is ideal for evaluating the curved structures of the hip. Each plane taken (13 total for 360° circumference) goes through the center of the joint. Thus, the obtained plane is perpendicular to the curvature of the joint, providing a cross section of the articular cartilage and labrum [79]. This reduces the partial volume-averaging effect seen with conventional planar imaging. Axial oblique MRI has been the gold standard reference for measurement of alpha angle, quantifying the degree of proximal femoral asphericity [80]. The images pass through the center of the femoral head parallel to the plane of the femoral neck. It essentially provides a view that corresponds to a lateral hip radiograph. In addition to the osseous and chondrolabral anatomy, MRI provides useful information on the capsule, musculotendinous units, and other extra-articular, but relevant, structures (lumbosacral spine [46], core muscle injury [81], and other gastrointestinal, genitourinary, obstetric, and gynecologic structures [82, 83]). The addition of intra-articular gadolinium dye (magnetic resonance arthrogram [MRA]) distends the joint capsule, separating the capsule, labrum, and articular cartilage and increasing spatial resolution for improved diagnosis of chondrolabral injury [84]. Although MRA improves the sensitivity (63–100 %), specificity (44–100 %), and accuracy (65–96 %), it is highly resource intensive, requiring both fluoroscopy (for the arthrogram) and MRI at the same time, temporal coordination of each appointment, and direct physician performance of the arthrogram. Further, there are risks associated with intra-articular hip dye injection [84].

With reference to femoral neck stress fractures, if plain radiographs do not reveal a fracture line or evidence of healing (periosteal thickening and elevation, cortical sclerosis), then MRI has a sensitivity and specificity of up to 100 % [85]. Technetium-99 m-labeled methylene diphosphonate bone scan (Triple-Phase Bone Scintigraphy) is a sensitive exam to detect femoral neck stress fracture, but has poor specificity [86]. Further, anatomic delineation of fracture location is poor with bone scan. Computed tomography (CT) scans are associated with significant radiation exposure and low sensitivity of detecting stress fracture, but do have high specificity [86].

CT scan is the optimal osseous evaluation of the hip joint, providing a patient-specific three-dimensional picture, evaluation of femoral and acetabular version, and precise acetabular coverage parameters [87]. CT is the best preoperative evaluation of the proximal femoral head-neck junction. However, intraoperatively, CT is not utilized. A combination of six fluoroscopic views (AP neutral, AP in 30° internal rotation, AP in 30° external rotation, 50° flexion view in neutral, 50° flexion view in 40° external rotation, 50° flexion view in 60° external rotation) can reproducibly characterize the topography of the cam deformity from the 11:45 to 2:45 position, covering the most commonly observed maximum alpha angles [88]. Because the most common reason for revision hip arthroscopy is residual FAI, the potential for inadequate resection should be mitigated as much as possible [89]. On the acetabular side, CT has shown that normal femoral head coverage was $40 \pm 2\,\%$ in an asymptomatic cohort, with the mean lateral coverage corresponding to a lateral center-edge angle of $31 \pm 1°$ [90].

Differential Diagnosis Evaluation

The clinician must combine the subjective history with the objective physical examination with the objective imaging studies to determine a differential diagnosis (Table 13.2). The first step in the evaluation and management of hip pain in the endurance athlete is determining if the pain is intra- or extra-articular. The magnitude and potential severity of intra-articular diagnoses merit priority over most extra-articular sources (Table 13.2). However, the clinician must always be aware that these diagnoses are not mutually exclusive and frequently may coexist either as two distinct entities or one as a result of another. Intra-articular sources include most commonly FAI, labral tear, dysplasia, arthritis, and stress fracture, among other much less common causes. Athletes with intra-articular sources of symptoms typically have a chief complaint of deep groin pain.

Table 13.2 Subjective and objective evaluation pearls in endurance athletes with hip pain

	History	Physical examination	Imaging—plain radiographs	Imaging—advanced—MRI/CT
Femoral neck stress fracture	Groin pain, rapid training increase, female athlete triad	Pain with axial load, hop, log roll, and impingement testing	Compression versus tension side, frequently negative	Edema, discrete fracture line, 100% sensitivity, 100% specificity
FAI, labral tear	Groin pain, worse with deep flexion and rotational sports	Positive impingement testing, decreased flexion and rotation	Cam (increased alpha angle, loss of head-neck offset); Pincer (lateral CEA >40°, crossover, posterior wall, ischial spine signs, protrusio)	Labral tear, articular cartilage injury, subchondral edema "herniation pit"/"impingement cyst"
Dysplasia	Groin pain, worse with deep flexion and rotational sports; frequent "abductor fatigue"	Positive impingement testing, increased abduction, pain with resisted abduction	Lateral CEA <20°, anterior CEA <20°, Tönnis angle >15°, femoral head extrusion index >25%	Labral tear (hypertrophic size), articular cartilage injury
Osteoarthritis	Groin pain, worse with deep flexion and rotational sports; crepitus	Positive impingement testing, decreased flexion and rotation	Loss of joint space (<2 mm), subchondral sclerosis, cysts, osteophytes	Articular cartilage narrowing, subchondral cysts, sclerosis, effusion, capsular thickening
Extra-articular impingement—AIIS	Groin pain, worse with straight hip flexion, prior "groin strain"—likely rectus femoris avulsion	Subspine impingement, decreased hip flexion	Type II or III AIIS, prior rectus avulsion with calcification or ossification	Labral tear (2:00–3:00), subspine edema
Extra-articular impingement—ischiofemoral	Posterior hip or buttock pain, especially in "turnout" position in dancers	Posterolateral hip pain with extension and external rotation	Decreased ischiofemoral distance	Quadratus femoris edema and narrowed ischiofemoral space
Extra-articular impingement—trochanteric-pelvic	Deep lateral or anterior groin pain, especially in hyperabducted position, either in IR or ER	Abduction >90°, positive trochanteric-pelvic impingement test	"Splits" radiograph illustrating trochanteric-pelvic impingement, vacuum sign, coxa vara	Labral tear, extra-articular edema at site of impingement
Extra-articular impingement—iliopsoas	Groin pain, worse with active hip flexion, worse with deep flexion and rotational sports, audible internal snapping	Positive anterior impingement, positive Ludloff, iliopsoas test, iliopsoas snap	Increased femoral anteversion, type II or III AIIS	3:00 labral tear, edema at iliopsoas-AIIS interval, increased femoral anteversion
Peritrochanteric pain syndrome	Lateral hip pain, superficial, visible snapping	Peritrochanteric tenderness, positive Ober test, abductor weakness	Coxa valga, calcification at abductor insertion	Edema at bursa, abductor tendinopathy, partial tear
Deep gluteal (aka "piriformis") syndrome	Non-discogenic "sciatica" posterior hip or buttock pain, poor sitting tolerance	Posterolateral hip, gluteal, retro-trochanteric tenderness, worse with hip rotation in flexion with knee extended, antalgic sitting position	Decreased ischiofemoral distance, ischiofemoral impingement	Sciatic neural enlargement, loss of normal fascicular appearance, fibrous bands over piriformis
Proximal hamstring syndrome	Posterior hip, proximal hamstring pain, worse with running	Ischial tuberosity tenderness, worse with resisted hamstring	Prior ischial tuberosity avulsion, calcification at hamstring origin	Proximal hamstring tendinopathy, partial tear
Core muscle injury (aka "athletic pubalgia")	Groin pain, worse with Valsalva and high-intensity sport	Tenderness at pubis, adductor, rectus abdominis, no direct or indirect hernia	Frequent with FAI, osteitis pubis	Edema at pubis, adductor origin, conjoined tendon, rectus abdominis, labral tear
Lumbosacral spine	Low back pain, sciatica	Lumbosacral tenderness, positive straight-leg raise	Lumbosacral spondylosis, degenerative disk/facet	Herniated nucleus pulposus, spondylolisthesis

The clinician should be cognizant that these diagnoses are not mutually exclusive and may frequently coexist. *AIIS* anterior inferior iliac spine, *CEA* center-edge angle, *IR* internal rotation, *ER* external rotation

The pain is most frequently perceived deep in the hip, unable to be touched superficially. Sitting tends to exacerbate the pain more than standing. Deep flexion and rotational maneuvers also exacerbate. Sports that involve high-intensity or high-frequency hip flexion and rotation are frequent culprits. In patients with any degree of concern for femoral neck stress fracture, every diagnostic step necessary must be taken to ensure a correct diagnosis is made, as missed diagnoses may be catastrophic with displacement of the fracture and significantly increased risk of femoral head avascular necrosis, even with timely prompt and anatomic reduction (up to 30 %) [91]. These patients often complain of groin pain that begins early in the activity (e.g., running), progressively worsens during the activity, and may progress to the point of activity cessation due to pain. Endurance athletes with a previous stress fracture, females, amenorrhea, disordered eating, and low bone mineral density warrant a stress fracture evaluation. On physical examination, pain with weight bearing, axial load, single-leg stance, squat, hop, and positive impingement testing is a characteristic of femoral neck stress fracture. If plain radiographs reveal no sign of fracture, then MRI is indicated. In athletes with similar symptomatology with negative stress fracture evaluation, plain radiographs frequently reveal FAI, and an MRI is then indicated to evaluate for chondrolabral injury. In athletes with similar symptomatology with negative stress fracture evaluation, dysplasia may also be a cause of deep hip pain. However, frequently this is secondary to abductor fatigue. Dysplasia induces a component of femoral head translation (in addition to rotation) with motion [30, 92]. This microinstability requires greater abductor activity to keep the femoral head center of rotation centered in the acetabulum ("abductor fatigue"). In athletes with groin pain, loss of motion, and crepitus, plain radiographs should be critiqued for osteoarthritis (joint space narrowing, subchondral sclerosis, cysts, osteophytes).

If the symptoms and examination are consistent with an extra-articular source of symptoms, then the differential diagnosis is very different from that of intra-articular sources. Extra-articular impingement, similar to traditional FAI, involves a mechanical conflict that inhibits hip motion and places extra stress on tissues unequipped to handle the stress. This can occur at the AIIS in straight hip flexion with the distal anterior femoral neck contacting a prominent type II or III AIIS [93]. Despite this being an extra-articular phenomenon, labral pathology is frequently observed, and the AIIS may be surgically treated with "intra-articular" arthroscopy [94, 95]. Further, despite being extra-articular FAI, AIIS subspine impingement symptoms are frequently perceived deep in the groin, similar to cam and pincer FAI. Straight hip flexion subspine impingement testing combined with false-profile radiographs and three-dimensional CT scan can reliably diagnose subspine impingement [66]. Trochanteric-pelvic impingement may be observed in high range of motion endurance sports (ballet, gymnastics, mixed martial arts, figure skating). Patients frequently complain of pain in the lateral splits (grand écart facial) and front splits positions (grand écart lateral) [96]. Additionally, in dancers, "turnout" (extension and external rotation) frequently may induce lesser trochanter impingement on the lateral ischium and proximal hamstring origin (ischiofemoral impingement) [97]. This presents as posterior hip and buttock pain in provocative positions and maneuvers. It is important to evaluate the proximal hamstring and gluteus maximus function in this situation for concurrent proximal hamstring tendinopathy or partial tearing. This deep gluteal syndrome (formerly known as piriformis syndrome) is a commonly encountered source of posterior hip pain with a rapidly evolving and still incompletely understood etiology [82]. Iliopsoas impingement is frequently seen as an internal snapping hip, with complaints of deep groin pain with active hip flexion and rotation, inducing snapping and far anteromedial labral tears [33]. In patients with lateral hip pain, superficial tenderness is frequently diagnosed as "bursitis" [98]. However, patients with discrete abductor weakness and insignificant iliotibial band tightness warrant MRI for evaluation of abductor tendinopathy and possible tear.

Treatment

The management of most conditions causing hip pain in endurance athletes is not emergent or urgent (Table 13.3). The only potentially urgent diagnosis necessary to be made is that of potential femoral neck stress fracture and its inherent risk of displacement. In non-displaced compression-sided femoral neck stress fractures, immediate non-weight bearing is instituted with crutch-assisted ambulation for 6 weeks. If the fracture heals, the patient's pain with weight bearing resolves, and a slow return to sport (with recognition and address of underlying risk factors)

is commenced. Persistent pain warrants MRI to evaluate for fracture persistence or worsening (Fig. 13.10a). In this situation of failed nonsurgical measures, percutaneous screw fixation (Fig. 13.10b–d), followed by weight bearing as tolerated ambulation (6 weeks) and gradual return to sport (6–12 weeks), is commenced. In non-displaced tension-sided stress fractures, percutaneous screw fixation is indicated, as nonsurgical treatment is not indicated due to the unfavorable biomechanics of fracture location. Any stress fracture displacement requires prompt (same day) anatomic reduction (closed or open means) and fixation (percutaneous screw or

Table 13.3 Treatment and outcomes for endurance athletes with hip pain

	Nonsurgical treatment	Surgical treatment
Femoral neck stress fracture	Compression side, non-displaced: NWB × 6 weeks	Tension side or failed nonsurgical treatment compression side: In situ percutaneous screw fixation Displaced fracture: anatomic reduction, screw fixation
FAI, labral tear	Limited evidence; activity modification, oral NSAID, ± intra-articular injection, PT	Labral preservation, pincer acetabuloplasty, cam osteoplasty
Dysplasia	Activity modification, oral NSAID, ± intra-articular injection, PT	Borderline dysplasia: arthroscopic hip preservation; dysplasia: periacetabular osteotomy
Osteoarthritis	Rest, activity modification, oral NSAID, intra-articular injection, PT, nutraceutical	Total hip arthroplasty
Extra-articular impingement—AIIS	Limited evidence; activity modification, oral NSAID, ± intra-articular injection, PT	Arthroscopic subspine decompression osteoplasty
Extra-articular impingement—ischiofemoral	Limited evidence; activity modification, oral NSAID, PT	Endoscopic or open ischiofemoral decompression (lesser trochanter)
Extra-articular impingement—trochanteric-pelvic	Limited evidence; activity modification, oral NSAID, ± intra-articular injection, PT	Open trochanteric osteotomy advancement
Extra-articular impingement—iliopsoas	Limited evidence; activity modification, oral NSAID, ± iliopsoas tendon sheath injection, PT	Arthroscopic subspine decompression and/or iliopsoas tenotomy
Peritrochanteric pain syndrome	Rest, activity modification, oral NSAID, bursal injection, PT	Endoscopic or open bursectomy and iliotibial band window, abductor repair
Deep gluteal (aka "piriformis") syndrome	Rest, activity modification, oral NSAID, infiltration injection test (corticosteroid, anesthetic)	Endoscopic or open sciatic neurolysis, lysis of fibrous adhesions
Proximal hamstring syndrome	Rest, activity modification, oral NSAID, PRP injection, PT (emphasize eccentric)	Proximal hamstring repair
Core muscle injury (aka "athletic pubalgia")	Rest, activity modification, oral NSAID, PT (core muscle activation, strengthening)	Open repair, decompression of adductor/rectus/conjoined tendon complex as indicated by pathology
Lumbosacral spine	Rest, activity modification, oral NSAID, injection, PT	Open decompression and fusion (if indicated)

NWB non-weight bearing, *NSAID* nonsteroidal anti-inflammatory, *PT* physical therapy

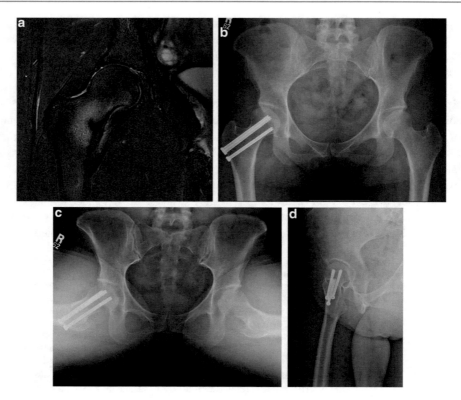

Fig. 13.10 (a) Coronal T2-weight MRI of a 28-year-old female runner with a compression-sided right femoral neck fracture. This patient had failed 6 weeks of nonsurgical treatment consisting of non-weight-bearing crutch-assisted ambulation. (b) Same patient as Fig. 13.10a, 1 day after the MRI, illustrating postoperative AP pelvis X-ray with three partially threaded 7.3-mm-diameter screws traversing the femoral neck. Key surgical pearls include avoidance of a proximal femoral stress riser effect by keeping the screw entry point on the lateral proximal femoral cortex proximal to the superior aspect of the lesser trochanter. (c) Same patient as in Fig. 13.10a, illustrating postoperative Dunn 90° lateral radiograph with three partially threaded screws. (d) Same patient as in Fig. 13.10a, illustrating postoperative false-profile radiograph with three partially threaded screws

plate/screw fixation). Fracture displacement on any imaging modality is an indication to immediately abandon nonsurgical treatment and anatomically reduce and fix the fracture.

In patients with symptomatic FAI and labral tear, initial nonsurgical management consists of activity modification (avoidance of deep flexion and rotation), oral anti-inflammatory medications, and physical therapy (core, hip, pelvis strengthening and flexibility; dynamic reduction in anterior impingement by improving posterior pelvic tilt). Intra-articular anesthetic and corticosteroid injections may be used both diagnostically and therapeutically. However, the clinician and patient should always be cognizant of the fact that neither medications nor injections

can change the pathoanatomy of the hip morphology or heal the labral tear (Fig. 13.11a–d). Thus, nearly all of the current evidence focuses on surgical treatment of FAI and labral pathology [99]. Both arthroscopic and open techniques are successful, with a high rate of good to excellent outcomes at short- and midterm follow-up. No long-term outcomes of either open or arthroscopic hip preservation yet exist [100].

Conclusions

Evaluation and management of the endurance athlete with hip pain require a thorough knowledge of the layered structure of normal anatomy

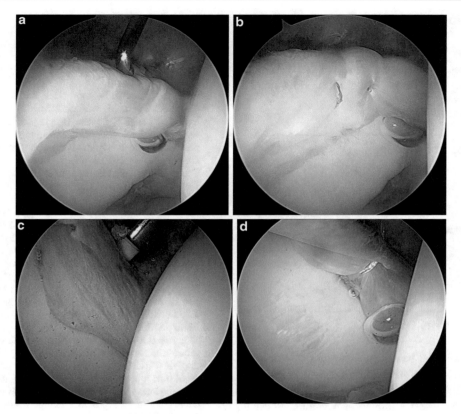

Fig. 13.11 (a) Arthroscopic right hip preservation surgery in a 27-year-old female volleyball player. Viewing from anterolateral portal with 70° arthroscope. Probe instrumenting from mid-anterior portal pushing on acetabular labrum at 1:30 on clockface. The chondrolabral disruption is clearly visible at the chondrolabral junction. (b) Same patient as Fig. 13.11a after two suture anchors have been placed in the acetabular rim with a pierced vertical mattress configuration. The typical labral repair follows acetabuloplasty rim trimming to eliminate pincer impingement (when indicated). Two to four suture anchors are typically used. (c) Arthroscopic right hip preservation surgery in an 18-year-old female collegiate rower. Viewing from anterolateral portal with 70° arthroscope. Radiofrequency device is localizing an iliopsoas-induced acetabular labral tear at 3:00 on clockface. Erythema at the location of impingement, in addition to the chondrolabral disruption, is visible on this image. (d) Same patient as Fig. 13.11c after suture anchor repair in the acetabular rim with a pierced vertical mattress configuration

and abnormal pathoanatomy in and around the hip joint. The subjective history and objective physical examination must be combined with any imaging to properly "treat the athlete and not the X-ray." Patients with intra-articular pathology report deep groin pain, worse with the offending sporting activity, deep flexion, and rotational maneuvers. Physical examination typically reveals a loss of hip flexion and rotation with positive impingement findings. Risk factors for femoral neck stress fracture must be sought, evaluated, and promptly managed as this is an unmissable diagnosis. Femoroacetabular impingement and labral tears are likely the most common diagnoses in endurance athletes. Plain radiographs are very useful in endurance athletes with hip pain. However, advanced imaging with MRI and CT has a distinct and growing role in appropriate evaluation. Sources of pain around the hip joint frequently coexist, and the clinician must systematically assess all potential diagnoses, as they are not mutually exclusive.

Location of Investigation

Houston Methodist Hospital, Department of Orthopedics and Sports Medicine, 6550 Fannin Street, Smith Tower, Suite 2500, Houston, TX 77030, USA.

Source of Funding

None.

Statement of Originality

All data, figures, tables, and text are original and previously unpublished.

Disclosures

JDH: Editorial board: *Arthroscopy: The Journal of Arthroscopic and Related Surgery*; *Frontiers in Surgery*; Research Support: Smith and Nephew; Depuy Synthes; Publication royalties: SLACK, Inc. Committees: AOSSM Self-Assessment Committee; AAOS Osteoarthritis Pain and Function Workgroup.

References

1. Nawabi DH, et al. The demographic characteristics of high-level and recreational athletes undergoing hip arthroscopy for femoroacetabular impingement: a sports-specific analysis. Arthroscopy. 2014; 30(3):398–405.
2. Lloyd-Smith R, et al. A survey of overuse and traumatic hip and pelvic injuries in athletes. Phys Sportsmed. 1985;13(10):131–41.
3. Rankin AT, Bleakley CM, Cullen M. Hip joint pathology as a leading cause of groin pain in the sporting population: a 6-year review of 894 cases. Am J Sports Med. 2015;43(7):1698–703.
4. Draovitch P, Edelstein J, Kelly BT. The layer concept: utilization in determining the pain generators, pathology and how structure determines treatment. Curr Rev Musculoskelet Med. 2012;5(1):1–8.
5. Silvers-Granelli H, et al. Efficacy of the FIFA 11+ Injury Prevention Program in the Collegiate Male Soccer Player. Am J Sports Med. 2015;43(11): 2628–37.
6. Tonnis D, Heinecke A. Acetabular and femoral anteversion: relationship with osteoarthritis of the hip. J Bone Joint Surg Am. 1999;81(12):1747–70.
7. Gebhart JJ, et al. Correlation of pelvic incidence with cam and pincer lesions. Am J Sports Med. 2014;42(11):2649–53.
8. Harris J, Chahal J. Femoral Neck Stress Fractures. Oper Tech Sports Med. 2015;23(3):241–7.
9. Speirs AD, et al. Bone density is higher in cam-type femoroacetabular impingement deformities compared to normal subchondral bone. Osteoarthritis Cartilage. 2013;21(8):1068–73.
10. Speirs AD, Beaulé PE, Rakhra KS, Schweitzer ME, Frei H.Osteoarthritis Cartilage. 2013 Apr;21(4): 551–8.
11. Les CM, et al. Estimation of material properties in the equine metacarpus with use of quantitative computed tomography. J Orthop Res. 1994;12(6):822–33.
12. Philippon MJ, et al. An anatomical study of the acetabulum with clinical applications to hip arthroscopy. J Bone Joint Surg Am. 2014;96(20):1673–82.
13. Philippon MJ, et al. Surgically relevant bony and soft tissue anatomy of the proximal femur. Orthop J Sports Med. 2014;2(6):1–9.
14. Philippon MJ, et al. Arthroscopic management of femoroacetabular impingement: osteoplasty technique and literature review. Am J Sports Med. 2007;35(9):1571–80.
15. Ilizaliturri Jr VM, et al. A geographic zone method to describe intra-articular pathology in hip arthroscopy: cadaveric study and preliminary report. Arthroscopy. 2008;24(5):534–9.
16. Lee WA, Saroki AJ, Løken S, Trindade CA, Cram TR, Schindler BR, LaPrade RF, Philippon MJ.Am J Sports Med. 2016 Jan;44(1):67–73.
17. Philippon MJ, et al. The hip fluid seal—Part I: The effect of an acetabular labral tear, repair, resection, and reconstruction on hip fluid pressurization. Knee Surg Sports Traumatol Arthrosc. 2014;22(4): 722–9.
18. Dwyer MK, et al. Femoroacetabular impingement negates the acetabular labral seal during pivoting maneuvers but not gait. Clin Orthop Relat Res. 2015;473(2):602–7.
19. Kilicarslan K, et al. Immunohistochemical analysis of mechanoreceptors in transverse acetabular ligament and labrum: a prospective analysis of 35 cases. Acta Orthop Traumatol Turc. 2015;49(4):394–8.
20. Gerhardt M, et al. Characterisation and classification of the neural anatomy in the human hip joint. Hip Int. 2012;22(1):75–81.
21. Alzaharani A, et al. The innervation of the human acetabular labrum and hip joint: an anatomic study. BMC Musculoskelet Disord. 2014;15:41.
22. Haversath M, et al. The distribution of nociceptive innervation in the painful hip: a histological investigation. Bone Joint J. 2013;95-b(6):770–6.
23. Harris J, et al. Routine complete capsular closure during hip arthroscopy. Arthrosc Tech. 2013;2(2): e89–94.

24. Myers CA, et al. Role of the acetabular labrum and the iliofemoral ligament in hip stability: an in vitro biplane fluoroscopy study. Am J Sports Med. 2011;39(Suppl):85S–91.
25. Martin HD, et al. The function of the hip capsular ligaments: a quantitative report. Arthroscopy. 2008;24(2):188–95.
26. Hewitt JD, et al. The mechanical properties of the human hip capsule ligaments. J Arthroplasty. 2002;17(1):82–9.
27. Bayne CO, et al. Effect of capsulotomy on hip stability-a consideration during hip arthroscopy. Am J Orthop (Belle Mead NJ). 2014;43(4):160–5.
28. Frank RM, et al. Improved outcomes after hip arthroscopic surgery in patients undergoing T-capsulotomy with complete repair versus partial repair for femoroacetabular impingement: a comparative matched-pair analysis. Am J Sports Med. 2014;42(11):2634–42.
29. Walters BL, Cooper JH, Rodriguez JA. New findings in hip capsular anatomy: dimensions of capsular thickness and pericapsular contributions. Arthroscopy. 2014;30(10):1235–45.
30. Harris JD, Gerrie BJ, Lintner DM, Varner KE, McCulloch PC.Orthopedics. 2016 Jan 1;39(1): e169–75.
31. Mitchell RJ, Gerrie BJ, McCulloch PC, Murphy AJ, Varner KE, Lintner DM, Harris JD. Arthroscopy. 2016 Mar 1. pii: S0749-8063(16)00015-3. doi: 10.1016/j.arthro.2015.12.049. [Epub ahead of print]. PMID: 26944667.
32. Hammoud S, et al. The recognition and evaluation of patterns of compensatory injury in patients with mechanical hip pain. Sports Health. 2014;6(2): 108–18.
33. Domb BG, et al. Iliopsoas impingement: a newly identified cause of labral pathology in the hip. HSS J. 2012;7(2):145–50.
34. Austin DC, Horneff 3rd JG, Kelly JDT. Anterior hip dislocation 5 months after hip arthroscopy. Arthroscopy. 2014;30(10):1380–2.
35. Sansone M, et al. Total dislocation of the hip joint after arthroscopy and iliopsoas tenotomy. Knee Surg Sports Traumatol Arthrosc. 2013;21(2):420–3.
36. Fabricant PD, et al. Clinical outcomes after arthroscopic psoas lengthening: the effect of femoral version. Arthroscopy. 2012;28(7):965–71.
37. Miller SL, Webb GR. The proximal origin of the hamstrings and surrounding anatomy encountered during repair. Surgical technique. J Bone Joint Surg Am. 2008;90(Suppl 2 Pt 1):108–16.
38. Philippon MJ, et al. A qualitative and quantitative analysis of the attachment sites of the proximal hamstrings. Knee Surg Sports Traumatol Arthrosc. 2015;23(9):2554–61.
39. Fredericson M, et al. High hamstring tendinopathy in runners: meeting the challenges of diagnosis, treatment, and rehabilitation. Phys Sportsmed. 2005;33(5):32–43.
40. White KE. High hamstring tendinopathy in 3 female long distance runners. J Chiropr Med. 2011; 10(2):93–9.
41. Ross JR, Stone RM, Larson CM. Core muscle injury/sports hernia/athletic pubalgia, and femoroacetabular impingement. Sports Med Arthrosc. 2015;23(4):213–20.
42. Farber AJ, Wilckens JH. Sports hernia: diagnosis and therapeutic approach. J Am Acad Orthop Surg. 2007;15(8):507–14.
43. Rivera CE. Core and lumbopelvic stabilization in runners. Phys Med Rehabil Clin N Am. 2016;27(1): 319–37.
44. Philippon M, et al. Decreased femoral head-neck offset: a possible risk factor for ACL injury. Knee Surg Sports Traumatol Arthrosc. 2012;20(12): 2585–9.
45. Bullock-Saxton JE, Janda V, Bullock MI. The influence of ankle sprain injury on muscle activation during hip extension. Int J Sports Med. 1994;15(6):330–4.
46. Redmond JM, et al. The hip-spine syndrome: how does back pain impact the indications and outcomes of hip arthroscopy? Arthroscopy. 2014;30(7):872–81.
47. Redmond JM, et al. The hip-spine connection: understanding its importance in the treatment of hip pathology. Orthopedics. 2015;38(1):49–55.
48. Van Dillen LR, et al. Hip rotation range of motion in people with and without low back pain who participate in rotation-related sports. Phys Ther Sport. 2008;9(2):72–81.
49. Harris-Hayes M, Sahrmann SA, Van Dillen LR. Relationship between the hip and low back pain in athletes who participate in rotation-related sports. J Sport Rehabil. 2009;18(1):60–75.
50. Vad VB, et al. Hip and shoulder internal rotation range of motion deficits in professional tennis players. J Sci Med Sport. 2003;6(1):71–5.
51. Murray E, et al. The relationship between hip rotation range of movement and low back pain prevalence in amateur golfers: an observational study. Phys Ther Sport. 2009;10(4):131–5.
52. Deshmukh AJ, et al. Accuracy of diagnostic injection in differentiating source of atypical hip pain. J Arthroplasty. 2010;25 Suppl 6:129–33.
53. Crawford RW, et al. Diagnostic value of intra-articular anaesthetic in primary osteoarthritis of the hip. J Bone Joint Surg (Br). 1998;80(2):279–81.
54. Martin RL, Irrgang JJ, Sekiya JK. The diagnostic accuracy of a clinical examination in determining intra-articular hip pain for potential hip arthroscopy candidates. Arthroscopy. 2008;24(9):1013–8.
55. Ayeni OR, et al. Pre-operative intra-articular hip injection as a predictor of short-term outcome following arthroscopic management of femoroacetabular impingement. Knee Surg Sports Traumatol Arthrosc. 2014;22(4):801–5.
56. Khan W, et al. Utility of intra-articular hip injections for femoroacetabular impingement: a systematic

review. Orthop J Sports Med. 2015;3(9): 2325967115601030.

57. Temme KE, Hoch AZ. Recognition and rehabilitation of the female athlete triad/tetrad: a multidisciplinary approach. Curr Sports Med Rep. 2013;12(3):190–9.

58. Peeler J, Anderson J. Reliability of the Thomas test for assessing range of motion about the hip. Phys Ther Sport. 2007;8(1):14–21.

59. Ober F. The role of the iliotibial band and fascia lata as a factor in the causation of low-back disabilities and disabilities in sciatica. J Bone Joint Surg Am. 1936;18:105–10.

60. Council MR. Aids to the examination of the peripheral nervous system, vol. 45. London: Her Majesty's Stationery Office; 1981.

61. Garrett Jr WE. Muscle strain injuries. Am J Sports Med. 1996;24 Suppl 6:S2–8.

62. Holmich P. Long-standing groin pain in sportspeople falls into three primary patterns, a "clinical entity" approach: a prospective study of 207 patients. Br J Sports Med. 2007;41(4):247–52. Discussion 252.

63. Laible C, et al. Iliopsoas syndrome in dancers. Orthop J Sports Med. 2013;1(3):2325967113500638.

64. Mozes M, et al. Iliopsoas injury in soccer players. Br J Sports Med. 1985;19(3):168–70.

65. Reiman MP, et al. Diagnostic accuracy of clinical tests for the diagnosis of hip femoroacetabular impingement/labral tear: a systematic review with meta-analysis. Br J Sports Med. 2015;49(12):811.

66. Larson CM, Kelly BT, Stone RM. Making a case for anterior inferior iliac spine/subspine hip impingement: three representative case reports and proposed concept. Arthroscopy. 2011;27(12):1732–7.

67. Philippon MJ, et al. Prevalence of increased alpha angles as a measure of cam-type femoroacetabular impingement in youth ice hockey players. Am J Sports Med. 2013;41(6):1357–62.

68. Maslowski E, et al. The diagnostic validity of hip provocation maneuvers to detect intra-articular hip pathology. PM R. 2010;2(3):174–81.

69. Blakey CM, et al. Secondary capsular laxity of the hip. Hip Int. 2010;20(4):497–504.

70. Larson CM, Stone RM. Current concepts and trends for operative treatment of FAI: hip arthroscopy. Curr Rev Musculoskelet Med. 2013;6(3):242–9.

71. Philippon M, et al. Hip instability in the athlete. Oper Tech Sports Med. 2007;15:189–94.

72. Boykin RE, et al. Hip instability. J Am Acad Orthop Surg. 2011;19(6):340–9.

73. Suter A, et al. MR findings associated with positive distraction of the hip joint achieved by axial traction. Skeletal Radiol. 2015;44(6):787–95.

74. Frank JM, Harris JD, Erickson BJ, Slikker W 3rd, Bush-Joseph CA, Salata MJ, Nho SJ.Arthroscopy. 2015 Jun;31(6):1199–204.

75. Kaeding CC, Miller T. The comprehensive description of stress fractures: a new classification system. J Bone Joint Surg Am. 2013;95(13):1214–20.

76. Devas MB. Stress fractures of the femoral neck. J Bone Joint Surg (Br). 1965;47(4):728–38.

77. Blickenstaff LD, Morris JM. Fatigue fracture of the femoral neck. J Bone Joint Surg Am. 1966;48(6):1031–47.

78. Fullerton Jr LR. Femoral neck stress fractures. Sports Med. 1990;9(3):192–7.

79. Petchprapa CN, et al. Demystifying radial imaging of the hip. Radiographics. 2013;33(3):E97–112.

80. Notzli HP, et al. The contour of the femoral head-neck junction as a predictor for the risk of anterior impingement. J Bone Joint Surg (Br). 2002;84(4):556–60.

81. Coker DJ, Zoga AC. The role of magnetic resonance imaging in athletic pubalgia and core muscle injury. Top Magn Reson Imaging. 2015;24(4):183–91.

82. Hernando MF, et al. Deep gluteal syndrome: anatomy, imaging, and management of sciatic nerve entrapments in the subgluteal space. Skeletal Radiol. 2015;44(7):919–34.

83. Hansen A, et al. Postpartum pelvic pain—the "pelvic joint syndrome": a follow-up study with special reference to diagnostic methods. Acta Obstet Gynecol Scand. 2005;84(2):170–6.

84. Rakhra KS. Magnetic resonance imaging of acetabular labral tears. J Bone Joint Surg Am. 2011;93 Suppl 2:28–34.

85. Kiuru MJ, et al. MR imaging, bone scintigraphy, and radiography in bone stress injuries of the pelvis and the lower extremity. Acta Radiol. 2002;43(2):207–12.

86. Gaeta M, et al. CT and MR imaging findings in athletes with early tibial stress injuries: comparison with bone scintigraphy findings and emphasis on cortical abnormalities. Radiology. 2005;235(2):553–61.

87. Massey PA, Nho SJ, Larson CM, Harris JD. Osteoarthritis Cartilage. 2014 Dec;22(12):2093–4.

88. Ross JR, et al. Intraoperative fluoroscopic imaging to treat cam deformities: correlation with 3-dimensional computed tomography. Am J Sports Med. 2014; 42(6):1370–6.

89. Cvetanovich GL, et al. Revision hip arthroscopy: a systematic review of diagnoses, operative findings, and outcomes. Arthroscopy. 2015;31(7):1382–90.

90. Larson CM, et al. Are normal hips being labeled as pathologic? A CT-based method for defining normal acetabular coverage. Clin Orthop Relat Res. 2015;473(4):1247–54.

91. Ehlinger M, et al. Early prediction of femoral head avascular necrosis following neck fracture. Orthop Traumatol Surg Res. 2011;97(1):79–88.

92. Harris JD, Gerrie BJ, Varner KE, Lintner DM, McCulloch PC.Am J Sports Med. 2016 Jan;44(1): 20–7.

93. Hetsroni I, et al. Anterior inferior iliac spine morphology correlates with hip range of motion: a classification system and dynamic model. Clin Orthop Relat Res. 2013;471(8):2497–503.

94. Hetsroni I, et al. Anterior inferior iliac spine deformity as an extra-articular source for hip impingement: a series of 10 patients treated with arthroscopic decompression. Arthroscopy. 2012;28(11): 1644–53.

95. Amar E, Warschawski Y, Sharfman ZT, Martin HD, Safran MR, Rath E. Surg Radiol Anat. 2015 Nov 30. [Epub ahead of print]. PMID: 26620219.

96. Mitchell R, et al. Radiographic evidence of hip microinstability in elite ballet. Arthroscopy. 2016;32:1–8.

97. Gómez-Hoyos J, Schröder R, Reddy M, Palmer IJ, Martin HD.Arthroscopy. 2016 Jan;32(1):13–8.

98. Ho GW, Howard TM. Greater trochanteric pain syndrome: more than bursitis and iliotibial tract friction. Curr Sports Med Rep. 2012;11(5):232–8.

99. Harris JD, et al. Treatment of femoroacetabular impingement: a systematic review. Curr Rev Musculoskelet Med. 2013;6(3):207–18.

100. Nwachukwu BU, Rebolledo BJ, McCormick F, Rosas S, Harris JD, Kelly BT.Am J Sports Med. 2016 Apr;44(4):1062–8.

Exercise and Osteoarthritis: The Effect of Running with Aging in the Masters-Level Athlete

14

Jason P. Zlotnicki, Aaron Mares, and Volker Musahl

Introduction

Participation in long-distance running events has increased across athletes of all ages, sex, and activity levels in recent years. Per the Annual US Marathon Report, a 140 % increase in US Marathon finishers has been observed (224,000 vs. 541,000) with an additional 40 % increase over the last 10 years alone (386,000 vs. 541,000) [1]. Per the same report, 47 % of all finishers were 40 years and older (47 %), which includes all classes of runners, including recreational runners as well as masters athletes. Per the World Association of Masters Athletes, an organization designated by the International Association of Athletics Federations (IAAF), a masters athlete is defined as man or woman of not less than 35 years of age that participates in a wide array of track and field and longer-distance aerobic sports [2]. As the definition of masters athletics infers a level of expertise and veteran status, these runners often demonstrate a high level of fitness with numerous years (and miles) of running and exercise experience. This increase at both the masters and recreational levels is widely supported by physicians of all specialties, as well as multiple federal health organizations, given the association between physical activity and a decreased lifetime risk for developing obesity, hypertension, type 2 diabetes mellitus, and thromboembolic stroke among others [3, 4]. More specifically participating in high-impact sports positively influences bone density scores and overall bone health, decreasing the risk for osteoporosis and fracture [5]. Despite these known health benefits, a persistent dogma and entrenched belief exist in a link between runners and chronic musculoskeletal injuries with the eventual "worn-out knees."

Recent epidemiologic data states that approximately 46 million people in the United States have symptomatic arthritis [6], with recent figures suggesting knee osteoarthritis (OA) affecting 250 million people worldwide [7]. The main studies demonstrate that from 1990 to 2010, OA has been shown to be the fastest increasing health condition, with knee pain limiting activity and impairing quality of life. While the health benefits for aging masters athletes, and all recreational runners, are well documented, there is little evidence to document the relationship between high-mileage runners and the development or worsening of knee OA. Studies have demonstrated knee OA as the most prevalent musculoskeletal disease in the masters athlete and has been well documented as a common complication of sports injury [8]. This chapter will serve to discuss the relationship between masters running and OA in three dimensions. This chapter will highlight:

J.P. Zlotnicki • A. Mares • V. Musahl (✉)
Department of Orthopaedic Surgery, University of Pittsburgh Medical Center, 3471 Fifth Avenue, Suite 1010, Kaufmann Medical Building, Pittsburgh, PA 15213, USA
e-mail: musahlv@upmc.edu

© Springer International Publishing Switzerland 2016
T.L. Miller (ed.), *Endurance Sports Medicine*, DOI 10.1007/978-3-319-32982-6_14

1. The currently accepted mechanisms for the development and progression of OA in masters runners and likewise all aging athletes, with presentation of current literature review for associations between running and disease prevalence
2. A proper evaluation and treatment paradigm for an aging runner with OA-associated knee pain and other running maladies
3. The current dogma and recommendations regarding runner activity, cross-training principles, and adequate nutrition associated with prolonged running health

Pathophysiology of Disease, At-Risk Populations, and the Modifiable Lifestyle Factors

In order to discuss the potential effects of long-distance running and high-impact mechanical loading of the articular cartilage in an osteoarthritic knee, the anatomy, mechanisms, and pathophysiology of OA must be addressed. From a mechanical standpoint, the knee joint is a diarthrodial, mobile hinge joint between the distal aspect of the femur, proximal tibia, and patella. This articulation permits flexion and extension as well as rotation to a lesser degree, all of which play a role in various athletic movements. The static and dynamic stabilizers of the joint allow for high amounts of motion throughout the kinetic chain of movement while providing the needed stability during explosive maneuvers associated with running, jumping, and rapid change of direction. These stabilizers include the ligaments (both intracapsular and extracapsular), menisci, muscle tendons that cross the joint, and the joint capsule and retinaculum itself. When in appropriate balance, these stabilizers allow for a relatively even distribution of contact forces throughout the joint surfaces of the femur, tibia, and patella and allow for smooth gliding of the hyaline cartilage-covered articular surfaces during movement. Comprised of chondrocytes, type 2 collagen fibers, negatively charged proteoglycans, and water, hyaline cartilage provides a surface that is resilient to wear, compressible, and sufficiently strong and stiff to tolerate high biomechanical loads and shear stresses during motion at the joint. This all serves to protect the subchondral bone from impact, while also facilitating smooth and energy efficient motion during movement. However, injury to these static and dynamic stabilizers and load-sharing structures can lead to rapid rates of injury and increased predisposition to arthritis. Injury, inflammation, and the degradation of cartilage with resultant pain, effusion, and loss of motion are the hallmark of OA [9].

From a clinical standpoint, the development of OA is broken into two main classifications: primary or secondary OA. Primary OA is initiated and propagated by an imbalance between synthesis and degradation of the articular surface matrix, driven by a complex milieu of pro-inflammatory cytokines [10]. Conversely, a mechanical disruption or direct insult to the joint via trauma can damage the extracellular matrix, causing cartilage fissures and defects that lead to secondary OA [11–13]. Despite this dichotomy, it is generally accepted that OA is a combination of genetic susceptibility and excessive mechanical stress [14–16]. Likewise, the majority of OA observed in aging athletes is a combination of high levels of mechanical stress with an underlying predisposition. As stated by Neogi et al., this predisposition may be genetic, age related, nutritional, or the presence of poor mechanical stability caused by joint malalignment and weak kinetic chain [17]. Aging has been demonstrated as the primary risk factor for OA [18], with common dogma that increased mechanical stresses (via high-impact exercise such as long-distance running) would accelerate this process over time and lead to painful, debilitated joint. This is certainly the case in cohorts of subjects who have sustained a known, traumatic injury to the articular cartilage [19–22]. While it has been shown that moderate, consistent mechanical loading of joints is necessary for maintenance of healthy articular cartilage [23], repetitive abnormal loading of joints is associated with injury and rapid decline of the articular surface [24]. This degradation appears even more rapid in unhealthy, obese individuals due to a combination of mechanical and inflammatory processes, with obesity acting as a major modifiable lifestyle factor in the development and treatment of knee arthritis.

Obesity is a common medical comorbidity in all patient populations. According to a recent study presented in JAMA, 36 % of all American adults are "obese," while 69 % are "overweight" by current BMI standards [25]. As previously discussed, the development and clinical morbidity seen with OA is a combination of mechanical forces and systemic susceptibility, with recent research highlighting obesity as a major modifiable factor. Biomechanical studies have documented that force loads across the knee joint reach levels approximately 4 times the body weight during walking [26] and that obese individuals experience higher vertical ground reaction forces than normal weight individuals [27]. Likewise, studies have also documented that obese individuals have a four- to tenfold higher risk of developing OA than normal weight counterparts [26]. Additional to excessive mechanical force, a component of systemic inflammation induced by the large reserves of adipose tissue is observed in obese individuals [26, 28]. These effects are confirmed by the induction of OA in non-weight-bearing joints, where cartilage destruction is propagated by inflammation rather than mechanical force [29]. Therefore in an event to reduce mechanical stress, as well as the systemic effects of obesity, targeted weight loss and exercise are a mandatory recommendation by clinicians. Weight loss alone has been shown to curtail symptoms of existing knee OA in obese patients [30]. In addition to the health benefits associated with running and mild-moderate cardiovascular exercise, an overall anti-inflammatory and anti-catabolic systemic response has been documented with exercise to aid against joint destruction. A recent review of the literature by Gleeson et al. discusses three possible mechanisms for the anti-inflammatory effect of exercise, each outline in specific review [31]. These include (1) reduction in visceral fat mass, which reduces inflammatory cytokine signaling, (2) increased

production of anti-inflammatory cytokines from active skeletal muscle, and (3) decreased expression of toll-like receptors (TLRs) on monocytes and macrophages, exhibiting an overall downregulation of the body's innate immune activity [32–34]. Overall, though mechanisms continue to be elucidated, multiple review and meta-analyses confirm that exercise reduces pain and improves function and that aerobic exercise (compared to strengthening) is superior for longterm functional improvement [35–38].

With all of these findings, persistent theories exist that long-distance, endurance running causes acute, repetitive microtrauma to the cartilage extracellular matrix, and this, combined with normal aging and loss of cartilage resiliency, accelerates the joint toward arthritis. Advanced imaging techniques, when used in the acute setting following rigorous training or marathon distance events, have demonstrated abnormal marrow signals as well as cartilage abnormalities prior to running marathon distance [39], but these lesions were not significantly altered on repeat imaging after completing the marathon. Even in asymptomatic running knees, studies have demonstrated a large amount of knee lesions, especially in runners with higher training levels, suggesting repetitive trauma and the stigmata associated with early arthritic injury [39, 40]. However, often these abnormal findings are alterations in bone marrow edema (BME) signal, with some intrasubstance meniscal lesions, that fluctuate during the season and most of which are asymptomatic in professional distance runners. The authors of this recent study concluded that this fluctuation of BME during the season, not necessarily related to development of clinical complaint, suggests an active remodeling process that does not require acute intervention without further surveillance and monitoring, though future study is certainly warranted [41]. Acute injury to the ligaments, menisci, or kinetic chain musculature has been shown in biomechanical studies to increase the forces on specific regions of the joint surface, accelerating wear and progression to arthritis [42–44]. In this population, timely operative management (discussed later) is important in restoring congruency and effective motion of the articular surface if return to a prior level of activity is the goal. This notion of timely diagnosis and management is further confirmed by risk assessment studies, which document findings that a major risk factor for a running-related injury is injury in the past 12 months [45, 46].

Despite the aforementioned evidence, longitudinal clinical studies have failed to document an increased prevalence of OA in runners [47, 48] nor a significant association between running and OA [49]. On the contrary, aging runners appear to have less pain, better function, and lower rate of death than their non-running, elderly counterparts. A 13-year progressive study following overall health and disability in members of a running club and controls showed a 3.3 times higher rate of death in the control population, with runners boasting decreased disability over that time period [50]. Newer studies searching for mechanisms for the avoidance of OA in runners are examining biomechanical factors, such as the amount of contact pressure divided by strides, such that a decreased stride length or increased frequency of stride reduces the total biomechanical force across the joint [51, 52], though this requires further investigation and will be discussed later in discussion. Due to this breadth of clinical evidence, there is more importance on the musculoskeletal examination and diagnosis than ever before. A new wave of masters-aged, active patients will be presenting with a host of lower extremity orthopedic complaints, and the clinical implications of the expansive research are clear. There are no current associations between running and the development of arthritis, aerobic activity in the presence of existing arthritis is beneficial for pain relief and function, and an articular injury requires immediate medical intervention as continued running will lead to rapid development of post-traumatic arthritis. Therefore a clinician should continue to encourage running activity for its well-known health benefits but must be vigilant in the setting of acute injury and timely intervention.

Evaluation of Masters Athlete with Lower Extremity/Knee Pain Associated with Running

The effective treatment of a masters endurance athlete starts with timely and thorough evaluation. An accurate diagnosis allows for early, focused treatment protocols and provides the athlete the best chance at returning to sport in a timely fashion with preserved pre-injury function. In order to properly assess symptoms about the knee joint, a complete history and physical examination must be performed with the presentation of any new masters athlete with lower extremity symptoms. This should include discussion regarding history of the spine, hip, knee or foot, and ankle pain or past injuries, as all may present with referral pain to the knee or serve as a primary mechanism for deficient knee biomechanics. Inconsistencies observed with perceived mechanism of injury, constellation of symptoms, and response to previous treatment should direct clinicians to alternative diagnoses and work-up for this patient perceived pain about the knee.

Evaluation of the masters runner with lower extremity pain must begin with a thorough patient history. It is also critical for the physician to garner an accurate assessment of the present (and past) activity level of the presenting individual. Whether the patient is a masters-aged athlete attempting to start running or an experienced masters athlete with training goals has large implications on their injury risk, according to recent studies. Videbaek et al. demonstrated in a recent literature review that novice runners face a significantly greater risk of injury per 1000 h (frequency/1000 h) of running, with an average of 17.8 injuries (95 % CI 16.7–19.1) compared to 7.7 (95 % CI 6.9–8.7) for more experienced peers. Even more significant was that of a wide range of reported values from a minimum of 2.5 per 1000 h in long-distance track and field athletes to a maximum of 33.0 per 1000 h in a study of novice runners [53]. This reiterates that all populations can experience a running-related injury, and a focused clinical acumen must be applied to each presenting patient.

Specific information regarding onset of symptoms, accompanying symptoms, time since onset, alleviating or aggravating factors, and any history of traumatic mechanism are critical in directing patient evaluation and eventual treatment. One of the most important pieces of information obtained from the history is localization of pain. This can establish laterality and often locate a specific structure that is injured and acting as an active pain trigger. Failure to localize pain to a specific location may be suggestive of a global inflammatory process, neuropathic condition, or a multifactorial injury to knee joint and surrounding components (the muscle, tendon, ligament, etc.). Subjective patient complaints such as clicking, popping, and mechanical instability (i.e., "knee buckles and gives out") are suggestive of ligamentous or meniscal pathology, with resulting ineffective static knee stabilization. However, this clicking and popping can be confounded by crepitus. Crepitus, defined as the subjective cracks or pops around and within a synovial joint, present in two basic varieties: (1) painless condition best explained as a synovial fluid phase transformation or (2) painful, common condition that accompanies the osteoarthritic changes of a joint and represents bone on bone collision and grinding. Specific information regarding patient age, history of injury, and/or location of discomfort can help to elucidate between true mechanical instability, healthy crepitus, and osteoarthritic crepitus.

Radiography and advanced imaging modalities are also an effective way to screen for underlying degenerative changes or acute injuries to the articular surface. Plain film study is critical in establishing a reproducible objective comparison of joint health over time and across various symptom presentations. Standing, weight-bearing, anteroposterior radiographs should be a first step in the work-up of any knee pain in a masters runner. In addition, a 45° flexion weight-bearing posteroanterior radiograph may be more sensitive and superior in demonstrating early and subtle joint space narrowing [54]. The presence of osteophytes, flattening of the femoral condyles, sharpening of the tibial spines, chondrocalcinosis, and narrowing of the notch are several radiographic findings suggestive of an arthritic joint, which can be documented over time in the aging masters athlete. In addition, radiographic view of all the joint surfaces from the hip to foot, or the "long cassette view," can provide valuable information regarding the mechanical and anatomic axes of the lower extremities. Though unilateral articular joint space narrowing, and likewise varus or valgus joint alignment, has been seen as a manifestation of OA and joint pain, this is seen most commonly in chronic meniscal pathology or after a partial/total meniscectomy with or without accompanying ligamentous injury [42–44]. Therefore, specific questioning regarding past operative intervention, including obtaining specific operative reports, is critical to ascertain prior to establishing a plan of treatment. Despite these studies regarding post-traumatic narrowing, multiple studies have shown that baseline alignment patterns, either varus or valgus, in the setting of normal, healthy knees do not predispose runners to injury or arthritic changes [55, 56]. However, these imaging studies and an overall assessment of alignment are important and may provide context for lateral or medial-sided knee pain in the masters athlete, especially if a past surgical history exists. Advanced imaging modalities, such as MRI and CT scan, are often indicated for the work-up of soft tissue (cartilage, ligament, meniscus, etc.) injuries about the joint when minimal radiographic findings of OA are noted. Advanced imaging may also be obtained early for preoperative planning, if an operative condition exists. For the purpose of this text, advanced imaging should be reserved for situations where there are mechanical symptoms about the joint and gross instability or after nonoperative regimens have failed and an impending operative plan is developing.

The physical examination, often the last part of the patient visit, will direct the clinician's decision to pursue specific treatment or advanced imaging modalities. Close side-to-side comparisons should be made between limbs, to evaluate for subtle muscle weakness, effusion, muscle atrophy, or alignment issues as result of chronic injury or past operative intervention. In the event of long-standing unilateral medial or lateral knee joint OA, genu varum (or genu valgum, respectively) may be readily noticeable on exam of lower extremity alignment. This patient may be a candidate for mechanical, off-loading brace technology, the indications for which are collected only on close examination with radiographic support. As mentioned, specific attention should be paid to the specific location of pain over the knee. Focused examination, and knowledge of anatomic landmarks, can differentiate insertional hamstring pain from true medial joint line tenderness. This will prevent an unnecessary and costly imaging work-up and can start the athlete back on the path to recovery and return to sport in a more timely fashion. However, confirmation of joint line tenderness on examination is an important aspect of the exam and important in the early diagnosis of articular surface or meniscal pathology, both of which may need operative intervention and an immediate cessation of activity per treatment recommendations. An arthritic knee will typically present with warmth and swelling on observation and palpation of the joint. Examination of strength and motion will demonstrate weakness, often secondary to pain and/or atrophy of the quadriceps, and restricted range of motion secondary to incomplete flexion and extension in normal activity. However, this loss of motion may be less in active, persevering individuals. In some patients with intermediate to advance OA, significant crepitus and "locking" may be noticeable on testing of knee motion. Though this can mimic a meniscus injury, initial work-up radiographs that demonstrate significant arthritis will preclude the need for MRI and isolate OA as a causative factor for the mechanical symptoms. Though degenerative meniscus tears can accompany OA, the presence of joint space narrowing on 45-degree flexion weight-bearing X-rays removes an indication for advanced MRI imaging [13]. In the running athlete, a thorough examination of patellofemoral mechanics during motion can elucidate a major generator of anterior knee pain while active. Evaluation includes tilt, glide, and palpation for tenderness and can be correlated with patella-specific radiographic tests

(i.e., "sunrise" or 45-degree axial Merchant view). With patella testing, comparisons of movement, crepitus, and tenderness to palpation must be associated with contralateral leg testing and can be used in the diagnosis of subtle osteochondral lesions or injury of the patella. Often, these patients will complain of anterior knee pain while going up or down stairs, while the extensor mechanism applies the largest amount of compression of the patella into the femoral notch. Unifying patient history and physical exam is the most important part of the orthopedic examination of the aging runner in the clinic.

Treatment of Masters Athlete: Nonoperative vs. Operative Management

Once thorough evaluation is complete, the clinician must produce a treatment plan that addresses both the functional level and the expectations of the patient. Often, this will present with an initial decision algorithm regarding the need for advanced imaging modalities and the likelihood of operative versus nonoperative treatment. As mentioned, an aging runner that presents with effusion and mechanical symptoms that have minimal findings of OA on plain radiograph would be a good candidate for an MRI. An older athlete, with documented radiographic changes suggestive of progressing OA and history of significant pain with activity despite lifestyle modifications and therapeutics, may not need advanced imaging, rather an early discussion regarding the role of arthroplasty in the active patient. Despite the slow progression and predictable, stepwise progression of OA, aging athletes need personalized care decisions from their healthcare providers in order to preserve activity and level of function into their older years. Recent reviews of diagnosis and treatment recommendations in the aging athlete population document that optimal outcomes are achieved when activity is preserved, with personalized training protocols and medical management of the aging athlete [18, 57]. Therefore in this chapter section, the algorithmic approach to the clinical management of early and advanced OA will be discussed while remembering that all treatment decisions are a balance between level of function, pain, and risk of progressive disease in this population.

In the aging population with knee OA, the paradigm for the management has been symptom management, with the goal of delaying surgery (i.e., arthroplasty) for as long as the patient can tolerate. This approach consists of exercise modification, targeted muscle training, bracing and orthoses, pharmaceuticals, intra-articular corticosteroids, and viscosupplementation. Some newer paradigms include the use of biologically active compounds, such as platelet-rich plasma (PRP), bone marrow aspirate concentrate (BMAC), and mesenchymal stem cells (MSCs), in an effort to stimulate the growth and regeneration of new articular cartilage. Though MSCs and BMAC have shown some anti-inflammatory effect and ability to aid in disease progression in animal models, translation to clinical use is lacking [58]. The current state of biologics advancement will be discussed later in this section.

Initial treatment paradigms for an aging athlete with knee pain, and findings suggestive of early arthritis without anatomic pathology, typically start with physical therapy and a brief stint of rest/activity modification. This should be paired with anti-inflammatory therapy with nonsteroidal anti-inflammatory medications (NSAIDs), for a multi-targeted approach of care. At this current time, large review studies have revealed no evidence for a specific NSAID as superior in the management of early OA and therefore recommend that NSAID selection be guided by relative safety, patient preference, and cost [59]. For therapy, multiple large RCTs have demonstrated that muscle-strengthening exercises in addition to low weight-bearing exercise is effective in relieving pain and also restoring kinetic chain balance. Patient cooperation and persistence with scheduled therapy are related to this success, as studies have demonstrated that beneficial effects of therapy can be lost as early as 6 months [36]. In patients that desire to continue running and participate in athletic competitions despite early symptoms of arthritis, knee bracing and orthoses are a common treatment

with the main goal of reducing symptoms, not necessarily eliminating symptoms, and therefore improving athletic function. Though there are a large variety of neoprene knee sleeves available for stabilization and relief of minor symptoms, review articles have shown these to be no superior to placebo for the alleviation of pain and symptoms [60]. However, some patients will present to clinic having already tried over-the-counter sleeves and braces, and if these are providing comfort, there is no harm in continuation of this therapy. As mentioned in the evaluation section, the best patient population most suited for bracing therapy is the symptomatic, passively correctable varus or valgus disease of less than 10 degrees [61]. The mechanical goal of these braces is the shift the axis of force transfer through an unaffected region of joint, decreasing symptoms without restricting activity. With this concept, there is evidence from gait analysis that shoe orthoses, specifically lateral wedge orthoses, have been effective in reducing pain and increasing function in patients with isolated medial compartment knee OA [62]. Despite these findings, there is insufficient data for the endorsement or recommendation by the American Association of Orthopaedic Surgeons (AAOS), and this evaluation is presented within the current guideline for non-arthroplasty management of OA [63]. Therefore, in an attempt to achieve return to sport for a presenting aging athlete, a trial of bracing or orthotics when properly indicated may achieve successful results, but expectations must be shaped accordingly given inconclusive literature-based efficacy.

After attempted physical therapy and bracing with concomitant NSAID therapy, the next line of therapy is intra-articular injection therapy, either with viscosupplementation or corticosteroid. Within a healthy joint, hyaluronate is a main component of synovial fluid and articular cartilage [64]. It provides the lubrication and shock-absorbing capacity of the articular fluid and surface. In the pathologic process of OA, the hyaluronate becomes depolymerized from its native structure and cleared at a faster rate which puts the joint at a biomechanical disadvantage by reducing the viscoelasticity of the synovial fluid

[65–67]. Based on these documented changes in an arthritic joint, exogenous intra-articular hyaluronate is available for supplementation aimed at alleviating the symptoms of knee OA. Several meta-analyses have been performed to assess the efficacy of this treatment, but a combination of variable findings, study heterogeneity, and publication bias has led to inconclusive evidence for clinical use. In addition to highlighting this evidence, most recent conclusions published in the *New England Journal of Medicine* document a range of modest effectiveness to minimal effect when compared to placebo [65]. As mentioned previously, inflammation is a major characteristic of the OA joint, leading to prolonged cytokine and innate immune reaction which is implicated in the progressive destruction of articular cartilage. Likewise, intra-articular corticosteroid was identified as a means to dampen the immune reaction, decrease synovial inflammation, and promote relief of OA symptoms. Recent systematic reviews of the clinical efficacy of corticosteroid (triamcinolone) have shown fast-acting but short-lasting clinically significant improvements in pain and function [68]. Past studies comparing corticosteroid to hyaluronic acid injection have concluded that steroid injection produced a rapid maximum benefit (within 2 weeks), while pain reduction and functional improvement were significantly better at the 3- and 6-month follow-up period [69]. A recent publication has documented the promising clinical effect of an extended-release formulation of triamcinolone, which was found to be superior to current standard over a range of 1–12 weeks [70]. More future study is needed to better quantify the clinical effect of longer-lasting, extended-release formulations of these intra-articular pharmaceuticals. As it stands currently, corticosteroid injections are a valuable clinical tool for rapid, short-lasting clinical relief from symptoms associated with early to advanced OA of the knee. However, long-term symptomatic management is dependent upon other treatment modalities, as the effect of intra-articular is only temporary and has not been shown to stop or slow disease progression.

Outside of the widely used corticosteroid and hyaluronate injections, the use of biologically active intra-articular therapies has gained significant momentum in athletic and recreational populations. However, the clinical use of biologic therapy with platelet-rich plasma (PRP) or mesenchymal stem cells (MSCs) has been plagued by significant study heterogeneity and variable results across studies, making conclusions and clinical advancement difficult. Aside from high cost of therapy, the standardization of therapy across research studies is lacking, with specific information regarding ideal platelet concentration in PRP and ideal dosing schedule, and long-term safety data have not been well characterized [71]. However, recent meta-analyses state that intra-articular PRP shows improvement in patient outcomes at 6 months that are maintained for up to a year. From the studies, these improvements were noted as clinically relevant development for decreased pain and increased function compared to control therapy [72]. There is a need for more prospective studies with multicenter collaboration to advance the role of biologic therapies for articular cartilage injury and early arthritis into the active, aging population. In an attempt to evaluate the main injectable therapies for early OA, the most recent randomized control trial comparing intra-articular PRP injections to viscosupplementation (hyaluronic acid injections) showed that PRP did not provide a superior clinical improvement when compared to hyaluronic acid therapy [73]. In regard to intra-articular MSCs for the treatment of early OA, animal studies have shown significant progress in restoring articular cartilage, with improvement in both histologic and radiographic studies when compared to controls [74]. When compared to surgical interventions, such as autologous chondrocyte implantation (ACI) or microfracture, intra-articular MSCs have shown similar efficacy. However, additional review shows that no human studies have compared intra-articular MSCs to non-MSC techniques in the absence of surgery [75]. Future prospective, multicenter studies comparing PRP, MSCs, and other intra-articular injectable therapies for the symptomatic relief of

OA are needed for biologics to emerge as a viable therapy for relief with quick return to sport and activity.

In the treatment of the aging, masters-level athlete, surgical intervention is often warranted when nonoperative management of symptoms no longer reduces pain or restores function. However, there are instances where a presentation of suspected arthritic knee pain has an acute surgical indication. For example, acute or symptomatic meniscal lesions, osteochondral defects, loose bodies, and ligamentous injuries, appropriately confirmed with MRI testing, are several pathologies that indicate an operative management paradigm. These are the variety of injuries that are most prevalent in athletic, sport-participating populations and have the highest documented rate of progress to post-traumatic arthritis [19, 76]. It is these types of intra-articular injury that disrupt the stability of articulation and the distribution of contact forces, serving to propagate cell death, inflammation, and a cyclic pattern of cartilage destruction. Therefore, it is critical that ligament and meniscal repair surgeries, with the goal of restoring normal anatomic biomechanics, be performed in a prophylactic manner to prevent repetitive trauma and early onset arthritic processes. In the event that meniscal and ligamentous stability is intact in an early or advanced OA knee, other surgical options remain for the preservation of function and activity level. These include arthroscopy, high tibial osteotomy, and arthroplasty. Each of these procedures has specific indications and must first begin with a discussion between athlete and clinician to clarify expectations for postoperative outcome and return to sport. Arthroscopic intervention is a common but controversial technique for an osteoarthritic knee. Studies have shown that approximately 50–75 % of patients have an initial benefit post debridement. However, this same study documents that 15 % of patients experience progression to total knee arthroplasty (TKA) within 1 year of arthroscopic debridement [77]. Other studies that support arthroscopy argue that the degree of disease (mild vs.

severe) is an independent predictor of outcome and that there is much clinical benefit to be obtained when patients are properly selected, while others (i.e., end-stage OA or mechanical alignment) are contraindicated from the procedure [78, 79]. However, other recent studies report unfavorably upon arthroscopic debridement of the early osteoarthritic joint, stating that this "clean-out procedure" has not been shown to have any beneficial effect or prevention of disease progression and that it provides no additional benefit to an otherwise optimized patient [80, 81]. Though not shown to be beneficial in slowing the progression of disease, the aforementioned studies that suggest benefit in mild, early arthritis knees will continue to keep the option of arthroscopic knee surgery available for competitive yet aging athletes as they strive to preserve their competitive function. However, the risks of surgical intervention and future need for arthroplasty must be discussed with patients prior to this treatment. Along the same lines in preserving athletic function, high tibial osteotomy (HTO) is a popular operative procedure for the patient with isolated, unicompartmental disease. As the surgical counterpart of mechanical braces, the goal of these procedures is to shift the mechanical axis of the knee to an area that is not affected by degenerative changes (i.e., remove the arthritic area from the zone of weight bearing). The significant benefit of this procedure is that while the weight-bearing zone is ideally located to a healthy area of articular cartilage, there is no modification of activity level needed once healed from the initial operation. It is most commonly implicated in treatment of unicompartment varus or valgus OA and is emerging as a technique used in conjunction with biologic cartilage restoration procedures [61]. It will not be effective in global arthritic degeneration and therefore must be reserved for the ideal active patient. Multiple studies suggest positive results, with one such study stating good to excellent function in 77 % at 17 years [82], while another reports survivorship of 98 % and 90 % at 10- and 15-year follow-up, respectively, for HTO [83]. A recent review summarizes the risk factors that contribute to the deterioration of an osteotomy procedure, citing time (i.e., continued wear and tear), increasing age, and obesity as factors shown by the literature to decrease the long-term effectiveness of this procedure [61]. However, if an osteotomy procedure can provide 10–15 years of high functional ability (i.e., continued ability to run) prior to mandatory arthroplasty procedure, among the running population, it would be difficult not to call this a great success. After osteotomy, unicondylar knee arthroplasty (UKA) and total knee arthroplasty (TKA) are typically a last resort option for runners despite their effectiveness in relieving pain and symptoms of OA, mainly due to the propensity for wearing out of polyethylene spaces and loosening of components in high-demand individuals. However, due to advances in design and increased durability of polyethylene, documented survivorship rates continue to increase. A study performed by Pennington et al. focused on UKA in the younger (<60) high-demand active patients and demonstrated an HSS score of excellent in 93 % of patients and good in 7 % [84]. Multiple studies in younger patients document high survival rates and low revision rates; however, the activity level is not well documented [85, 86]. Although it has been consistently shown that TKA is highly regarded and superior for the relief of symptoms, studies without documentation of activity level provide little benefit for the active, running population who may require TKA. Therefore, as the amount of arthroplasty performed in the future decades increases, more focused studies are needed to elucidate how aggressive runners can be in attempting return to sport after arthroplasty procedure. In conclusion to these operative options, it is clear that clinicians must present the risks of significant activity loss in a population of athletes focused upon return to sport. Surgical options for OA should be reserved until all nonoperative treatment paradigms have been attempted. Though runners can continue high levels of activity with osteotomy, and in most cases a UKA, important discussions regarding the expectations of return to preoperative function levels are needed to achieve satisfactory patient-reported outcomes.

Conclusion (Summary of Evaluation and Treatment, "Barefoot" Running, Role of Diet, and Cross-Training for Healthy Running)

The development of OA of the knee is a multifactorial issue. Clinicians must be able to understand and discuss a wide array of approaches to manage this disease in an active, aging population. Genetic susceptibility, aging, and past injury to the articular surface are well-defined risk factors, which accompany biomechanical principles in our ability to predict the development of joint pathology. Focused evaluation of all aging runners that present with knee complaints and any range of documented OA is needed to provide optimal treatment recommendations. Modifiable lifestyle factors, including diet, level of activity, and weight, have been shown to be effective in the modification of arthritis symptoms and the maintenance of function. The use of neoprene sleeves, off-loader braces, and supportive footwear has been shown in certain studies to be equal to or better than placebo in the relief of symptoms. The strongest conclusion that can be drawn is that there are specific circumstances (i.e., isolated medial unicompartmental OA) where unloader braces will be of best utility and other times where a brace may facilitate confidence if only to start activity and movement of the afflicted joint. The use of biologic compounds has enormous potential for the preservation of joint physiology and slowing of OA progression, but more study is needed before this potential can be realized and applied in clinical setting. Viscosupplementation and corticosteroid injections have their role in management to provide periods of symptom-free activity, but are not effective in slowing or preventing disease progression. Surgical intervention can be effective in a selected population of patients but is accompanied by serious risk of decreased function and inability to return to previous level of activity. Specifically, more data will need to be collected in order to recommend arthroplasty procedures to runners who continue to strive for high-demand activity as wear-out rates and aseptic loosening have been directly linked to activity levels. There is no supported increase risk in the development of OA in the knees of healthy aging runners, but clinicians should not recommend running as a primary mode of exercise in severe, advance knee osteoarthritis. For this patient population, alternative lower-impact modalities (biking, swimming, low contact weight training) should be recommended.

A recent Cochrane review by Yeung et al. [60] evaluated a broad set of interventions, including specific exercises, modification of training schedules, orthotics, and specific footwear and socks intended to prevent or reduce the incidence of running-related overuse injuries. Of the reviewed studies, 19/25 involved service personnel, while only three focused on general population athletes. Though this likely does not address the masters athlete or recreational runner, the findings concluded that the clinical evidence for most interventions is weak, with few prospective, low-bias studies [60]. Based on previous discussion within this chapter, this type of review is not surprising as it is difficult to evaluate the subjective effectiveness in such a high-demand, heterogeneous population of athletes. This lack of evidence will not stop athletes from pursuing their craft, and therefore clinicians must be accepting of a multi-tooled approach to this multifactorial disease. The emergence of "medically based running analysis" and designated sports performance centers are focused on tailoring training plans and injury prevention techniques to the individual runner [87]. In order to work in concert with these emerging concepts, clinicians must familiarize themselves with the newest trends in running. Given the high percentage of all-aged individuals that use running as aerobic exercise and the high proportion who suffer running-related injury, the running community is frequented by trends and new technologies that promise faster recovery and pain-free running. An example of this would be the minimalist, or barefoot, running movement that has spread rapidly across the running and fitness community. With less structure, less arch support, and lower heel drop (distance in height between heel and forefoot) profiles and softer, more forgiving fabrics, running shoes have sought to create a "barefoot" sensation that forces the

foot, ankle, and knee to absorb shock in a natural, biomechanically favorable way. Though shoe companies are quick to state that progression to these shoes must be scheduled and gradual, so as to not overload the knee, midfoot, and heel-cord structures, there are minimal longitudinal studies to document the effect of this barefoot phenomenon. A recent study, seeking to evaluate the biomechanical and runner adaptations to the barefoot or minimalist running shoe, documented some of the first literature regarding the topic. This study by Perkins et al. found moderate evidence to state that barefoot apparel results in overall less maximum vertical ground reaction forces, less extension moment and power absorption at the knee, less ground contact time, shorter stride length, and increased stride frequency among other variables [88]. Coupled with findings from other recent research in *The American Journal of Sports Medicine*, shorter stride length and increased stride frequency may decrease or at least not increase propensity for running injuries. However, the same study stated that one stride length does not appear to be clearly superior and that different foot strike styles may predispose runners to injury [89]. Not surprisingly, it can be concluded that the need for future well-designed RCTs testing the biomechanical effect of shoes, stride length, and running cadence is important to delineate recommendations and find a regimen to suit runners of all sizes and ability levels.

Regardless of the age or experience level of the masters-aged runners that present, time must be spent in the clinical visit discussing the importance of balanced diet and role of strength and resistance exercise in running at optimal health. Full dietary recommendations for athletic performance are available through multiple government resources, such as the US Anti-Doping Agency   (www.usada.org/resources/nutrition). Optimal dietary and hydration methods, in addition to balanced training and recovery, are global principles that can be reinforced by clinicians for all athletes. Even though running requires a combination of flexibility and strength, runners can achieve improved form and function by employing a full-body fitness regimen. The following recommendations are derived directly from the

US Department of HHS and should be a rubric for a clinical exercise protocol. Adults should participate in a balance of strength and training exercises in addition to >150 min/week of moderate-intensity or >75 min/week of vigorous-intensity aerobic activity. Strength training should be incorporated approximately 2–4 day/week, for approximately 30 min per session. In order to allow for adequate recovery and to avoid injury, 48 h of rest are recommended in between strength sessions. This type of routine can achieve an increase of approximately 2–3 times in strength in a period of only 4 months and can help improve the dynamics of the kinetic chain, making a faster and more efficient runner. In the event of an injury, prior to presentation in a medical clinic, first aid principles that include rest, ice, and anti-inflammatories should always be reiterated by clinicians to their practicing athletes. And lastly, athletes must have a sense of appropriate level of exertion based on their current level of fitness. Overtraining and inability to perform a mixture of strength and cardio exercises increase the risk of an injury, which will only set an athlete back in terms of performing at optimum function.

Overall, prolonged healthy running in the aging athlete is dependent upon a balance of injury-free running, intermittent cross-training, and the practice of healthy dietary principles. Practice of these concepts will increase the ability of an aging runner to participate at a high level of function. In order to promote injury-free running, clinicians must employ prompt diagnosis and accurate management aimed at relieving symptoms and preserving articular function. Prompt referral to a surgical specialist is needed when an intra-articular injury exists, as these are the most likely cause of post-traumatic OA and a premature decline in running function. Clinicians should encourage continued participation in running for the known health benefits and to preserve function in the presence of early OA of the knee. Health professionals should always address the goal of staying active and healthy and may explore other recommended activity options in patients with severe OA for whom high-impact running is no longer recommended.

References

1. Running USA. 2014 Running USA annual marathon report. 2015. runningusa.org
2. World Association of Masters Athletes, International Association of Athletics Federation (IAAF). 2015. www.world-masters-athletics.org
3. Wright VJ. Masterful care of the aging triathlete. Sports Med Arthrosc. 2012;20(4):231–6.
4. Foster C, Wright G, Battista RA, Porcari JP. Training in the aging athlete. Curr Sports Med Rep. 2007;6(3):200–6.
5. Leigey D, Irrgang J, Francis K, Cohen P, Wright V. Participation in high-impact sports predicts bone mineral density in senior Olympic athletes. Sports Health. 2009;1(6):508–13.
6. Helmick CG, Felson DT, Lawrence RC, Gabriel S, Hirsch R, Kwoh CK, et al. National Arthritis Data Workgroup. Estimates of the prevalence of arthritis and other rheumatic conditions in the United States. Part I. Arthritis Rheum. 2008;58(1):15–25.
7. Murray CJ, Vos T, Lozano R, et al. Disability-adjusted life years (DALYs) for 291 diseases and injuries in 21 regions, 1990–2010: a systematic analysis for the Global Burden of Disease Study 2010. Lancet. 2012;380(9859):2197–223.
8. Lawrence RC, Felson DT, Helmick CG, Arnold LM, Choi H, Deyo RA, et al. National Arthritis Data Workgroup. Estimates of the prevalence of arthritis and other rheumatic conditions in the United States. Part II. Arthritis Rheum. 2008;58(1):26–35.
9. Dieppe PA, Lohmander LS. Pathogenesis and management of pain in osteoarthritis. Lancet. 2005;365(9463):965–73.
10. Goldring MB, Goldring SR. Osteoarthritis. J Cell Physiol. 2007;213(3):626–34.
11. Buckwalter JA, Mow VC, Ratcliffe A. Restoration of injured or degenerated articular cartilage. J Am Acad Orthop Surg. 1994;2(4):192–201.
12. Buckwalter JA, Brown TD. Joint injury, repair, and remodeling: roles in post-traumatic osteoarthritis. Clin Orthop Relat Res. 2004;423:7–16.
13. Cole BJ, Harner CD. Degenerative arthritis of the knee in active patients: evaluation and management. J Am Acad Orthop Surg. 1999;7(6):389–402.
14. Amoako AO, Pujalte GG. Osteoarthritis in young, active, and athletic individuals. Clin Med Insights Arthritis Musculoskelet Disord. 2014;7:27–32.
15. Hunter DJ. Osteoarthritis. Best Pract Res Clin Rheumatol. 2011;25(6):801–14.
16. Kirkendall DT, Garrett Jr WE. Management of the retired athlete with osteoarthritis of the knee. Cartilage. 2012;3 Suppl 1:69S–76.
17. Neogi T, Zhang Y. Epidemiology of osteoarthritis. Rheum Dis Clin North Am. 2013;39(1):1–19.
18. Huleatt JB, Campbell KJ, Laprade RF. Nonoperative treatment approach to knee osteoarthritis in the master athlete. Sports Health. 2014;6(1):56–62.

19. Buckwalter JA. Sports, joint injury, and posttraumatic osteoarthritis. J Orthop Sports Phys Ther. 2003; 33(10):578–88.
20. Buckwalter JA. The role of mechanical forces in the initiation and progression of osteoarthritis. HSS J. 2012;8(1):37–8.
21. Anderson DD, Chubinskaya S, Guilak F, Martin JA, Oegema TR, Olson SA, et al. Post-traumatic osteoarthritis: improved understanding and opportunities for early intervention. J Orthop Res. 2011;29:802–9.
22. Brown TD, Johnston RC, Saltzman CL, Marsh JL, Buckwalter JA. Posttraumatic osteoarthritis: a first estimate of incidence, prevalence, and burden of disease. J Orthop Trauma. 2006;20(10):739–44.
23. Arokoski JP, Jurvelin JS, Väätäinen U, Helminen HJ. Normal and pathological adaptations of articular cartilage to joint loading. Scand J Med Sci Sports. 2000;10(4):186–98.
24. Griffin TM, Guilak F. The role of mechanical loading in the onset and progression of osteoarthritis. Exerc Sport Sci Rev. 2005;33(4):195–200.
25. Ogden CL, Carroll MD, Kit BK, Flegal KM. Prevalence of childhood and adult obesity in the United States, 2011-2012. JAMA. 2014;311(8):806–14.
26. Felson DT. Does excess weight cause osteoarthritis, and if so, why? Ann Rheum Dis. 1996;55(9):668–70.
27. Messier SP, Pater M, Beavers DP, Legault C, Loeser RF, Hunter DJ, et al. Influences of alignment and obesity on knee joint loading in osteoarthritic gait. Osteoarthritis Cartilage. 2014;22(7):912–7.
28. Issa RI, Griffin TM. Pathobiology of obesity and osteoarthritis: integrating biomechanics and inflammation. Pathobiol Aging Age Relat Dis. 2012;2(2012). pii: 17470.
29. Griffin TM, Fermor B, Huebner JL, et al. Diet-induced obesity differentially regulates behavioral, biomechanical, and molecular risk factors for osteoarthritis in mice. Arthritis Res Ther. 2010;12(4):R130.
30. Henriksen M, Christensen R, Danneskiold-Samsøe B, Bliddal H. Changes in lower extremity muscle mass and muscle strength after weight loss in obese patients with knee osteoarthritis: a prospective cohort study. Arthritis Rheum. 2012;64(2):438–42.
31. Gleeson M, Bishop NC, Stensel DJ, Lindley MR, Mastana SS, Nimmo MA. The anti-inflammatory effects of exercise: mechanisms and implications for the prevention and treatment of disease. Nat Rev Immunol. 2011;11(9):607–15.
32. Petersen AM, Pedersen BK. The anti-inflammatory effect of exercise. J Appl Physiol. 2005;98(4):1154–62. Review.
33. Mathur N, Pedersen BK. Exercise as a mean to control low-grade systemic inflammation. Mediators Inflamm. 2008;2008:109502. doi:10.1155/2008/109502. Epub 11 Jan 2009.
34. Flynn MG, McFarlin BK. Toll-like receptor 4: link to the anti-inflammatory effects of exercise? Exerc Sport Sci Rev. 2006;34(4):176–81.
35. Bennell K, Hinman R. Exercise as a treatment for osteoarthritis. Curr Opin Rheumatol. 2005;17(5):634–40.
36. van Baar ME, Dekker J, Oostendorp RA, Bijl D, Voorn TB, Bijlsma JW. Effectiveness of exercise in patients with osteoarthritis of hip or knee: nine months' follow up. Ann Rheum Dis. 2001;60(12): 1123–30.
37. Pelland L, Brosseau L, Wells G. Efficacy of strengthening exercises for osteoarthritis (part I): a meta-analysis. Phys Ther Rev. 2004;9:77–108.
38. Brosseau L, Pelland L, Wells G. Efficacy of aerobic exercises for osteoarthritis (part II): a meta-analysis. Phys Ther Rev. 2004;9:125–45.
39. Stahl R, Luke A, Ma CB, Krug R, Steinbach L, Majumdar S, et al. Prevalence of pathologic findings in asymptomatic knees of marathon runners before and after a competition in comparison with physically active subjects-a 3.0 T magnetic resonance imaging study. Skeletal Radiol. 2008;37(7):627–38.
40. Schueller-Weidekamm C, Schueller G, Uffmann M, Bader T. Incidence of chronic knee lesions in long-distance runners based on training level: findings at MRI. Eur J Radiol. 2006;58(2):286–93.
41. Kornaat PR, Van de Velde SK. Bone marrow edema lesions in the professional runner. Am J Sports Med. 2014;42(5):1242–6.
42. Neuman P, Englund M, Kostogiannis I, Fridén T, Roos H, Dahlberg LE. Prevalence of tibiofemoral osteoarthritis 15 years after nonoperative treatment of anterior cruciate ligament injury: a prospective cohort study. Am J Sports Med. 2008;36(9):1717–25.
43. Magnussen RA, Duthon V, Servien E, Neyret P. Anterior cruciate ligament reconstruction and osteoarthritis: evidence from long-term follow-up and potential solutions. Cartilage. 2013;4 Suppl 3:22S–6.
44. Ajuied A, Wong F, Smith C, Norris M, Earnshaw P, Back D, et al. Anterior cruciate ligament injury and radiologic progression of knee osteoarthritis: a systematic review and meta-analysis. Am J Sports Med. 2014;42(9):2242–52.
45. Saragiotto BT, Yamato TP, Hespanhol Jr LC, Rainbow MJ, Davis IS, Lopes AD. What are the main risk factors for running-related injuries? Sports Med. 2014;44(8):1153–63.
46. Wen DY. Risk factors for overuse injuries in runners. Curr Sports Med Rep. 2007;6(5):307–13.
47. Buckwalter JA, Lane NE. Athletics and osteoarthritis. Am J Sports Med. 1997;25(6):873–81.
48. Chakravarty EF, Hubert HB, Lingala VB, Zatarain E, Fries JF. Long distance running and knee osteoarthritis. A prospective study. Am J Prev Med. 2008; 35(2):133–8.
49. Willick SE, Hansen PA. Running and osteoarthritis. Clin Sports Med. 2010;29(3):417–28.
50. Wang BW, Ramey DR, Schettler JD, Hubert HB, Fries JF. Postponed development of disability in elderly runners: a 13-year longitudinal study. Arch Intern Med. 2002;162(20):2285–94.
51. Miller RH, Edwards WB, Brandon SC, Morton AM, Deluzio KJ. Why don't most runners get knee osteoarthritis? A case for per-unit-distance loads. Med Sci Sports Exerc. 2014;46(3):572–9.

52. Schubert AG, Kempf J, Heiderscheit BC. Influence of stride frequency and length on running mechanics: a systematic review. Sports Health. 2014;6(3):210–7.

53. Videbæk S, Bueno AM, Nielsen RO, Rasmussen S. Incidence of running-related injuries per 1000 h of running in different types of runners: a systematic review and meta-analysis. Sports Med. 2015;45(7): 1017–26.

54. Rosenberg TD, Paulos LE, Parker RD, Coward DB, Scott SM. The forty-five-degree posteroanterior flexion weight-bearing radiograph of the knee. J Bone Joint Surg Am. 1988;70(10):1479–83.

55. Wen DY, Puffer JC, Schmalzried TP. Lower extremity alignment and risk of overuse injuries in runners. Med Sci Sports Exerc. 1997;29(10):1291–8.

56. Wen DY, Puffer JC, Schmalzried TP. Injuries in runners: a prospective study of alignment. Clin J Sport Med. 1998;8(3):187–94.

57. Tayrose GA, Beutel BG, Cardone DA, Sherman OH. The masters athlete: a review of current exercise and treatment recommendations. Sports Health. 2015;7(3):270–6.

58. Wolfstadt JI, Cole BJ, Ogilvie-Harris DJ, Viswanathan S, Chahal J. Current concepts: the role of mesenchymal stem cells in the management of knee osteoarthritis. Sports Health. 2015;7(1):38–44.

59. Watson M, Brookes ST, Faulkner A, Kirwan J. WITHDRAWN: non-aspirin, non-steroidal anti-inflammatory drugs for treating osteoarthritis of the knee. Cochrane Database Syst Rev. 2007;1, CD000142.

60. Yeung SS, Yeung EW, Gillespie LD. Interventions for preventing lower limb soft-tissue running injuries. Cochrane Database Syst Rev. 2011;(7):CD001256.

61. Feeley BT, Gallo RA, Sherman S, Williams RJ. Management of osteoarthritis of the knee in the active patient. J Am Acad Orthop Surg. 2010;18(7):406–16.

62. Krohn K. Footwear alterations and bracing as treatments for knee osteoarthritis. Curr Opin Rheumatol. 2005;17(5):653–6.

63. Sanders JO, Murray J, Gross L. Non-arthroplasty treatment of osteoarthritis of the knee. J Am Acad Orthop Surg. 2014;22(4):256–60.

64. Balazs EA, Watson D, Duff IF, Roseman S. Hyaluronic acid in synovial fluid. I. Molecular parameters of hyaluronic acid in normal and arthritis human fluids. Arthritis Rheum. 1967;10(4):357–76.

65. Hunter DJ. Viscosupplementation for osteoarthritis of the knee. N Engl J Med. 2015;372(11):1040–7.

66. Conrozier T, Chevalier X. Long-term experience with hylan GF-20 in the treatment of knee osteoarthritis. Expert Opin Pharmacother. 2008;9(10):1797–804.

67. Balazs EA, Denlinger JL. Viscosupplementation: a new concept in the treatment of osteoarthritis. J Rheumatol Suppl. 1993;39:3–9.

68. Hepper CT, Halvorson JJ, Duncan ST, Gregory AJ, Dunn WR, Spindler KP. The efficacy and duration of intra-articular corticosteroid injection for knee osteoarthritis: a systematic review of level I studies. J Am Acad Orthop Surg. 2009;17(10):638–46.

69. Caborn D, Rush J, Lanzer W, Parenti D, Murray C. A randomized, single-blind comparison of the efficacy and tolerability of hylan G-F 20 and triamcinolone hexacetonide in patients with osteoarthritis of the knee. J Rheumatol. 2004;31(2):333–43.

70. Bodick N, Lufkin J, Willwerth C, Kumar A, Bolognese J, Schoonmaker C, et al. An intra-articular, extended-release formulation of triamcinolone acetonide prolongs and amplifies analgesic effect in patients with osteoarthritis of the knee: a randomized clinical trial. J Bone Joint Surg Am. 2015;97(11):877–88.

71. Everts PA, Brown Mahoney C, Hoffmann JJ, Schönberger JP, Box HA, van Zundert A, et al. Platelet-rich plasma preparation using three devices: implications for platelet activation and platelet growth factor release. Growth Factors. 2006;24(3):165–71.

72. Campbell KA, Saltzman BM, Mascarenhas R, Khair MM, Verma NN, Bach BR Jr, Cole BJ. Does Intra-articular Platelet-Rich Plasma Injection Provide Clinically Superior Outcomes Compared With Other Therapies in the Treatment of Knee Osteoarthritis? A Systematic Review of Overlapping Meta-analyses. Arthroscopy. 2015;31(11):2213–21.

73. Filardo G, Di Matteo B, Di Martino A, Merli ML, Cenacchi A, Fornasari P, et al. Platelet-rich plasma intra-articular knee injections show no superiority versus viscosupplementation: a randomized controlled trial. Am J Sports Med. 2015;43(7):1575–82.

74. Mokbel AN, El Tookhy OS, Shamaa AA, Rashed LA, Sabry D, El Sayed AM. Homing and reparative effect of intra-articular injection of autologus mesenchymal stem cells in osteoarthritic animal model. BMC Musculoskelet Disord. 2011;12:259.

75. Counsel PD, Bates D, Boyd R, Connell DA. Cell therapy in joint disorders. Sports Health. 2015;7(1):27–37.

76. Luyten FP, Denti M, Filardo G, Kon E, Engebretsen L. Definition and classification of early osteoarthritis of the knee. Knee Surg Sports Traumatol Arthrosc. 2012;20(3):401–6.

77. Dervin GF, Stiell IG, Rody K, Grabowski J. Effect of arthroscopic débridement for osteoarthritis of the knee on health-related quality of life. J Bone Joint Surg Am. 2003;85-A(1):10–9.

78. Day B. The indications for arthroscopic debridement for osteoarthritis of the knee. Orthop Clin North Am. 2005;36(4):413–7.

79. Aaron RK, Skolnick AH, Reinert SE, Ciombor DM. Arthroscopic débridement for osteoarthritis of the knee. J Bone Joint Surg Am. 2006;88(5):936–43.

80. Kirkley A, Birmingham TB, Litchfield RB, Giffin JR, Willits KR, Wong CJ, et al. A randomized trial of arthroscopic surgery for osteoarthritis of the knee. N Engl J Med. 2008;359(11):1097–107.

81. Howell SM. The role of arthroscopy in treating osteoarthritis of the knee in the older patient. Orthopedics. 2010;33(9):652.

82. Omori G, Koga Y, Miyao M, Takemae T, Sato T, Yamagiwa H. High tibial osteotomy using two threaded pins and figure-of-eight wiring fixation for medial knee osteoarthritis: 14 to 24 years follow-up results. J Orthop Sci. 2008;13(1):39–45.

83. Akizuki S, Shibakawa A, Takizawa T, Yamazaki I, Horiuchi H. The long-term outcome of high tibial osteotomy: a ten to 20-year follow-up. J Bone Joint Surg Br. 2008;90(5):592–6.

84. Pennington DW, Swienckowski JJ, Lutes WB, Drake GN. Unicompartmental knee arthroplasty in patients sixty years of age or younger. J Bone Joint Surg Am. 2003;85-A(10):1968–73.

85. Spahn G, Mückley T, Kahl E, Hofmann GO. Factors affecting the outcome of arthroscopy in medial-compartment osteoarthritis of the knee. Arthroscopy. 2006;22(11):1233–40.

86. Dalury DF, Ewald FC, Christie MJ, Scott RD. Total knee arthroplasty in a group of patients less than 45 years of age. J Arthroplasty. 1995;10(5):598–602.

87. Vincent HK, Herman DC, Lear-Barnes L, Barnes R, Chen C, Greenberg S, et al. Setting standards for medically-based running analysis. Curr Sports Med Rep. 2014;13(4):275–83.

88. Perkins KP, Hanney WJ, Rothschild CE. The risks and benefits of running barefoot or in minimalist shoes: a systematic review. Sports Health. 2014;6(6):475–80.

89. Boyer ER, Derrick TR. Select injury-related variables are affected by stride length and foot strike style during running. Am J Sports Med. 2015;43(9):2310–7.

Part III

Special Considerations

Clinical Aspects of Running Gait Analysis

15

Amanda Gallow and Bryan Heiderscheit

Introduction

An increased desire for a healthy lifestyle and awareness of the multiple health benefits associated with running has resulted in a sustained popularity for the activity in the United States and other countries. From 2002 to 2015, the number of individuals finishing running events increased 300 % to nearly 20,000,000 race finishers each year [1]. The annual rate of running-related injuries ranges from 24 to 65 %, with the most commonly injured joint being the knee [2, 3]. Among runners training for a marathon, the injury rate has been reported as high as 90 % [3]. Novice runners, defined as individuals with little to no running experience, comprise a growing portion of runners and may be at greatest risk. For example, novice runners (17.8 injuries per 1000 h of running) are more than twice as likely than recreational runners (7.7 injuries per 1000 h) to sustain a lower extremity musculoskeletal injury [4].

A. Gallow
Sports Rehabilitation Clinic, UW Health
at The American Center, 4602 Eastpark Blvd,
Madison, WI 53718, USA

B. Heiderscheit (✉)
Departments of Orthopedics and Rehabilitation and
Biomedical Engineering, UW Runners' Clinic,
Badger Athletic Performance Research, University of
Wisconsin-Madison, 1300 University Ave., Madison,
WI 53706, USA
e-mail: heiderscheit@ortho.wisc.edu

A variety of specific factors have been associated with an increased risk for a running-related injury including previous running injury, age, gender, mileage per week, BMI, and shoe age [2, 3, 5, 6]. However, injuries can generally occur secondary to four main factors: musculoskeletal impairment [7], extrinsic causes such as running surface or shoes [8], training error [9], and faulty running mechanics [10, 11]. Traditionally, management of running injuries has emphasized factors that are easily assessed by taking a thorough history or performing a complete physical examination. However, as measurement technology has improved, our ability to capture running mechanics as part of a routine clinical exam has increased, as well as our ability to integrate this information into our clinical decision-making process.

In this chapter, we will describe a standardized approach to assess running mechanics using high-speed video analysis. While recognizing that many options exist regarding equipment and procedure, it is our intent to provide the reader with a framework of the essential elements needed to conduct a video assessment of a runner as it relates to injury recovery and prevention.

Getting Started

Clinical video analysis of running enables the clinician to characterize the patient's running biomechanics, estimate the resulting joint and muscle loads, and identify aspects that may be associated with injury risk. However, this information is of limited value in isolation and therefore should always be combined with a thorough history and physical examination. In doing so, the relationship between individual physical impairments and altered running mechanics is better understood, especially as it relates to the individual's injury. The information gathered can then be utilized to develop the patient's plan of care and route of treatment.

Computerized three-dimensional (3-D) motion capture is considered the gold standard for movement analysis, providing the most accurate and comprehensive means to assess running mechanics. However, most clinics lack the necessary equipment or personnel for this approach, thereby limiting its use in general practice. As such, more feasible alternatives have been sought; likely the most commonly used approach is observational video analysis.

In its simplest form, observational video analysis typically involves the use of a video camera to record the runner's mechanics during either treadmill or overground running. Two-dimensional (2-D) views from the frontal and sagittal planes are typically obtained; multiple cameras may be used to provide a synchronized recording across planes of interest. The recordings are then played back directly to a monitor or through video analysis software and reviewed with regard to normative biomechanical values and to the amount of side-to-side asymmetry.

Comparisons between 2-D and 3-D analyses of running mechanics have been limited to frontal plane motions of the rearfoot [12] and hip [13], with both demonstrating comparable values when a strict measurement procedure is followed. It is important for the clinician to remember that there are distinct limitations with a 2-D analysis that will prevent the measurement accuracy and precision possible with a 3-D approach. As a result, the interpretation of the 2-D video must be made with this in mind.

To maximize measurement accuracy and reliability of a clinical video analysis, several factors must be considered. First, observational video analysis can have questionable reliability. Utilizing a consistent and systematic approach to the video analysis and developing experience in conducting video analysis will increase examiner reliability [14]. Second, to accurately identify specific events of the gait cycle (e.g., initial contact, mid stance), a camera with sufficient frame rate is necessary. Most commonly available video cameras record at 30 or 60 frames per second (fps). Although adequate for walking, these frame rates are insufficient for faster motions such as running where 100–120 fps is needed to more accurately capture the motions of the lower extremity, especially those which occur during foot-ground contact. Finally, placement of the tripod-mounted video camera needs to be perpendicular to the plane of interest. This is concerning for frontal plane measures, where out-of-plane motion can be substantial relative to that occurring within plane [15]. Unless a ceiling-mounted camera is available, motions occurring in the transverse plane are least accurate as they are inferred from the frontal and sagittal plane views.

The presence of these limitations should not prevent one from utilizing observational video analysis. Instead, knowledge of the limitations should enable one to avoid potential errors, such as trying to quantify rather subtle motions or interpreting minor changes (<5°) as real. While a variety of video analysis software is available and makes such measures seemingly possible, the software cannot overcome the inherent limitations of a 2-D video capture.

Patient Setup and Video Capture

The choice between analyzing running mechanics on a treadmill and overground is often determined based on practicality and feasibility. For example, treadmill analysis requires much less physical space than overground and can oftentimes be the determining factor. Performing an overground analysis offers greater ecological validity; that is, most runners run most of their miles overground and not on a treadmill, making overground running the more natural setting. This is an important consideration, as the analysis needs to capture the runner's typical running mechanics to determine if they may be contributing to injury. However, overground running presents with its own set of challenges that can increase measurement error including monitoring and maintenance of a constant running speed, perspective and parallax errors as the runner moves in and out of the field of view, and ability to record a limited number of gait cycles to represent the runner's typical mechanics. While the use of a treadmill can address all of these issues, additional factors need to be considered such as the runner being comfortable on a treadmill, sufficient stiffness of the treadmill deck to mimic overground running, and adequate motor power to ensure a constant speed of the treadmill belt. Although it is often assumed that biomechanics are dramatically different when running on a treadmill compared to overground, if the prior list of factors is addressed, the differences are generally minor [16].

The patient should wear contrasting colors with the shirt tucked into the level of the posterior superior iliac spines (PSIS) to improve the identification of pelvic alignment. If the patient is comfortable running without a shirt, then he or she should be encouraged to do so as it further improves the visual assessment of trunk and pelvis motion. Because runners are generally more comfortable running overground, treadmill familiarization is important and may involve walking for a couple of minutes prior to running. The treadmill should be set to a 0° incline (level), unless uphill or downhill running is of particular interest. It is recommended that the patient be allowed to run for at least 5 min at a self-selected speed before video recording begins to allow for the running form to normalize [17]. The patient's choice of running speed should reflect the conditions in which the symptoms are provoked and may include easy, moderate, or racing speeds. Depending on the chosen speed, only 10–15 s of recording from each movement plane is typically needed to obtain well over 20 strides for each limb.

Analysis of the Recorded Video

Understanding the running gait cycle is imperative for proper clinical gait analysis and communication with runners. The running gait cycle can be broken down into loading response (initial contact to mid stance), push-off, and swing (Table 15.1). The factor that distinguishes running from walking is the period of double float when both feet are off the ground. Important temporal spatial gait parameters that assist with clinical gait analysis are listed in Table 15.2.

While preparing the patient and capturing the video can quickly become a simple, routine aspect of performing a clinical running gait analysis, learning to break down the video and identify specific mechanics associated with injury is generally more complicated. The specific approach to reviewing and interpreting the video can widely vary; however, several basic parameters are worth noting to characterize the running mechanics. These will assist in determining biomechanical faults and imbalances that may be contributing to the runner's dysfunction and provide insights into the ground reaction force and joint loading. Please note that all values provided are estimates and reflect running at preferred, comfortable speed.

Sagittal Plane

Sagittal plane body postures have been found to estimate ground reaction forces and joint kinetics [18]. This is important to understand when working with runners because a common risk factor for running-related injuries is increased joint loads and ground reaction forces [19]. It's helpful to develop a systematic top-down or bottom-up approach to analyze the sagittal plane with particular attention paid to initial contact and mid stance.

Initial Contact

Initial contact, the instant at which the foot first makes contact with the running surface, can be clearly identified in the sagittal plane allowing

Table 15.1 Events within the running cycle

	Definition
Initial contact 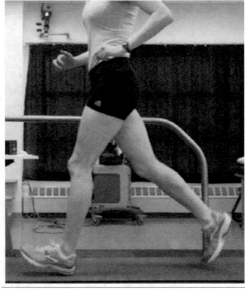	Instant at which the foot first makes contact with the ground and is best identified in the sagittal plane
Mid stance	Instant when the body's center of mass (COM) is directly over the foot and at its lowest vertical position of the gait cycle. This can be identified both in the frontal and sagittal planes
Frontal plane 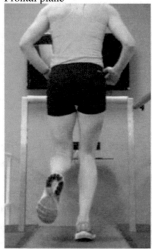 Sagittal plane 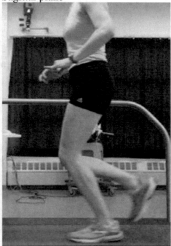	

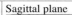

(continued)

Table 15.1 (continued)

	Definition
Mid-float 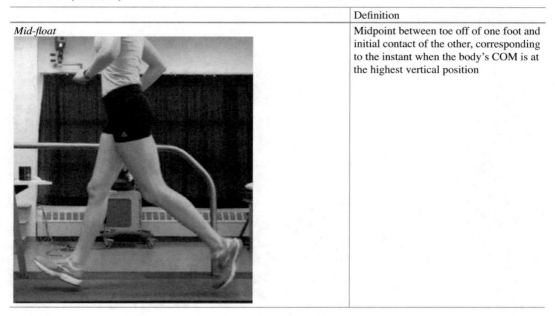	Midpoint between toe off of one foot and initial contact of the other, corresponding to the instant when the body's COM is at the highest vertical position

Table 15.2 Temporal spatial gait parameters

	Definition
Stride duration (s)	Time between successive initial contacts of the same foot
Step duration (s)	Time between initial contact of one foot to initial contact of the other foot
Stride length (m)	Distance from initial contact of one foot to the same foot
Step length (m)	Distance from initial contact of one foot to initial contact of the other foot
Speed (m/s)	Distance traveled per unit of time. Can be calculated as stride length divided by stride time
Cadence (steps/min)	Number of steps within a minute of running

for the assessment of the lower extremity posture. This posture at initial contact is associated with the resulting ground reaction forces and loads to the lower extremity joints and muscles [18]. The following kinematic parameters are of particular importance: foot inclination angle, foot to center of mass (COM) horizontal distance, leg inclination angle, and knee flexion angle.

Foot Inclination Angle The foot inclination angle is the angle between the running surface and the sole of the runner's shoe and allows for the determination of foot-strike pattern (Fig. 15.1). A heel-strike pattern occurs when the runner lands on the posterior aspect of their heel and is evident by a more steep foot inclination angle. A rearfoot-strike pattern involves the runner landing more on the anterior aspect of the heel, generally with a foot inclination angle of 10° or less. A mid foot strike is characterized by both the rearfoot and forefoot making contact nearly simultaneously, with a foot inclination angle near 0°. A forefoot-strike pattern occurs when a runner makes initial contact on the forefoot resulting in a negative foot inclination angle. As foot inclination angle increases, so does peak vertical ground reaction force, braking impulse, knee extensor moment, and negative work performed by the knee extensors, all of which have been associated with various running-related injuries [18]. A large proportion of runners are unable to accurately determine their foot-strike pattern by simply asking them [20], requiring the clinician to directly assess this in clinic.

Horizontal Distance from Foot to COM The horizontal distance from a runner's foot placement

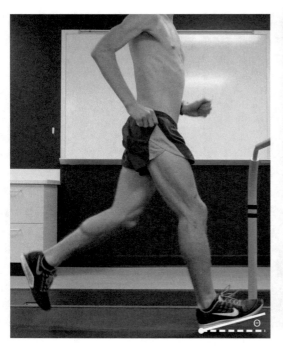

Fig. 15.1 Foot inclination angle is the angle between the running surface and the sole of the runner's shoe and allows for the determination of foot-strike pattern

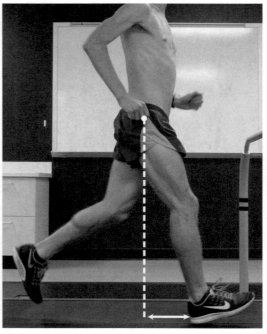

Fig. 15.2 Horizontal distance from the foot to body's center of mass (COM) is measured at initial contact from the point of foot-ground contact to the body's line of gravity, estimated as the center of the pelvis

at initial contact to the whole body's COM (estimated at S2) will influence the resulting ground reaction forces (Fig. 15.2). Specifically, a greater distance between the foot's point of contact and the COM increases the braking impulse and resulting knee extensor moment during the loading response [18].

Leg Inclination Angle The leg inclination angle is the angle of the midline of the leg in relationship to true vertical (Fig. 15.3). This angle can play a role in the amount of loading that occurs to the tibia during running. Increased instantaneous and average vertical loading rates and tibial peak accelerations were found in runners with a history of tibial stress fracture [11]. The leg inclination angle is altered with a reduction in stride length to a more vertical position. Specifically, a reduction in tibial contact force while running was observed when stride length was reduced by 10 %, which may have implications for preventing tibial stress injuries [21].

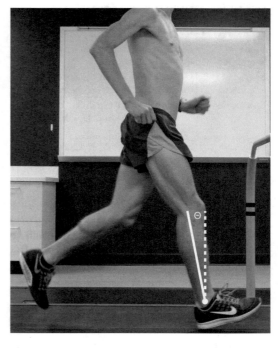

Fig. 15.3 Leg inclination angle is the angle between the midline of the leg and true vertical

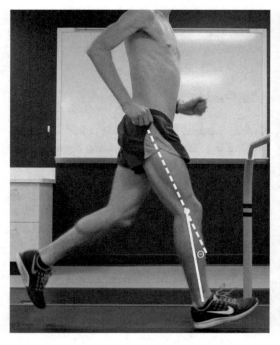

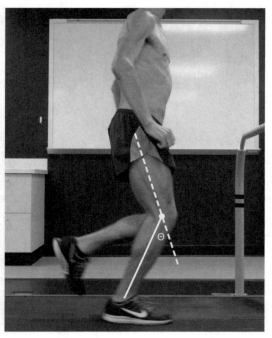

Fig. 15.4 Knee flexion angle at initial contact is measured between the midline of the thigh and the midline of the leg

Fig. 15.5 Peak knee flexion angle at mid stance is defined by the midline of the thigh and the midline of the leg

Knee Flexion Angle Knee flexion angle at initial contact is measured as the angle between the midline of the thigh and the midline of the leg (Fig. 15.4). A more extended knee is commonly observed in individuals who overstride and have an aggressive heel-strike pattern. Knee flexion angles near 20° are generally recommended.

The combination of these measures determines whether an individual is overstriding. For example, a lower extremity posture at initial contact comprised of decreased knee flexion angle, increased leg inclination angle, increased horizontal distance from heel to COM, and increased foot inclination angle is reflective of an overstriding pattern and is associated with increased ground reaction forces and loading to the hip and knee joints [22].

Mid Stance

Two joint alignment measures are of particular importance and occur near mid stance (the instant

when the body's COM is directly over the foot): peak knee flexion angle and peak ankle dorsiflexion angle.

Peak Knee Flexion Angle Peak knee flexion angle is defined in the same manner as knee flexion at initial contact, i.e., the angle between the midline of the thigh and the midline of the leg (Fig. 15.5). This angle is highly predictive of peak patellofemoral joint force, such that peak force increases as knee flexion angle increases [18, 23]. Peak knee flexion angles near 45° are generally recommended, although like all joint kinematic values, this will vary with running speed.

Peak Ankle Dorsiflexion Angle Ankle dorsiflexion is defined by the midline of the leg relative to vertical (Fig. 15.6), with peak values typically occurring shortly after mid stance. Assessing peak ankle dorsiflexion during stance may provide insights into calf muscle load and Achilles tendon strain. For example, greater peak ankle dorsiflexion requires the calf muscle-tendon units to undergo greater stretch, possibly

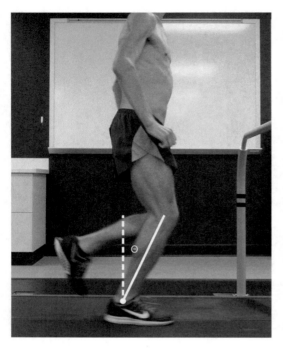

Fig. 15.6 Peak ankle dorsiflexion angle at mid stance is defined by the midline of the foot and the midline of the leg

requiring the muscle fibers to operate at longer lengths. These muscle-tendon kinematics have been associated with increased risk of injury [24].

Additional Sagittal Measures

COM Vertical Excursion Vertical displacement of the runner's COM during the gait cycle can impact both performance and joint loading. This important measure is determined by estimating the linear displacement of the COM from its highest point (mid flight) to its lowest (mid stance) (Fig. 15.7). If the COM undergoes a large excursion, an increase in several kinetic variables will occur including peak vertical ground reaction force, braking impulse and peak knee extensor moment [18]. Greater COM vertical excursion is also associated with an increase in oxygen consumption and reduced running economy [25, 26]. While a specific optimum value for COM excursion has not been defined, 6–10 cm is a generally acceptable range with the higher values more typical for novice runners.

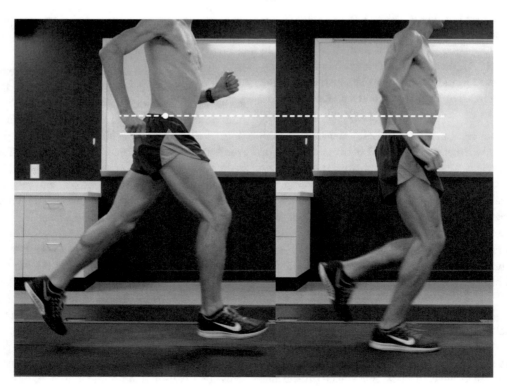

Fig. 15.7 Center of mass (COM) vertical excursion is determined by estimating the linear displacement of the COM from its highest point at (**a**) mid flight to its lowest at (**b**) mid stance

Hip Extension and Pelvic Tilt Hip extension and pelvic tilt are assessed during the push-off phase of the running cycle, although the amount of pelvic tilt may also be evaluated during mid stance. Hip extension is the angle between the midline of the thigh and midline of the pelvis, while pelvic tilt is defined by the midline of the pelvis relative to vertical. Although there is limited research regarding lumbopelvic positioning in the sagittal plane in runners, it's an important feature to assess especially in those with low back or hip pain and in the postpartum running population. Throughout the running cycle, the pelvis demonstrates an average anterior tilt position of 15–20° [27]. Anterior pelvic tilt and hip extension ROM are coordinated motions, as runners who display decreased hip extension ROM during push-off often show an increase in anterior pelvic tilt [28]. Excessive anterior pelvic tilt can be associated with high hamstring tendinopathy, as well as low back pain secondary to the associated increase in lumbar lordosis. As running speed increases, runners appear to achieve the necessary stride length by compensating at the pelvis and lumbar spine rather than simply through hip extension [29].

Forward Trunk Lean Trunk lean is the angle between the midline of the trunk and the vertical. A small degree (5–10°) of forward trunk lean may place the lower spine in a more neutral position and facilitate placing one's foot closer under the COM at initial contact.

Frontal Plane

The frontal plane captures the runner best in the mid stance position of the gait cycle. Mid stance in the frontal plane allows for analysis of trunk side bending, lateral pelvic drop, hip adduction angle, knee center position, foot COM position, and rearfoot and forefoot positions.

Mid Stance

Mid stance is of key interest for assessing frontal plane measures as it reflects the end of loading response and the time in which the vertical ground

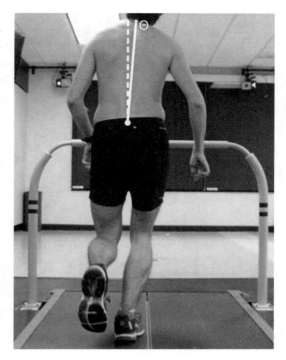

Fig. 15.8 Trunk side bend is defined as the midline of the trunk relative to vertical

reaction forces have peaked. The corresponding position of the lower extremity provides insights into the neuromuscular systems' ability to effectively control joint and limb position.

Trunk Side Bend Trunk side bend, defined as midline of the trunk relative to the vertical, can demonstrate motion in either the ipsilateral or contralateral directions (Fig. 15.8). The total amplitude of motion is approximately 10° with 5° in each direction [27]. Increased ipsilateral trunk lean is found in runners with both patellofemoral pain and iliotibial band syndrome [30, 31], often times associated with increased motion of the pelvis in the frontal plane. Whether this is secondary to hip abductor weakness, spinal deformity, low back pain, poor neuromuscular control, or other compensatory factors would need to be determined through further testing.

Lateral Pelvic Drop Lateral pelvic drop is defined by a line connecting the iliac crests relative to the horizontal (Fig. 15.9). During the first half of stance phase, the iliac crest on the stance

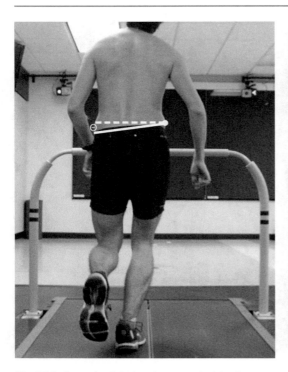

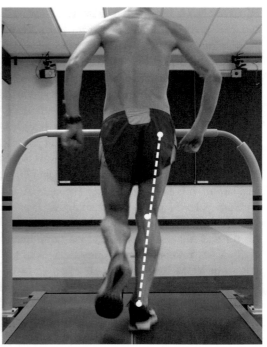

Fig. 15.9 Lateral pelvic drop is assessed with a line connecting both iliac crests relative to horizontal

Fig. 15.10 Knee center position is measured as the position of the knee joint center relative to a line connecting the hip and ankle joint centers

limb is slightly elevated relative to the contralateral iliac crest, with this position commonly referred to as contralateral pelvic drop, i.e., the pelvis is laterally tilted toward the contralateral (swing) side. Contralateral pelvic drop reaches a maximum position of 5–7° near mid stance, with females at the higher end of the range.

Knee Center Position The knee joint center position is identified relative to a line connecting the hip and ankle joint centers (Fig. 15.10). The knee joint center should be located on this line, indicative of the three major lower extremity joints to be in alignment with each other. If the knee center is located medial to the line, it would indicate the presence of a dynamic valgus, with a lateral location being a dynamic varus. Dynamic valgus has been associated with knee joint injuries including patellofemoral pain [32].

Mediolateral Distance from Foot to COM This distance is determined from the heel relative to the vertical line originated at the body's COM (line of

gravity) (Fig. 15.11). This distance is dependent on running speed, such that as speed increases toward sprinting, the foot approximates and even crosses over the line. However, at common recreational running speeds (slower than 8:00 min/mile), the foot will typically remain lateral to the line. A crossover position at slower running speeds may increase the risk for iliotibial band syndrome and medial tibial injuries [33–35].

Rearfoot and Forefoot Position Rearfoot position is defined by the midline of the heel relative to the midline of the lower leg (Fig. 15.12). Forefoot position is actually a transverse plane alignment that can be assessed from the frontal angle and involves determining how much of the forefoot is visibly lateral to the rearfoot (Fig. 15.13). In combination, these measures are useful in characterizing the amount of foot pronation that is occurring during running, which may influence recommendations regarding shoes and shoe inserts.

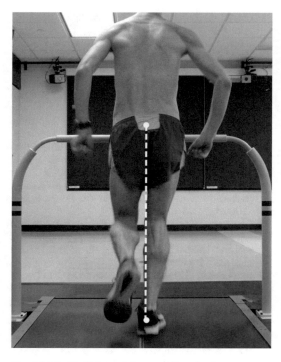

Fig. 15.11 Mediolateral distance from the foot to center of mass (COM) is determined from the position of the heel relative to the body's line of gravity, estimated as the center of the pelvis

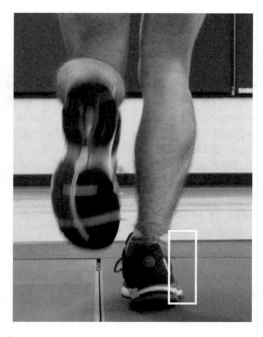

Fig. 15.13 Forefoot position involves determining how much of the forefoot is visibly lateral to the rearfoot

Other Variables

Arm swing and trunk rotation should be also assessed, especially as when a runner complains of abdominal pain or breathing difficulties. Transient abdominal pain during running occasionally occurs for most runners, while some experience it on a fairly consistent basis. At times this abdominal pain can be debilitating to the runner. Although this is an area of limited research, trunk rotation and side bending with corresponding rib approximation could be a component of the problem. In a case study of two female runners with recurrent transient abdominal pain, decreasing this side bending motion while running, in addition to various other trunk and breathing exercises, resulted in resolution of their symptoms [36]. Arm swing while running helps maintain balance and posture while counterbalancing the effects of reciprocal leg swing, helping to reduce the metabolic cost of running [37]. Further, when arm swing is eliminated, the trunk appears to compensate with increased rotation, which may affect breathing and abdominal discomfort as described previously.

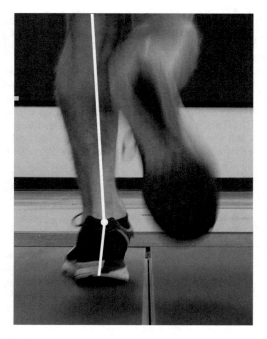

Fig. 15.12 Rearfoot angle is defined as the midline of the heel relative to the midline of the leg

Summary

Becoming efficient and competent in clinical video gait analysis takes time, effort, and practice. As the number of runners continues to grow, the need for clinical video gait analysis as part of a comprehensive injury management plan will also increase. While this chapter has focused on the importance of clinical video gait analysis for the injured, a thorough history and physical examination including review of training, nutrition, and sleeping habits are important. The integration of these different factors will hopefully lead to improved injury management and prevention strategies for all runners.

Disclosure

Drs. Heiderscheit and Gallow do not have any commercial or financial conflicts of interest to disclose.

References

1. Running USA Statistics. 2015. http://www.runningusa.org/statistics.
2. Macera CA, Pate RR, Powell KE, Jackson KL, Kendrick JS, Craven TE. Predicting lower-extremity injuries among habitual runners. Arch Intern Med. 1989;149(11):2565–8.
3. van Gent RN, Siem D, van Middelkoop M, van Os AG, Bierma-Zeinstra SM, Koes BW. Incidence and determinants of lower extremity running injuries in long distance runners: a systematic review. Br J Sports Med. 2007;41(8):469–80. Discussion 80. Epub 3 May 2007.
4. Videbæk S, Bueno AM, Nielsen RO, Rasmussen S. Incidence of running-related injuries per 1000 h of running in different types of runners: a systematic review and meta-analysis. Sports Med. 2015;45(7):1017–26.
5. Buist I, Bredeweg SW, van Mechelen W, Lemmink KA, Pepping GJ, Diercks RL. No effect of a graded training program on the number of running-related injuries in novice runners: a randomized controlled trial. Am J Sports Med. 2008;36(1):33–9.
6. Hootman JM, Macera CA, Ainsworth BE, Martin M, Addy CL, Blair SN. Predictors of lower extremity injury among recreationally active adults. Clin J Sport Med. 2002;12(2):99–106.
7. Dierks TA, Manal KT, Hamill J, Davis IS. Proximal and distal influences on hip and knee kinematics in runners with patellofemoral pain during a prolonged run. J Orthop Sports Phys Ther. 2008;38(8):448–56. Epub 6 Aug 2008.
8. Taunton JE, Ryan MB, Clement DB, McKenzie DC, Lloyd-Smith DR, Zumbo BD. A prospective study of running injuries: the Vancouver Sun Run "In Training" clinics. Br J Sports Med. 2003;37(3):239–44.
9. Lysholm J, Wiklander J. Injuries in runners. Am J Sports Med. 1987;15(2):168–71.
10. Ferber R, Noehren B, Hamill J, Davis IS. Competitive female runners with a history of iliotibial band syndrome demonstrate atypical hip and knee kinematics. J Orthop Sports Phys Ther. 2010;40(2):52–8.
11. Milner CE, Ferber R, Pollard CD, Hamill J, Davis IS. Biomechanical factors associated with tibial stress fracture in female runners. Med Sci Sports Exerc. 2006;38(2):323–8.
12. Nakagawa TH, Moriya É, Maciel CD, Serrão AF. Frontal plane biomechanics in males and females with and without patellofemoral pain. Med Sci Sports Exerc. 2012;44(9):1747–55.
13. Maykut JN, Taylor-Haas JA, Paterno MV, DiCesare CA, Ford KR. Concurrent validity and reliability of 2d kinematic analysis of frontal plane motion during running. Int J Sports Phys Ther. 2015;10(2):136–46. Epub 18 Apr 2015.
14. Brunnekreef JJ, van Uden CJ, van Moorsel S, Kooloos JG. Reliability of videotaped observational gait analysis in patients with orthopedic impairments. BMC Musculoskelet Disord. 2005;6:17.
15. Areblad M, Nigg BM, Ekstrand J, Olsson KO, Ekstrom H. Three-dimensional measurement of rearfoot motion during running. J Biomech. 1990;23(9): 933–40.
16. Riley PO, Dicharry J, Franz J, Della Croce U, Wilder RP, Kerrigan DC. A kinematics and kinetic comparison of overground and treadmill running. Med Sci Sports Exerc. 2008;40(6):1093–100.
17. Lavcanska V, Taylor NF, Schache AG. Familiarization to treadmill running in young unimpaired adults. Hum Mov Sci. 2005;24(4):544–57.
18. Wille CM, Lenhart RL, Wang S, Thelen DG, Heiderscheit BC. Ability of sagittal kinematic variables to estimate ground reaction forces and joint kinetics in running. J Orthop Sports Phys Ther. 2014;44(10):825–30.
19. Messier SP, Legault C, Schoenlank CR, Newman JJ, Martin DF, DeVita P. Risk factors and mechanisms of knee injury in runners. Med Sci Sports Exerc. 2008;40(11):1873–9. Epub 11 Oct 2008.
20. Goss DL, Lewek M, Yu B, Ware WB, Teyhen DS, Gross MT. Lower extremity biomechanics and self-reported foot-strike patterns among runners in traditional and minimalist shoes. J Athl Train. 2015; 50(6):603–11.
21. Edwards WB, Taylor D, Rudolphi TJ, Gillette JC, Derrick TR. Effects of stride length and running mileage on a probabilistic stress fracture model. Med Sci Sports Exerc. 2009;41(12):2177–84.
22. Heiderscheit BC, Chumanov ES, Michalski MP, Wille CM, Ryan MB. Effects of step rate manipulation on

joint mechanics during running. Med Sci Sports Exerc. 2011;43(2):296–302.

23. Lenhart RL, Thelen DG, Wille CM, Chumanov ES, Heiderscheit BC. Increasing running step rate reduces patellofemoral joint forces. Med Sci Sports Exerc. 2014;46(3):557–64. Epub 7 Aug 2013.

24. Thelen DG, Chumanov ES, Best TM, Swanson SC, Heiderscheit BC. Simulation of biceps femoris musculotendon mechanics during the swing phase of sprinting. Med Sci Sports Exerc. 2005;37(11):1931–8.

25. Halvorsen K, Eriksson M, Gullstrand L. Acute effects of reducing vertical displacement and step frequency on running economy. J Strength Cond Res. 2012;26(8):2065–70. Epub 27 Oct 2011.

26. Cavanagh PR. The biomechanics of lower extremity action in distance running. Foot Ankle. 1987;7(4):197–217.

27. Schache AG, Bennell KL, Blanch PD, Wrigley TV. The coordinated movement of the lumbo-pelvic-hip complex during running: a literature review. Gait Posture. 1999;10(1):30–47. Epub 2 Sep 1999.

28. Schache AG, Blanch PD, Murphy AT. Relation of anterior pelvic tilt during running to clinical and kinematic measures of hip extension. Br J Sports Med. 2000;34(4):279–83.

29. Franz JR, Paylo KW, Dicharry J, Riley PO, Kerrigan DC. Changes in the coordination of hip and pelvis kinematics with mode of locomotion. Gait Posture. 2009;29(3):494–8. Epub 7 Jan 2009.

30. Noehren B, Pohl MB, Sanchez Z, Cunningham T, Lattermann C. Proximal and distal kinematics in female runners with patellofemoral pain. Clin Biomech (Bristol, Avon). 2012;27(4):366–71.

31. Foch E, Reinbolt JA, Zhang S, Fitzhugh EC, Milner CE. Associations between iliotibial band injury status and running biomechanics in women. Gait Posture. 2015;41(2):706–10.

32. Powers CM. The influence of altered lower-extremity kinematics on patellofemoral joint dysfunction: a theoretical perspective. J Orthop Sports Phys Ther. 2003;33(11):639–46.

33. McClay IS, Cavanagh PR. Relationship between foot placement and mediolateral ground reaction forces during running. Clin Biomech (Bristol, Avon). 1994;9(2):117–23.

34. Meardon SA, Campbell S, Derrick TR. Step width alters iliotibial band strain during running. Sports Biomech. 2012;11(4):464–72. Epub 25 Dec 2012.

35. Meardon SA, Derrick TR. Effect of step width manipulation on tibial stress during running. J Biomech. 2014;47(11):2738–44. Epub 18 Jun 2014.

36. Spitznagle TM, Sahrmann S. Diagnosis and treatment of 2 adolescent female athletes with transient abdominal pain during running. J Sport Rehabil. 2011;20(2):228–49. Epub 18 May 2011.

37. Arellano CJ, Kram R. The metabolic cost of human running: is swinging the arms worth it? J Exp Biol. 2014;217(Pt 14):2456–61. Epub 18 Jul 2014.

Clinical Considerations of Bike Fitting for the Triathlete

16

Matthew S. Briggs and Travis Obermire

Introduction

Triathlon began in 1978 with the inaugural triathlon held in Hawaii, USA [1]. In 1982, US Triathlon (USAT) was founded [the national governing body for triathlon in the USA] [2]. Over the last 40 years, the visibility and popularity of the sport of triathlon has grown tremendously, and it is now a major Olympic event. Triathlon is an individual multisport event consisting of three separate disciplines of swimming, biking, and running typically in that order held in competition on the same day. These events are separated by "transition" periods between each stage. In addition, there are many different distances associated with the sport of triathlon. These distances may vary but often are categorized as sprint (0.75 km swim, 20 km cycle, and 5 km run), Olympic (1.5 km swim, 40 km cycle, and 10 km run), half iron distance (1.9 km swim, 90 km cycle, and 21.1 km run), full iron distance (3.8 km swim,

180 km cycle, and 42.2 km run), and ultra-distance triathlons (10 km swim, 421 km cycle, and 84 km run) [1, 3, 4]. The cycling portion of any distance (sprint, Olympic, half iron, full iron, or ultra) comprises approximately 75–80 % of the total race. Thus, considerations pertaining to bike fit, injury, and performance are extremely important to the cycling aspect of the sport of triathlon regardless of any distance.

In 1982, USA Triathlon (USAT), the national governing body for triathlon in the USA, was founded [2]. Since then USAT membership growth has reflected the increased popularity of the sport, from 1500 members in 1982 to 140,000 in 2011 [2]. Triathlon became an Olympic event for the first time in Sydney in 2000. Approximately one million people participate in triathlon and/or related events (e.g., duathlon, aquabike, etc.) [2, 5, 6]. Older athletes participate in more races; 95 % participate for the personal challenge, while 87 % participate to stay in shape. On average, they participated in 4.2 triathlons during the previous 12 months; 86 % plan to do longer races in the future. Sprint triathlon remains the most popular, with those events attracting participation of more than three quarters of respondents [2]. According to data from the USAT, 78 % of triathletes participate in sprint, 58 % participate in Olympic, 39 % participate in half iron distance, and 17 % participate in full iron distance [2].

M.S. Briggs (✉)
OSU Sports Medicine and Sports Medicine Research Institute, The Ohio State University Wexner Medical Center, 2050 Kenny Road, Columbus, OH 43221, USA
e-mail: matt.briggs@osumc.edu

T. Obermire
Sports Rehabilitation Clinic, UW Health at The American Center, 4602 Eastpark Boulevard, Madison, WI 53718, USA

© Springer International Publishing Switzerland 2016
T.L. Miller (ed.), *Endurance Sports Medicine*, DOI 10.1007/978-3-319-32982-6_16

Injury Considerations in the Triathlete

The average triathlete will spend approximately 800 hours per year doing some type of training [5, 7]. Further, triathletes tend to average more time in sport participation per week and have a higher incidence of injury when compared to individual swimmers, cyclists, and runners [5, 8]. However, medical treatment is only sought by approximately 50 % of triathletes who report injuries [7]. Injury rates in triathlon have been shown to be as high as 91 % and most often occurring during training versus competition [1, 4, 9–11]. However, the types of injury appear to be different when comparing males and females. For example, Bertola et al. [3] conducted a cross-sectional study of 190 amateur athletes competing in a sprint distance triathlon (750 m swim, 20 km bike, and 5 km run) and recorded their self-reported injury history. The majority of injuries reported in males were muscle related (54 %), whereas women reported a more distributed injury profile with 32 % related to muscle, 32 % related to tendinous, and 32 % related to bone [3]. Thus gender should be considered as a factor in the evaluation and management of triathletes.

The running discipline of the triathlon has the highest prevalence of injury (79 % for males and 92 % for females) followed by cycling (16 % for males and 8 % for females) [3]. However, Zwingenberger et al. [11] conducted both a retrospective and prospective study evaluating injury patterns in over a period of 12 months in non-professional triathletes. Results from this study indicated that 50 % of injuries were related to running, 43 % related to cycling, and 7 % related to swimming, while between 45 % and 78 % of injuries were soft tissue in nature (e.g., ligament, muscle, and tendon). The neck and the knee are the two most common body regions associated with overuse injury during cycling [12, 13]. With the incorporation of aerobars in triathlon versus road cycling, the neck may be at even more vulnerable and at risk of pain and injury. However, overuse injury to the knee related to cycling has been shown to incurre the most time loss from training and competition

when compared to injury to other body regions [14]. Further, the number of overuse injuries in Olympic distance triathlon racing has been shown to inversely correlate with the percentage of training time and number of sessions doing bike hill repetitions ($r=-0.44$ and -0.39, respectively, $p<0.05$) [4]. For full iron distance triathletes, the number of "speed bike" training session positively correlated with injury ($r=0.56$, $p<0.05$) [4]. It is suggested that a vast majority of triathlon cycling injuries can be linked to sub-optimal bike fit and cycling mechanics [15].

Triathlon Bike Anatomy

Knowing and understanding triathlon bike anatomy (Figs. 16.1 and 16.2) helps to remove much of the mystery out of a bike discussion and is imperative in understanding patient/client demands, injuries, and concerns during a triathlon. Figure 16.1 illustrates the primary components and aspects of a representative triathlon bike frame and drive train, while Fig. 16.2 illustrates the primary components of the "cockpit" or the handlebar region of a traditional triathlon bike setup.

Clinical Considerations of Cycling Mechanics

Joint position and forces during cycling are affected by workload, seat/saddle height, foot position on the pedal, and seat tube angle [16]. Sagittal plane joint angles are typically the focus of most measurements during triathlon bike fittings. For example, changes in saddle height, power output, and foot position all have an effect on lower extremity joint movement during cycling [16, 17]. Understanding how these variables affect lower extremity joint movement and angles highlights the importance of individualizing the bike fit based on the athlete's ability, goals, training terrain, and potential injury. In general, lower extremity joint excursion during cycling is approximately 45° at the hip, 75° at the knee, and 20° at the ankle [18]. Changes in aero position

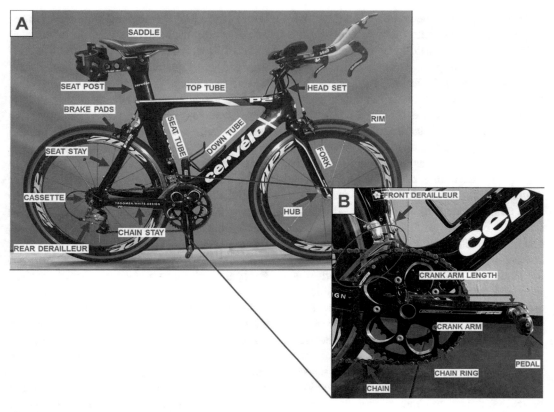

Fig. 16.1 Basic triathlon bike anatomy/components. (**a**) Sagittal view of a representative triathlon bike; (**b**) sagittal view of the drive train, bottom bracket, crank, and pedal region

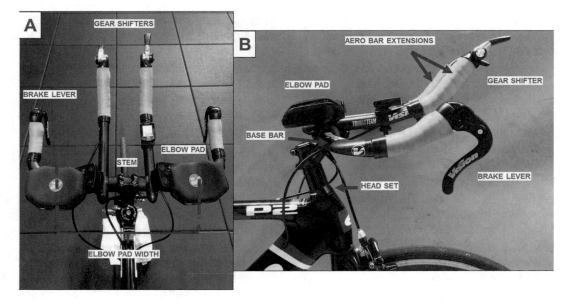

Fig. 16.2 Components of the "cockpit" or handlebar region. (**a**) Top view/rider's view and (**b**) Sagittal view

and cadence have not been shown to substantially alter these lower extremity joint excursion values [19]. However, seat/saddle height influences not only these sagittal plane values but frontal plane movement as well. Therefore, full consideration needs to be given to the inter-relationships of all of the upper and lower extremity joints with any change to the athlete/bike interface.

The knee joint has the greatest joint excursion during cycling, and as previously mentioned, knee pain is a common complaint in cyclists and triathletes [12, 13, 18]. It is thought that anterior knee pain is caused by an imbalanced relationship between knee joint forces and kinematics resulting in changes in patellofemoral force, contact area, and pressure [18, 20]. For example, increases in mechanically simulated knee moments have been shown to significantly increase patellofemoral contact area and forces during fixed pedal cycling [21]. However, it should be noted that patellofemoral contact stress did not significantly change [21]. Patellofemoral forces are almost entirely determined by seat/saddle height and force output while appearing to be less correlated to cleat position and cadence [16, 22]. For example, patellofemoral compressive forces have been shown to be inversely related to seat/saddle height [23]. Therefore, modifying these two fit parameters (saddle height and force output) in a triathlete with knee pain is critical. This does not mean that the other variables do not matter, but if the goal is to decrease stress or associated pain, decreasing the causal forces should be of focus during the fit. Subsequent adjustment of other parameters will then be used to optimize position. In addition, consideration of mediolateral and transverse movement and associated forces at the knee during the pedal stroke should also be evaluated when adjusting the saddle, cleat, and forefoot posting [24]. In general, "If the aim is to minimize the risk of patellofemoral joint injuries, the inverse relationship between saddle height and patellofemoral compressive force may be used as a reference" [18].

The foot-shoe-pedal interface is where the transfer of force occurs from the rider to the bike [25]. The tangential force (versus the centrifugal force) of the foot on the pedal during the downstroke of the pedal cycle is the most efficient force while cycling and propelling the bike forward [16, 26]. Common sense would suggest that these forces inherently change based on cycling conditions and terrain. For example, a 26% increase in torque occurs while cycling at the same cadence on level ground versus inclined ground at an 8% grade [27]. This increase in force at the foot-pedal interface ultimately requires a transfer of energy from the entire lower extremity. Further understanding these relationships will assist clinicians in both modifying bike fit and educating triathletes, patients, and clients on how simple changes in terrain may affect lower extremity loads and potentially injury risk. Foot pain is also a common occurrence in cyclists due to the high reactive forces and pressures being transferred to a small pedal [25]. Individuals with foot pain during cycling may consider the use of an insert orthosis in their cycling shoe. If foot pain persists after a proper bike fitting, then custom, contoured orthosis should be considered. Contoured orthoses have been shown to increase the contract area of the foot in the shoe and thus decreasing pressure when compared to flat inserts [25].

Getting Started: Basic Fit Setup and Equipment

A thorough understanding of any type of athlete's flexibility, stability, neuromuscular control, strength, endurance, cardiovascular characteristics, and any anatomic variations is imperative to optimizing treatment. Thus, a physical exam is imperative, and all of these factors should be considered in some capacity either when assisting in a triathlete's rehabilitation from injury and/or in attempt to optimize their performance on the bike. Although the purpose of this chapter is not to provide all of the tools necessary to develop the clinician into a bike fitter or a bike mechanic, a basic understanding of simple bike adjustments and/or recommendations may assist clinicians in their treatment and care of triathletes. This understanding will help to foster communication and understanding with the athlete, the bike mechanic, as well as the certified expert bike fitter, all of whom are essential players in the sports medicine team of a triathlete. There are many different types of bike fitting

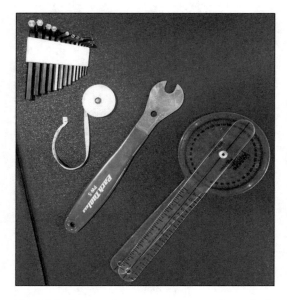

Fig. 16.3 Basic equipment necessary to perform a basic bike fit assessment [allen wrenches (ideally also a torque wrench), tape measure (also used as a make-shift plumb bob), pedal wrench, and goniometer] (bike trainer not shown)

techniques ranging from static to dynamic fittings. During static fittings, the athlete's joints are measured while not moving/pedaling. Dynamic fittings involve the measurement of joint angles and forces during the act of pedaling and typically require expensive three-dimensional motion analysis equipment and techniques. However, a basic, static bike assessment can quickly be performed in almost any clinic and/or office with the right equipment and space. Basic equipment includes a bike trainer, goniometer, tape measure, pedal wrench, a set of Allen wrenches, and obviously the athlete's bike (Fig. 16.3).

The Bike: Fit Window

Cycling position in triathlon is a balancing act between maximal power output, comfort, and aerodynamics to optimize cycling speed or velocity (Fig. 16.4) [28]. The primary concern of this chapter is understanding the rider's position on the bike and how it will affect both the athlete and cycling performance. It should be noted that dynamic bike fitting in the laboratory produces significantly different flexion angle for all joints in the lower extremity, when compared to angles on the open road [29]. Furthermore, evidence

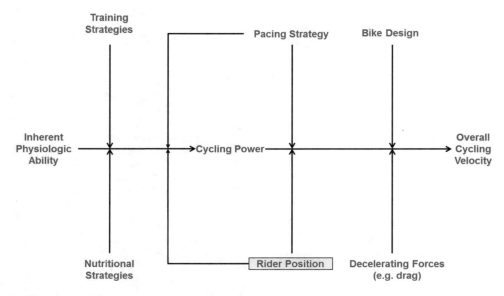

Fig. 16.4 Factors influencing cycling power and speed (modified and adapted with permission from Atkinson et al. (2003) [47] and Taylor & Francis Ltd. (http://www.tandfonline.com)

suggests there is significantly more variability in cycling kinematics when measured on the on the road versus on a stationary trainer [29]. Thus, the validity of bike fittings performed on a stationary trainer may limit the generalizability of the athlete's fit to the road. Clinicians should recognize this limitation and may require more than one fitting session to ensure a triathlete's bike fit is optimal and "dialed-in."

The rider's position on a triathlon bike is designed to decrease frontal area in efforts to improve aerodynamics and to improve running performance off of the bike. "At racing speeds greater than 14 m/s, with a classical racing bicycle, aerodynamic drag represents about 90% of the overall resistive forces" [30–33]. Overall, lower torso angle improves performance in the aero position in trained cyclists, but the lower you go, the greater the metabolic cost [34]. However, the "aero" position is less economical and requires a higher metabolic demand, but the aerodynamic benefits outweigh this metabolic and comfort cost (to a point), and the athlete is faster [34]. Thus, there is a trade-off between maximizing aerodynamic advantage and physiologic functioning [34]. In triathlon, especially long course, an aerodynamic position must be comfortable enough to maintain for a long period of time while optimizing the physiologic capacity. This is especially important for full iron distance races requiring athletes to maintain a position for 4–6+ hours.

The effect of aerodynamics plays a greater influence as velocity increases. In other words, the faster the athlete is that you are treating, the more important their aerodynamic position is. So what is the best aero position for triathlons? The answer is it depends on the athletes: race distance, flexibility, ability, goals, past medical history, comfort, financial resources for change, and safety. There are several schools of thought when it comes to triathlon fitting. The main systems out there are Dan Empfield's Fit Institute "Slowtwitch" [35], Serotta International Cycling Institute, Retul, Trek [36], Specialized [37], etc. However, a limitation to all of these methods is that they are based on mostly expert opinion versus strong empirical, scientific evidence. The correct fitting method is most likely a combination of several (if not all) of these methods.

To optimize a bike fit for a triathlete, it may be necessary to evaluate them immediately following a swim (swim-to-bike brick) as power output has been shown to change after swimming which may influence mechanics [38]. This sequencing may provide the most optimized event-specific position possible. The subsequent paragraphs will outline general "guidelines" for fitting or "fit window." In reality, most athletes can tolerate a fit within a few centimeters in several directions and can dial in their specific position based on the parameters listed above. When considering the biomechanics of triathlon fitting, the major elements include the following: seat tube angle, seat/saddle height, cleat position, forefoot posting, arch support, pedal/shoe selection, shoulder-hip-knee angle, shoulder angle/reach "cockpit distance," arm pad stack and reach, armrest width, crank length, saddle width/tilt, and helmet/sunglasses.

Seat Tube Angle (STA) (Fig. 16.5)

Understanding how changes in seat tube angle (STA) may affect other joint angles and perfor-

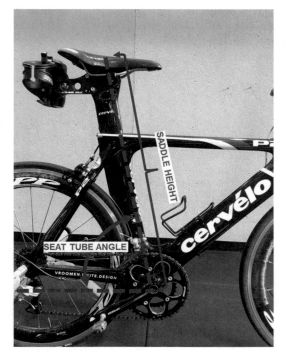

Fig. 16.5 Saddle height and seat tube angle

mance is important in triathletes as triathlon bikes typically have steeper STA when compared to road bikes: STA in triathlon bikes are typically between 78 and 80° [35, 39]. This essentially allows the rider to rotate their entire body forward on the bike, keeping a similar hip flexion angle and in turn decreasing frontal area and associated drag by bringing their torso more horizontal. Increasing the STA has been shown to increase anterior pelvic tilt but has limited to no influence on other lower extremity joint angles [39]. In addition, typically the steeper the STA, the lower the associated pad stack height/drop. This position allows a rider to use less power to go faster, as compared to an upright position on a road bike secondary to reduced drag [34]. Seat tube angle affects the riders positon, and thus moving the saddle position changes the effective seat tube angle of the riders actual position. This should be considered when adjusting saddle fore/aft or when changing out to a different kind of saddle.

Seat/Saddle Height (Fig. 16.5)

Seat/saddle height may be the most important part of a bike fit in optimizing mechanical work, pedaling efficiency, and joint stress [40]. Most often, seat/saddle height is the distance measured from the center of the bottom bracket to the midportion of the top of the saddle. Others may cite seat/saddle height as the distance between the top of the saddle to the top of the pedal axle with the pedal at dead bottom center (crank arm at the bottom of the pedal stroke aligned with STA) [17]. The goal with seat/saddle height is to achieve a knee flexion angle at dead bottom center to be approximately 25–40° (statically measured) as this range has been suggested to reduce the risk of knee injuries and optimize aerobic performance [40, 41].

There are three common methods of determining seat/saddle height including (1) the Greg LeMond method, (2) heel method, and (3) knee angle method [18]. The Greg LeMond method is performed by taking inseam measurement and multiplying it by 0.883 [18]. A limitation of this method includes that it does not account femur,

tibial, foot, or crank length which may be important factors depending on individual athlete body types and sizes. The heel method is performed by having the triathlete sit on the seat/saddle with heel on the pedal with cranks in line with seat tube [18]. In this position, optimal seat/saddle height would be indicated with the knees in full extension. Finally, the most commonly used technique for determining optimal seat/saddle height is the knee angle method [18]. This method is the most specific and considers crank, tibial, foot, and femur lengths, thus improving consistent knee kinematics between riders [18]. However, when utilizing the knee angle method, "ankling" (excessive plantar flexion at the bottom of the pedal stroke) at the bottom of the pedal stroke and/or lateral rocking of the hips should be minimized as these compensations may influence knee flexion angles by as much as 5–6° [40]. The knee angle method is most accurately measured during active cycling using video or three-dimensional motion analysis. However, static bike fit measurements (measurements taken at rest) of the knee have been shown to underpredict the dynamic measurements (measurements while riding) using two-dimensional and three-dimensional analyses [42].

Cleat Position (Fig. 16.6)

Most competitive and elite-level triathletes will opt for what is known as a "clipless pedal." This is somewhat a misnomer as "clipless pedal" is actually directly attached to a cleat at the bottom of the shoe, firmly securing the pedal and the shoe as one unit. This pedal-shoe interface improves cycling efficiency. There are many different types and versions of cleats and pedals (e.g., Speedplay, Look, SPD, etc.). Cleat position may assist in the accommodation for leg length discrepancies, knee/foot pain, and foot numbness. However, most often cleat adjustments are based on expert opinion and experience. Factors to consider when adjusting cleat position include fore/aft, medial/lateral placement, rotation or "float," cant, and shimming. The cleat rotation should mimic that of the way the individual walks

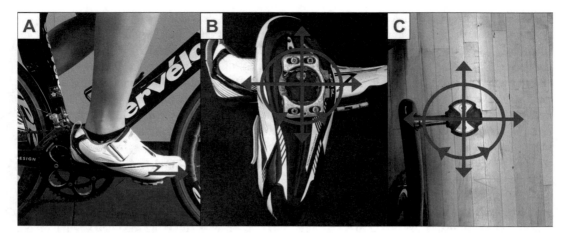

Fig. 16.6 Cleat position with a speed play © pedal/cleat. (**a**) Fore/aft position, (**b**) cleat position on shoe indicating the potential positioning and available float, (**c**) speedplay © pedal indicating the potential positioning and available float

and/or sits with their feet dangling from a table. The athlete should have some available medial and lateral rotation or "float" at the bottom and top of the pedal stroke. If this is not present at both of these points, cleat adjustment is warranted [37]. "The ideal rotational angle of the cleat on the sole of the shoe is the one where while pedaling under load; the rider has a more or less even degree of free movement either side of where their foot naturally sits on the pedal. If the foot is locked in place at a less than ideal rotational angle, stresses on the knee result; or, autonomic self-protection of the knee from stress shifts the load to other elements in the kinetic chain involved in pedaling or structures involved in stabilizing those elements" [43]. The cleat and the inside of the shoe of an injured triathlete may/should be adjusted for forefoot abnormalities such as forefoot varus and valgus with wedged shim(s) between the cleat and the shoe or in the shoe under the insole. This may also be achieved with custom orthotics.

Hip Angle (Fig. 16.7)

There are several different ways hip angle may be measured. However, for the purposes of this chapter, hip angle will be described as the angle from the lateral portion of the acromion to the greater trochanter and to the bottom bracket (Fig. 16.7).

The optimal range of hip flexion on the bike is approximately 90–105° [35]. An athlete's functional availability of hip flexion is critical with this measurement [37]. Functional hip flexion measured off the bike should be measured with their knee in approximately 30° of flexion to mimic aero position on the bike. If hip flexion is measured with the rider's knee fully flexed, their functional available hip flexion may be overpredicted. Therefore, this is one of the most important components of the pre-bike fit examination. Hip angle measure on the bike greater than 105° may predispose the athlete low back, hamstring, and anterior hip pain [15]. The bottom line here is that care must be taken not to place the athlete on the bike in a position that exceeds their functional and/or anatomical constraints found during a physical exam. The optimal hip angle can be achieved by raising and/or lowering the handlebars.

Shoulder Angle (Fig. 16.8)

The angle of the shoulder should be approximately 90° of flexion and is the angle measured between a line through the long axis of the humerus and line following the torso angle (e.g., same torso line used in the hip angle) [35]. This angle allows for the most comfortable position when aero and is closely linked to the reach of the aero bars as the elbow angle should also be at 90°

Fig. 16.7 Hip angle measured with subject positioned with pedal at dead bottom center

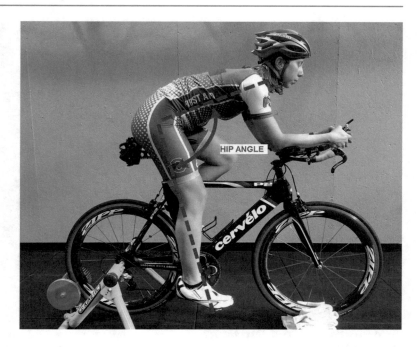

Fig. 16.8 Shoulder angle

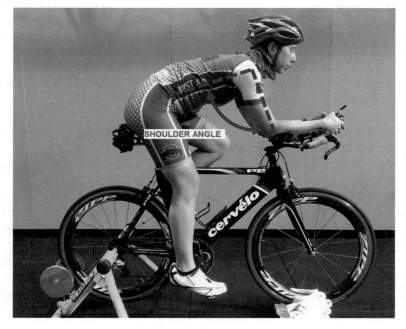

of flexion. An additional technique that may be used to evaluate and optimize shoulder angle is to drop a plumb line from the AC joint. This line should fall at the posterior aspect of the elbow [37, 44]. It should also be noted that the proximal portion of the elbow should be hanging off the aero pad to prevent compression of the ulnar nerve and to prevent the elbow from slipping off of the pad when hitting a bump. Both of which are a safety concern. However, even with these considerations, many triathletes prefer to have their elbows directly on the pads.

Fig. 16.9 Stack height/drop

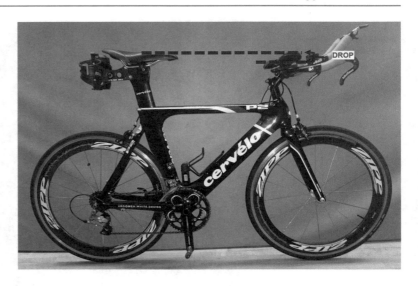

Arm Pad Stack/Drop and Reach (Fig. 16.9)

Arm pad stack or drop is the measurement taken from the top of the saddle where the rider sits in aero (not the highest point of the rear upslope of the saddle) to the center portion of the top of the pads and is the vertical distance. This measurement may also be measured as the vertical distance from the center of the bottom bracket to the top of the arm pad. Reach is the horizontal distance from the center of the bottom bracket to the center of the arm pad. The amount of drop needed can be determined by formulas that use seat/saddle height and seat angle to calculate. However, the most important parameter in this position is the rider's ability to sustain this position for a given distance/time. If the rider is in pain or is unable to maintain a particular stack height for the duration of the event, they are in the wrong position. The more drop an athlete has, the more cervical extension is required to maintain vision down the road. Often when a rider's drop is lowered to achieve a greater aerodynamic advantage, interventions may need to be prescribed to improve/optimize cervical mobility and stability to maintain this more aggressive position. Failure to give the athlete

interventions off the bike may make this position unsustainable in training and racing and subsequently limit performance and/or cause injury. The amount of drop should also keep the riders hip flexion angle the same/similar as it is on a road fit. This can be achieved by moving the seat fore as the bars are lowered [37].

Armrest Width (Fig. 16.2a)

In triathlon this is determined by comfort, flexibility, race distance, and the athlete's shoulder width. One way to determine their functional flexibility of the posterior shoulder is to perform an elbow touch test. This is performed by flexing shoulders and elbows to 90° and touching elbows together as in horizontal adduction [36]. Interventions focused on thoracic and shoulder mobility and stability may be warranted when adjusting armrest width.

Crank Length (Fig. 16.1b)

Ideal crank arm length is up for debate. It appears that a large change in crank length is required to cause a decrease in power output. "Crank length does not affect relative joint-specific power once the effects of pedaling rate and pedal speed are accounted for" [45]. When caring for an injured triathlete, shorter cranks may be another way to increase their hip angle and decrease stress on athlete's hips and knees. If crank length is significantly changed, the rest of the fit will have to be adjusted. Changing crank length can be very useful in riders with hip dysfunction and the aging triathlete with mobility issues. There are various tables you can find and/or formulas to use to predict ideal crank length. Bottom line, the shorter the triathlete the more important crank length is, because it affects their joint angles more.

Saddle Position

Triathletes participating triathlon should be educated in the need to evaluate multiple saddles to find the most comfortable one. This is very athlete dependent. Some fitting methods argue that the front of a triathlete's saddle should be tilted down to make the aero position more comfortable [37]. If the athlete complains of sliding forward, the seat/saddle should be tilted more toward the horizontal. If an athlete is having trouble getting comfortable on the saddle when in aero, then you may need to assess their sacral angle in aero and compare this to their sacral angle when doing a toe touch or standing hamstring stretch [36]. If a steeper angle is present, the saddle may be limiting the ability of the pelvis to rotate anteriorly. Furthermore, the rider's saddle width can be determined by measuring ischial tuberosity width, but this still requires testing on the bike to ensure comfort is achieved.

Helmets/Sunglasses

Riding in the aero position can put considerable strain on the cervical spine especially with lowering stack heights. The more of an aggressive aerodynamic position a rider achieves, the more cervical extension is required. Other components which may influence cervical position include helmet position and sunglasses. Thus, a triathlete with neck pain should have their helmet fit checked (i.e., is the helmet obstructing their vision and thus causing more cervical extension). It is also recommended that triathletes wear safety sunglasses that do not have a brim at the top, as this may also obstruct vision and further require additional cervical extension. Thus, poor helmet fit and suboptimal eyeglass wear may predispose the athlete to increased cervical pain and injury.

Other Fit Considerations for Different Triathlon Distances

As previously mentioned, there are several different types of triathlons all following the traditional swim-bike-run format (short course, long course, and draft legal). Although it is beyond the scope of this chapter to describe all of the considerations related to cycling for these different distances, attention to the following may be helpful to the clinician who is new to triathlon. In particular, for long course (e.g., half and full iron distance triathlons), raising the aerobars slightly may be helpful for longer events. This will increase the hip angle, allow more room for the diaphragm to move, and decrease tension on the hamstrings, low back, and perineum [46]. Although a small amount of aerodynamic advantage will be lost, this will be made up for with greater cycling comfort when training or racing for 2–7 h. Conversely for short-course training and racing, lowering the bars may provide more of an aerodynamic benefit. Although this position will likely be less comfortable, the shorter duration of the cycling leg of a short-course triathlon may allow the athlete to sustain this position for a short period of time. It should be noted that it is usually not recommended to make changes to bike fit close to or the day of a race.

Finally, most long-course (e.g., half and full iron distance) and short-course (e.g., sprint and Olympic distance) triathlons in the USA are non-draft legal racing. This means athletes must maintain a particular distance away from other triathletes during cycling to avoid any drafting benefit. However, draft legal triathlon racing is a growing trend in the USA and is common internationally and at the Olympics.

This type of racing typically follows the format of 1.5 km swim, 40 km cycle, and 10 km run and allows competitors to ride in the draft of others. This makes for very tight packs or pelotons of triathletes during the cycling portion of the race and requires quick handling in tight spaces similar to standard road races such as criteriums. For this reason, those participating in draft legal triathlons often ride with standard road drop handlebars with shorter clip-on aero bars versus full aerobars. Thus, there may be different considerations of the triathlete and their bike fit who race in draft legal events which are beyond the discussion of this chapter.

Summary

Becoming efficient and competent in understanding medical bike fitting for the triathlete requires substantial time, effort, and practice. As the number and types of triathletes (e.g., short-course versus long-course) continue to grow, the need for competent clinicians and medical professionals to perform medical bike fittings will be imperative to a comprehensive injury management plan. It is imperative to recognize that every bike fit is unique, and a one-size-fits-all approach to fitting will not meet the need of triathletes. While this chapter has focused on the importance of medical bike fittings for the triathlete, much of this information may also be extrapolated to other types of cyclists including time-trialists, road, cyclo-cross, and mountain. However, these types of cyclists have other unique considerations which are beyond the scope of this chapter. Finally, an integration of a thorough history and physical examination including review of training, nutrition, and sleeping habits is extremely important in the comprehensive management of the triathlete.

References

1. Egermann M, Brocai D, Lill C, Schmitt H. Analysis of injuries in long-distance triathletes. Int J Sports Med. 2003;24(4):271–6.

2. USA Triathlon. 2015. http://www.usatriathlon.org/. Accessed 31 Aug 2015.

3. Bertola IP, Sartori RP, Corrêa DG, Zotz TGG, Gomes ARS. Profile of injuries prevalence in athletes who participated in SESC Triathlon Caiobá-2011. Acta Ortop Bras. 2014;22(4):191–6.

4. Vleck VE, Bentley DJ, Millet GP, Cochrane T. Triathlon event distance specialization: training and injury effects. J Strength Cond Res. 2010;24(1):30–6.

5. Strock GA, Cottrell ER, Lohman JM. Triathlon. Phys Med Rehabil Clin N Am. 2006;17(3):553–64.

6. Wilk BR, Fisher KL, Rangelli D. The incidence of musculoskeletal injuries in an amateur triathlete racing club. J Orthop Sports Phys Ther. 1995;22(3): 108–12.

7. Cipriani DJ, Swartz JD, Hodgson CM. Triathlon and the multisport athlete. J Orthop Sports Phys Ther. 1998;27(1):42–50.

8. Levy C, Kolin E, Berson B. The effect of cross training on injury incidence, duration, and severity (part 2). Sports Med Clin Forum. 1986;3:1–8.

9. O'Toole ML, Hiller WDB, Smith RA, Sisk TD. Overuse injuries in ultraendurance triathletes. Am J Sports Med. 1989;17(4):514–8.

10. Galera O, Gleizes-Cervera S, Pillard F, Riviere D. Prevalence of injuries in triathletes from a French league. Apunts Med Esport. 2012;47(173):9–15.

11. Zwingenberger S, Valladares RD, Walther A, Beck H, Stiehler M, Kirschner S, et al. An epidemiological investigation of training and injury patterns in triathletes. J Sports Sci. 2014;32(6):583–90.

12. Dettori NJ, Norvell DC. Non-traumatic bicycle injuries. Sports Med. 2006;36(1):7–18.

13. Wilber C, Holland G, Madison R, Loy S. An epidemiological analysis of overuse injuries among recreational cyclists. Int J Sports Med. 1995;16(3):201–6.

14. Clarsen B, Krosshaug T, Bahr R. Overuse injuries in professional road cyclists. Am J Sports Med. 2010;38(12):2494–501.

15. Deakon RT. Chronic musculoskeletal conditions associated with the cycling segment of the triathlon; prevention and treatment with an emphasis on proper bicycle fitting. Sports Med Arthroscopy Rev. 2012;20(4):200–5.

16. Ericson MO, Nisell R, Németh G. Joint motions of the lower limb during ergometer cycling. J Orthop Sports Phys Ther. 1988;9(8):273–8.

17. Fonda B, Sarabon N. Biomechanics of cycling. Sport Sci Rev. 2010;19(1–2):187–210.

18. Bini MR, Hume PA, Croft JL. Effects of bicycle saddle height on knee injury risk and cycling performance. Sports Med. 2011;41(6):463–76.

19. Chapman AR, Vicenzino B, Blanch P, Knox JJ, Dowlan S, Hodges PW. The influence of body position on leg kinematics and muscle recruitment during cycling. J Sci Med Sport. 2008;11(6):519–26.

20. Bini RR, Hume PA, Kilding AE. Saddle height effects on pedal forces, joint mechanical work and kinematics of cyclists and triathletes. Eur J Sport Sci. 2014;14(1):44–52.

21. Wolchok JC, Hull M, Howell SM. The effect of intersegmental knee moments on patellofemoral contact mechanics in cycling. J Biomech. 1998;31(8): 677–83.
22. Ericson MO, Nisell R. Patellofemoral joint forces during ergometric cycling. Phys Ther. 1987;67(9): 1365–9.
23. Bressel E. The influence of ergometer pedaling direction on peak patellofemoral joint forces. Clin Biomech. 2001;16(5):431–7.
24. Ruby P, Hull M, Hawkins D. Three-dimensional knee joint loading during seated cycling. J Biomech. 1992;25(1):41–53.
25. Bousie JA, Blanch P, McPoil TG, Vicenzino B. Contoured in-shoe foot orthoses increase mid-foot plantar contact area when compared with a flat insert during cycling. J Sci Med Sport. 2013;16(1):60–4.
26. Hoes MJ, Binkhorst R, Smeekes-Kuyl AE, Vissers AC. Measurement of forces exerted on pedal and crank during work on a bicycle ergometer at different loads. Eur J Appl Physiol Occup Physiol. 1968; 26(1):33–42.
27. Bertucci W, Grappe F, Groslambert A. Laboratory versus outdoor cycling conditions: differences in pedaling biomechanics. J Appl Biomech. 2007;23(2):87.
28. Atkinson G, Peacock O, Gibson ASC, Tucker R. Distribution of power output during cycling. Sports Med. 2007;37(8):647–67.
29. Cockcroft SJ. An evaluation of inertial motion capture technology for use in the analysis and optimization of road cycling kinematics. Stellenbosch: University of Stellenbosch; 2011.
30. Candau RB, Grappe F, Ménard M, Barbier B, Millet GY, Hoffman MD, et al. Simplified deceleration method for assessment of resistive forces in cycling. Med Sci Sports Exerc. 1999;31:1441–7.
31. Di Prampero PE. Cycling on earth, in space, on the moon. Eur J Appl Physiol. 2000;82(5–6):345–60.
32. Martin JC, Milliken DL, Cobb JE, McFadden KL, Coggan AR. Validation of a mathematical model for road cycling power. J Appl Biomech. 1998;14:276–91.
33. Debraux P, Grappe F, Manolova AV, Bertucci W. Aerodynamic drag in cycling: methods of assessment. Sports Biomech. 2011;10(3):197–218.
34. Fintelman D, Sterling M, Hemida H, Li FX. Optimal cycling time trial position models: aerodynamics versus power output and metabolic energy. J Biomech. 2014;47(8):1894–8.
35. Empfield D. The F.I.S.T. Method for fitting triathletes to their bikes. 2007. http://www.slowtwitch.com/Bike_Fit/F.I.S.T._Tri_bike_fit_system/The_F.I.S.T._Method_for_fitting_triathletes_to_their_bikes_16.html.
36. Lohr J, Timmerman M. Trek ten-step triathlon fitting manual. Madison, WI: University of Wisconsin; 2013. Trek Fit Services.
37. Pruitt A. Body Geometry bicycle fit course. 5th ed. Morgan Hill: Specialized Bicycle Components, INC; 2008. p. 1–80.
38. Peeling P, Bishop D, Landers G. Effect of swimming intensity on subsequent cycling and overall triathlon performance. Br J Sports Med. 2005;39(12):960–4.
39. Silder A, Gleason K, Thelen DG. Influence of bicycle seat tube angle and hand position on lower extremity kinematics and neuromuscular control: implications for triathlon running performance. J Appl Biomech. 2011;27(4):297–305.
40. Ferrer-Roca V, Roig A, Galilea P, García-López J. Influence of saddle height on lower limb kinematics in well-trained cyclists: Static vs. dynamic evaluation in bike fitting. J Strength Cond Res. 2012;26(11): 3025–9.
41. Holmes J, Pruitt A, Whalen N. Lower extremity overuse in bicycling. Clin Sports Med. 1994;13(1): 187–205.
42. Fonda B, Sarabon N, Li FX. Validity and reliability of different kinematics methods used for bike fitting. J Sports Sci. 2014;32(10):940–6.
43. Hogg S. Footloose. 2010. http://bicyclingaustralia.com.au/content/2010/steve-hogg/footloose.
44. Pruitt AL, Matheny F. Andy Pruitt's complete medical guide for cyclists. Boulder: VeloPress; 2006.
45. Barratt PR, Korff T, Elmer SJ, Martin JC. Effect of crank length on joint-specific power during maximal cycling. Med Sci Sports Exerc. 2011;43(9):1689–97.
46. Zinn L, Telander T. Zinn & the art of triathlon bikes. Boulder: VeloPress; 2007.
47. Atkinson G, Davison R, Jeukendrup A, Passfield L. Science and cycling: current knowledge and future directions for research. J Sports Sci. 2003;21(9): 767–87.

Evaluation and Treatment of the Swimming Athlete

17

Katherine Wayman and Joshua Pintar

Introduction

Swimming as a competitive sport has archaeological evidence dating its origins back to the first century BCE in Japan [1, 2]. The popularity of competitive swimming grew between the seventeenth and nineteenth century and has evolved ever since the inclusion of swimming in the modern Olympic games in 1896 [1]. The sport has drastically changed over its competitive history, and it continues to mature into the twenty-first century with sports science developing evidence-based-driven coaching, injury prevention, and treatment. This sport evolution includes stroke and training technique, advancements in suit technology, the addition of goggles, and resistance/assistance training both in and out of the water. Competitions navigated from open water distances to natatoriums with meter/yard pools while have added starting blocks and wave-dampening lane lines and gutters over time. An example of this swimming revolution can be seen in one of the oldest competitive events, the 100 m freestyle, in which man has decreased his time by 18 s between the 1908 and 2008 Olympic games. Current event distances range between 50 and 1500 m with four distinct competitive strokes (freestyle, backstroke, breaststroke, and butterfly) and an event that combines them all, the individual medley [1–4].

The Four Competitive Strokes

Swimming is a unique sport in which ground reaction forces are rarely used during competition; the exception is off the walls/blocks for starts and turns. Instead, the core becomes a location of proximal stability to drive movement and propulsion for the upper and lower extremities. No matter the stroke, each is a balance of power and efficiency dependent on technique that is susceptible to fatigue. Swimming performance is strongly related to technique and swimming economy. Higher-level swimmers demonstrate better economy with less speed fluctuation, lower drag forces, and increased velocity during propulsion phases [5]. Each stroke will be discussed in detail later, but their link from the core will be

K. Wayman (✉) • J. Pintar
Department of Sports Medicine, The Ohio State University, 2050 Kenny Road, Suite 3100, Columbus, OH 43204, USA

Clinical Outcomes Research Coordinator (CORC) Program, Sports Medicine Research Institute, The Ohio State University, Columbus, OH 43204, USA
e-mail: katherine.wayman@osumc.edu

© Springer International Publishing Switzerland 2016
T.L. Miller (ed.), *Endurance Sports Medicine*, DOI 10.1007/978-3-319-32982-6_17

introduced to highlight the differences found between the elite international-level swimmers and those who pursue the sport recreationally.

During breaststroke and butterfly, core control occurs along a short axis, as the hips and lumbar spine undulate and develop power from sagittal plane movement [6]. A similar anterior and posterior movement is used off the wall for most strokes in a kicking sequence called a dolphin kick. Breaststroke allows only one underwater kick, whereas butterfly, freestyle, and backstroke allow as many underwater kicks as possible until the swimmer reaches the 15 m mark.

Freestyle and backstroke core control occurs along a long axis, with a hip and shoulder rotation along transverse plane along the spine [6]. The body rolls along this long axis to make arm recovery easier while allowing the opposite arm to pull more directly under the center of mass [7]. The hips rotate and kick to counter balance the sway of the swing of the arms and breathing action [8]. With proper body roll, a swimmer can decrease drag and improve efficiency [9]. There are differences found between the shoulder and hip roll during freestyle between skill levels [7]. The shoulder roll has been found to increase while breathing, which will increase drag and decrease speed. Elite skill levels adapt their technique by decreasing their shoulder roll, which increases speed [7]. Hip roll increases with fatigue creating additional drag that reduced speeds; however, no difference has been found in the hip roll while breathing in freestyle [7].

Freestyle Biomechanics

Phases of swimming have not clearly been defined in literature and vary depending on sources and audience. Current biomechanical literature breaks freestyle stroke into five phases, while literature more clinically based breaks the stroke into 3–4 phases [10]. For consistency of language, we divided the phases of swimming into four phases to best communicate with existing clinical literature (Fig. 17.1) [11]:

- Early pull-through
- Late pull-through
- Early recovery
- Late recovery

The optimal freestyle technique and a synopsis of key factors for this stroke as described by Pink et al. [12] and Spigelman et al. [10] are illustrated below.

Freestyle Upper Extremity Movement

- As the hand enters the water, the elbow should be located above the hand. The wrist should maintain slight flexion as this position appropriately engages the latissimus dorsi.
- The palm and forearm should face backward with fingertips pointing down toward the bottom of the pool for as long as possible to improve use of the forearm as a propulsive "paddle."

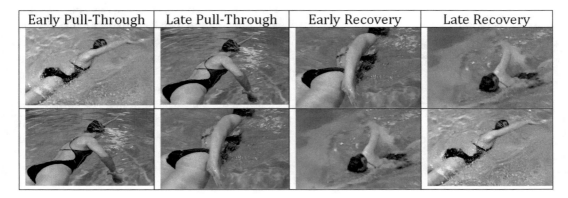

| Early Pull-Through | Late Pull-Through | Early Recovery | Late Recovery |

Fig. 17.1 Phases of the swimming stroke [11]

- The swimmer should not flick the wrist to exit the water as this causes the swimmer to lead with the hand (should be lead with the elbow) and increase impingement positions of the shoulder.
- Optimal body roll during the stroke should be approximately 30–45° along the longitudinal axis of the body.
- During recovery, the elbow should remain higher than the hand in preparation for entry as elbow should not contact the water first. Frequently, a dropped elbow position predisposes the swimmer to a thumb-first hand entry, which increases shoulder impingement and labral/bicep stress (Table 17.1).

Freestyle Lower Extremity Movement

- A six-beat kick is most commonly utilized as it promotes symmetry of stroke with regard to body roll and upper extremity stroke mechanics.
- The kick will have knees separated slightly with the hips slightly internally rotated (IR) and the ankles plantar flexed and relaxed. The kick should finish below the water surface.
- The lower extremity performs a repeated flutter kick during freestyle with legs alternating the flexion and extension movements. The knee should be slightly flexed (~10°), and ankles should be relaxed in a plantar-flexed and inverted position.

Freestyle Stroke Mechanics: General Notes

- Sprinters most commonly use a six-beat kick (three kicks per arm revolution), while distance swimmers most commonly utilize a four-beat kick (two kicks per arm revolution).
- The preferred breathing pattern is called the "alternate breathing pattern" and occurs when the swimmer breathes every three strokes. This encourages muscular symmetry and decreases risks of injury due to overexposure to impingement positions (Table 17.2).

Table 17.1 Freestyle upper extremity muscle activation [10, 12, 13]

Phases	Description	Muscle activity
Early pull-through	Begins with hand entry and ends at mid-pull-through, where arm is perpendicular to the body	Begins with upper trapezius, rhomboids, supraspinatus, anterior and middle deltoid, and serratus anterior and ends with pectoralis major, teres minor, and serratus anterior
Late pull-through	Begins as the hand and arm continue backward underwater toward the hip and ends as the hand exits water	Muscle activation transitions from above and ends with latissimus dorsi, subscapularis, and serratus anterior
Early recovery	Begins as the hand exits the water led by the elbow and ends at mid recovery as the arm is perpendicular to the body	Muscle activation transitions from above and adds middle and posterior deltoid, supraspinatus, subscapularis, and rhomboids
Later recovery	Begins as the arm moves past mid recovery and ends as the hand breaks the surface of the water for the next hand entry	Muscle activation transitions from above and ends with anterior and middle deltoid, supraspinatus, subscapularis, and rhomboids

Table 17.2 Freestyle lower extremity muscle activation [14]

Phases	Description	Muscle activity
Upbeat 1	Hip extension-knee extension	Biceps femoris (eccentric), gastrocnemius
Upbeat 2	Hip extension-knee flexion	Biceps femoris (concentric), gastrocnemius, and internal oblique during transition from upbeat to downbeat
Downbeat 1	Hip flexion-knee flexion positions	Rectus femoris (eccentric) and vastus medialis
Downbeat 2	Hip flexion-knee extension	Rectus femoris (concentric) and vastus medialis

Backstroke Biomechanics

In backstroke, the swimmer is supine while per-forming reciprocal arm strokes that are coupled with trunk rotation and an alternating leg kick [12]. The stroke is very similar to freestyle as propulsion is again impacted by stroke rate and length. Additionally, similar muscle activation patterns are used in both strokes [15]. The opti-mal backstroke technique and a synopsis of key factors for this stroke according to Pink et al. are described below [12].

Backstroke Upper Extremity Movement

- Hand entry should be pinkie first with internal rotation and full extension at shoulder. Entry is above the head, approximately shoulder width apart, and without crossing midline of the body.
- Hand entry should consist of trunk rotation ~20–40°, so the body is on the side during the catch (when the arm switches from recovery to propulsive phases). This rotation is to be timed with the underwater stroke finish of the opposite arm.
- The first motion of the underwater catch should be to flex the wrist to align direction of force toward the feet. The elbow flexion should immediately follow, to allow forearm water propulsion toward feet.
- The catch becomes the pull phase once the hand and forearm begin to pull down and backward toward the feet.
- The middle pull focuses on keeping upper arm aligned with the scapular plane with the elbow flexed between 110 and 120°; thus the hand is vertically under the shoulder without crossing midline of the body. The palm of the hand and the forearm continue to direct propulsion forces toward the feet.
- Once the hand passes the waist, the hand will pitch downward and inward as the shoulder internally rotates and the elbow extends. The hand should finish the stroke slightly deeper than the hips and wider than the shoulder. The hand should finish with the pinkie down, thumb up, and palm facing medially position
- The finish provides leverage to rotate the body toward the opposite hand's entry.
- Recovery should be driven from the shoulder, lifting arm out of the water with body rotation. The hand is positioned thumb up via shoulder external rotation (ER).
- The shoulder flexion that drives the recovery should allow for a relaxed arm to be straight as it transitions from shoulder external (ER) to internal rotation (IR) by the time of hand entry.

Backstroke: Lower Extremity Movement

- The kick should create most of the propulsion on the upbeat driven from the hips, similar to the freestyle downbeat.
- Most commonly, a six-beat kick is used to cre-ate propulsion, reduce drag, and aid in body rotation.
- The kick will have knees separated slightly with the hips IR and the ankles plantar flexed.
- The kick should finish below the water surface.

Backstroke Mechanics: General Notes

- The head throughout all phases should remain constant in an upward position toward the ceiling with a subtle tilt backward to keep water level at the ear (Table 17.3).

Butterfly Biomechanics

The butterfly stroke is a combination of freestyle and breaststroke mechanics. The stroke is a short-axis stroke, in that the swimmer moves in the frontal plane, the short axis of the body [12]. The optimal butterfly technique and a synopsis of key factors for this stroke according to Pink et al. are described below [12].

Table 17.3 Backstroke upper extremity muscle activation [12, 16]

Phases	Description	Muscle activity
Early pull-through	Begins with hand entry and ends at mid-pull-through, where the arm is perpendicular to the body	Begins deltoids supraspinatus, rhomboids, upper trap, and serratus anterior
Late pull-through	Begins as the hand and arm continue backward underwater toward the hip and ends as hand exits water	Muscle activation transitions from above and ends with latissimus dorsi, subscapularis, and teres minor
Recovery	Begins as the hand exits the water led by the elbow and ends as the hand breaks the surface of the water for the next hand entry	Rhomboids

Butterfly Upper Extremity Movement

- The hands should enter the water palms down to slightly outward about shoulder width apart. As the hands enter the water, they will travel laterally, just outside of shoulder width for the underwater catch.
- As the catch ends prior to propulsion phase, the wrists and elbows flex to direct the palms and forearms toward the feet, while the shoulder internally rotates into a high-elbow position.
- The propulsion phase begins once the swimmer has reached the high-elbow position. At this point, the hand and forearm are used in conjunction to direct propulsion forces toward the feet as the shoulders adduct.
- During the pull, there may be a slight in-sweep, bringing hands under body, but not crossing midline.
- The hands should accelerate through the entire pull to allow for efficient momentum between strokes. The final portion of the underwater pull is the ideal time to breathe during butterfly.
- The arms begin the recovery phase at the end of the propulsion phase. The arms should be straight during recovery with the palm facing the water.
- The head and arms will enter the water in conjunction with the kick to reinforce the undulation motion that drives the stroke (Table 17.4).

Butterfly Lower Extremity Movement

- The butterfly kick is executed with both legs beating at the same time with two beats per stroke cycle of the arms for sprints and sometimes one beat in distance butterfly.
- The first kick should occur as the hands enter the water.
- The second kick should occur as the hands end the propulsion phase to provide propulsion for the recovery phase. This kick should be more powerful than the first.
- The butterfly kick creates most of its propulsion during the downward sweep of the legs. It is driven by the hip flexors and core with the legs extending and driving force through separated, internally rotated, and plantar-flexed legs and ankles.

Butterfly Stroke Mechanics: General Notes

- A neutral spine posture should be maintained during breathing strokes by elevating the torso. The alignment between the head and torso remains the same with and without breath. The eyes should remain looking at the bottom of the pool with each stroke and breath (never looking forward toward the end of pool).

Breaststroke Biomechanics

The breaststroke is a unique stroke; it uses less propulsion by pushing the water toward the feet from the arms [12]. Instead it requires propulsion lift and drag from a sculling action with the arms, while greater propulsion forces are being driven

Table 17.4 Butterfly upper extremity muscle activation [12]

Phases	Description	Muscle activity
Early pull-through	Begins as the hands enter palms down just slightly wider than shoulders. The wrists and elbows will flex to face the palms and forearms toward the feet, while the shoulder internal rotates into a high-elbow position	Begins deltoids supraspinatus, rhomboids, upper trap, and serratus anterior
Late pull-through	Begins as the arms propel with a slight in-sweep bringing hands underbody, no further than midline, and continue to accelerate through the entire pull and round off into a scull to the outside	Muscle activation transitions from above and ends with latissimus dorsi, subscapularis, and teres minor
Recovery	Begins as the hands exit the water and continue until entry with straight arms facing palm	Rhomboids and deltoids

by the kick. The optimal breaststroke technique and a synopsis of key factors for this stroke according to Pink et al. are described below [12].

Breaststroke Upper Extremity Movement

- The stroke begins in a streamline position with the arms fully extended overhead and the legs streamlined and extended behind the body. The head should be aligned in a neutral position with eyes looking down to minimize drag.
- The upper extremity begins to separate into a pull position once the legs are in a streamline position. The hands will separate from the streamline position by pulling/sculling outward, slightly wider than shoulders, while the head remains in neutral position.
- Once in the widest pull position, the wrists and elbows flex for a high-elbow position as the shoulders internally rotate.
- As the body begins to pull, the torso should rise with neutral spine for breath as the hands sweep inward and adduct under the body but not crossing midline. The scooping motion of the pull should focus on pulling body forward and not upward.
- The arms continue to accelerate into the recovery, as the hands turn inward toward each other and upward during the scooping motion. The end position is when the arms return to the extended position of the streamline. The body should surge forward due to the force of the kick during the recovery with the elbows in a narrow elbow position (Table 17.5).

Breaststroke Lower Extremity Movement

- The kick begins as the legs are drawn up, with knee and hip flexion, toward the buttock during recovery.
- As the heels get closer to the buttock, the hips internally rotate to position and set up the feet for the kick. The feet should externally rotate outward, so the toes point laterally slightly and the plantar surface of the feet point behind the swimmer.
- As the kick propulsion begins, the arms should be in a streamline position overhead. Here, the legs will rapidly extend the legs rearward and slightly downward. Pressure should be felt in the heel and plantar surface with the feet laterally rotated for the majority for the kick. The downward motion of the kick will drive the hips upward into an undulation.
- At the end of the kick, the feet and legs are adducted rapidly together into a streamline position (Table 17.6).

Breaststroke Stroke Mechanics: General Notes

- Undulation should occur at the torso and chest with a neutral spine from the head to the trunk.
- The streamline position can be held for different lengths of time depending on the length of competition distance.
- The timing of the kick is crucial to an effective breaststroke. It should begin once the arms move to the recovered position.

Table 17.5 Breaststroke upper extremity muscle activation [12, 17, 18]

Phases	Description	Muscle activity
Early pull-through	Begins with upper and lower extremity in streamline position, with the hands separating and sculling out to a shoulder width position	Begins with triceps brachii, deltoids, serratus anterior, and teres minor
Late pull-through	Begins as the wrists and elbows flex for a high-elbow position as the shoulder internally rotates as the arms begin to pull, raise the torso, and sweep inward and forward under the body	Muscle activation transitions from above and ends with serratus anterior, teres minor, deltoid, bicep brachii, pectoralis major, and latissimus dorsi
Recovery	Begins as the arms accelerate and the hands turn medially and upward during the scooping motion and end back into the extended internally rotated position of the streamline	Ends with serratus anterior, teres minor, and deltoid

Table 17.6 Breaststroke lower extremity muscle activation [12, 17, 18]

Phases	Description	Muscle activity
Hip kick phase	Begins with hip extending out of the recovery position	Begins with biceps femoris and other hip extenders
Knee kick phase	Begins as the knee extends from the recovery position	Muscle activation transitions from above and ends with rectus femoris and other knee extenders
Ankle kick phase	Begins in dorsiflexion and extends to plantar-flexed positions	Muscle activation transitions from tibialis anterior to plantar flexors
Recovery	Begins as the ankle, hips, and knees flex during recovery	Ends with rectus femoris, biceps femoris, and tibialis anterior

Common Stroke Technique Error

Swim stroke modifications can occur as swimmers fatigue. Novice swimmers decrease speed when fatigued, and this can be demonstrated with decreased stroke rate and stroke length [19]. Conversely, expert swimmers show less speed reduction, but rather these swimmers increase stroke rate to make up for decreased stroke length. The expert swimmers spend more time in the propulsive phases of the stroke and shorten the recovery time to maintain speed [19].

Freestyle Errors

Pink and Tibone [20] reported most common shoulder injuries during freestyle occur in early pull-through (70%) or early recovery (18%). Virag et al. [21] performed an underwater and above-water video analysis on healthy individuals to investigate biomechanical errors found in swimming that increase the risk of shoulder pain.

Common Errors in Freestyle Are Found Below (% Prevalence in Subjects Tested) [21]

- Dropped elbow during the pull-through phase (61.3%)
- Dropped elbow during the recovery phase (53.2%)
- Eyes-forward head-carrying angle (46.8%)
- Incorrect hand entry (45.2%)
- Incorrect hand entry angle (38.71%)
- Incorrect pull-through pattern (32.3%) (Figs. 17.2, 17.3, 17.4, 17.5, 17.6, 17.7, and 17.8) [21]

The above errors can lead to anterior shoulder impingement, increased stress to the anterior labrum and bicep attachment, and shoulder impingement (both general impingement and

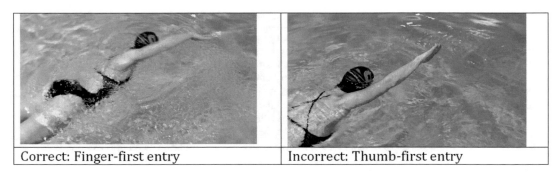

| Correct: Finger-first entry | Incorrect: Thumb-first entry |

Fig. 17.2 Hand entry angle [21]

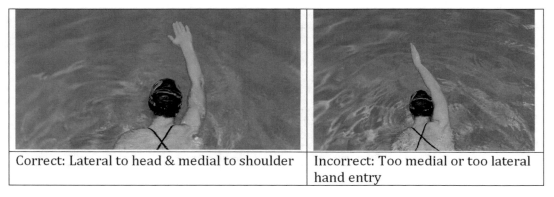

| Correct: Lateral to head & medial to shoulder | Incorrect: Too medial or too lateral hand entry |

Fig. 17.3 Hand entry position [21]

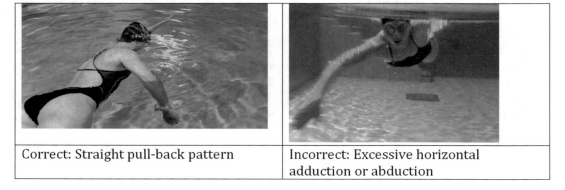

| Correct: Straight pull-back pattern | Incorrect: Excessive horizontal adduction or abduction |

Fig. 17.4 Pull-through pattern [21]

subacromial impingement). Furthermore, inappropriate positioning of the upper extremity in these biomechanical errors listed above can place the active muscles in positions of mechanical disadvantage leading to early fatigue of the swimmer and progressively earlier faulty mechanics during practice and/or competition.

An example of a mechanical position error that can create shoulder pain and impingement is called "humeral hyperextension" which is defined as "a combination of humeral abduction and extension (i.e., the humerus is behind the long axis of the body while the arm is abducted)" [12]. This position can frequently occur with inappro-

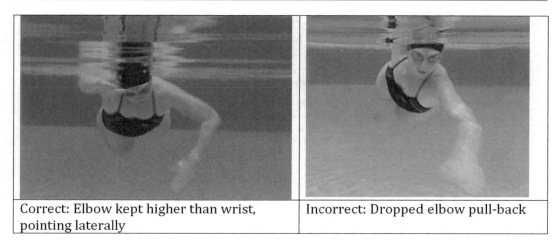

| Correct: Elbow kept higher than wrist, pointing laterally | Incorrect: Dropped elbow pull-back |

Fig. 17.5 Elbow position during pull-through [21]

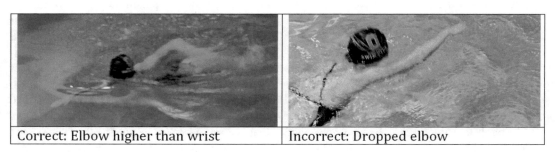

| Correct: Elbow higher than wrist | Incorrect: Dropped elbow |

Fig. 17.6 Elbow position during recovery [21]

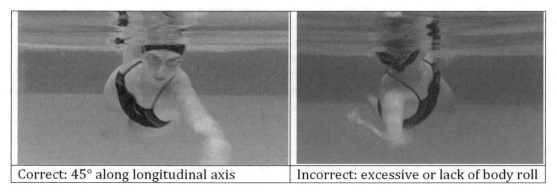

| Correct: 45° along longitudinal axis | Incorrect: excessive or lack of body roll |

Fig. 17.7 Body roll angle [21]

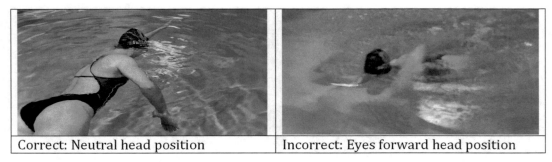

| Correct: Neutral head position | Incorrect: Eyes forward head position |

Fig. 17.8 Head-carrying angle [21]

priate hand entry (too wide or too narrow) as well as with inappropriate body roll (too much = greater than 45° or too little = less than 30°) [12].

Many of the errors demonstrate a pattern of being interrelated, suggesting one error may lead to other errors. Patterns found include the following: (a) dropped elbow during recovery phase can lead to thumb-first hand entry, (b) a dropped elbow during recovery phase can lead to incorrect hand entry position where the hand enters too wide from shoulders or crosses midline of the long axis of the body, and lastly, (c) eyes-forward head position can cause inappropriate underwater pull-through technique [21]. When coaches and athletes can identify these biomechanical errors, shoulder injury risk factors can be decreased and allow the athletes more opportunity for injury-free swimming.

Yanai et al. [22] also studied shoulder impingement with freestyle. Important findings include noting that healthy swimmers rated impingement during some trials and not others (approximately 25% of the swim trials), which suggests that impingement is not completely explained by only shoulder joint anatomy abnormalities but likely rather due to stroke technique abnormalities. These authors also found that unilateral breathing patterns are associated with shoulder impingement on the same side during the recovery phase of freestyle swimming [22]. This study suggests that by adopting a bilateral breathing pattern, the swimmer can reduce risk of shoulder impingement injury by reducing the scapular tilt, which can impinge the shoulder joint on the breathing side during recovery.

Injury Prevalence and Incidence

As aquatic endurance athletes, swimmers train beyond the recreational and therapeutic level for sport-specific adaptations. In 2012, two systematic reviews on the epidemiology, treatment, and rehabilitation in the competitive swimmer allowed insight for the health-care professional regarding musculoskeletal injuries to the shoulder, knee, and spine that can occur during this highly repetitive sport. Research highlights muscle fatigue, joint laxity/ ROM deficits, and improper or altered stroke kinematics as stressors that cause micro-damage to the static and dynamic stabilizers which are prone to injury in swimmers at all levels [13, 23].

And it appears injury rates are on the rise. During the 2012 Olympics, 5.4% of the swimmers reported injuries, which increased from 3.4% in 2008 [24, 25]. Injury rates were also found to increase between the 2009 and 2013 world championships from 2.7 to 6.1 per 100 swimmers [26, 27]. The incidence of injuries reported by the NCAA between 2009 and 2014 from swim training/competition include a proportion of 1.48/1000 for male athletes and 1.63/1000 for female athletes [28]. In 1996, a 7-year injury rate in female NCAA swimmers highlights an injury rate of 2.22/1000 swimmers when dryland weight training injury rates were included [29]. Research suggests a trend exists for both swim training and weight training injuries in the sport of swimming. Most injuries in the pool are from non-contact/overuse injuries, which occur in females more than males. Luckily, rarely are these overuse injuries severe enough for surgery with a recent occurrence rate of 2.7% in male and 2.9% in female swimmers [28]. For stroke-specific injury rates, swimmers specializing in breaststroke, backstroke, butterfly, or the individual medley (IM) are at a higher risk of injury as compared to the freestyle-only specialists [28, 30].

Performance Considerations

With regard to muscle endurance, strength, and range of motion (ROM), Evershed et al. [31] defined asymmetry as a difference between limbs greater than 10%. Evershed et al. found three categories of swimmers based on these clinical data: (1) symmetrical group with symmetrical clinical strength for all strength measures, (2) uniform asymmetrical group which represents the swimmers with strength deficits consistently on the same side, and (3) mixed asymmetrical group with swimmers that have strength deficits on both sides of the body [31]. Results from this study found that 84% ($n=27$) of the 32 subjects were asymmetrical with strength production, most commonly in internal rotation, shoulder adduction, and horizontal adduction. Interestingly, 60% of these swimmers demonstrated symmetrical hand force production (meaning equal underwater propulsive forces bilaterally despite asymmetries in the clinical strength tests). This is because 14 of the 27 asymmetrical swimmers were able to compensate for the asymmetries [31].

These results suggest that a swimmer that has a strength asymmetry in one of their prime movers may develop a compensatory strength imbalance in another muscle group (this was found in 86% of the swimmers), and the result is symmetrical hand force production. The example given is "Subject 16's left horizontal abduction is stronger than right, but right internal rotation and adduction are stronger than left. When these forces are summated, the overall force production reflects symmetry" [31]. When the strength compensations were not made by the swimmer, some swimmers found a way to compensate through kinematic strategy changes. The movement strategy changes most commonly noted in the study included significant changes in thoracic rotation (which likely contributes to asymmetrical body roll) [31].

Another example of these compensatory strategies is highlighted in a study by Hellard et al. [32] that demonstrated 200 m stroke-rate variability between Olympic and national semifinalists. They found Olympic swimmers exhibited faster backstroke rate and longer freestyle stroke length with less stroke-rate variability [32]. Both level of swimmers decreased stroke rate in butterfly, freestyle, and backstroke with fatigue in the second 100 m. Breaststroke swimmers demonstrated variability in performance based more upon stroke rate and length and less due to fatigue, suggesting greater ability to individualize technique based upon swimmer build [32].

Research regarding the underwater dolphin kick has described that the maximal thrust occurring with a downbeat kick is approximately twice that of the upbeat kick [33]. During the up- and downbeat of the kick, drag forces increase from 16 N gliding to 208 N and will grow in size and strength with each kick [33]. A case study found there may be an optimal kick cycle specific for each individual swimmer, as speed can eventually match the amount of drag a swimmer creates, making additional efforts inefficient for the energy costs [33]. A 15 m underwater kick time trial is frequently performed by coaches to help swimmers find their most efficient individualized kick rate.

The Pediatric Swimmer

Most scientific literature focuses on the high school swimmer and older. However, there are approximately 266,000 registered pediatric swimmers in the United States (USA) and approximately 2.5 million pediatric swimmers worldwide. Of US swimmers, 57% of these 266,000 swimmers are between ages of 6 and 12 years, and 37% are between 13 and 17 years of age [34]. With specialization in sport becoming more prevalent across all sports, coaches, parents, and athletes are always seeking ways to find a competitive edge. Several authors have investigated energy cost of swimming and parameters that may indicate success in swimming.

Energy cost of swimming has been defined as the total energy expenditure required for displacing the body over a given unit of distance [35]. It has been reported that pediatric athletes accumulate less blood lactate than adults with swimming [36, 37]. Van Praagh reported these energy cost differences could be attributed to hormonal effects, neuromotor maturation, and/or muscle fiber characteristic changes [38]. Another consideration includes the assumption that pubertal children can produce more energy-utilizing anaerobic pathways [38].

Jurimae et al. [39] studied 29 boys and divided them into two groups, 15 prepubertal boys (11.9 years ± 0.3; Tanner stages 1–2) and 14 pubertal boys (14.3 years ± 1.4; Tanner stages 3–4), and studied anthropometrics, body composition, peak oxygen consumption, stroking parameters, and energy cost in a 400 m freestyle event. These authors recognized two key patterns from their study. First, they found that backward extrapolation of 400 m freestyle at maximal effort is an appropriate mechanism to assess VO2peak in water as long as expired gas samples were collected in the first 20 s of recovery [39]. Second, the authors found the top predictive factors for swimming performance [39]:

- Best biomechanical factor → stroke index (SI)
- Best anthropometric factor → arm span
- Best bioenergetic factor → in-water VO2peak

These results were in agreement with another study by Lätt et al. (2010). Lätt et al. [35] were able to quantify how these performance predictors could account for variance between swimmers. This group reported that stroke index accounted for 90.3 % of variance, arm span accounted for 45.8 % of variance, and blood lactate accumulation accounted for 45.2 % of performance variance between youth swimmers [35]. Dormehl et al. [40] compared male and female swimmers in two age categories, ages 12–14 and 15–18. These authors studied video footage of these swimmers competing in 100 m

and 200 m events. It was found that the older age group demonstrated a higher velocity, longer stroke length, and greater stroke index than the younger swimmers. Additionally, as distance increased, stroke length decreased progressively with larger changes noted in the younger swimmers, which may indicate the role of physical immaturity and racing inexperience, which this may have a role in swimmers' pacing abilities and performance with longer distances [40]. Knowledge of the weight of these variables and parameters can help coaches create appropriate training loads for the pediatric swimmer to boast performance while minimizing overtraining and injury risk.

The Masters Swimmer

Even in healthy adults, physiological functional capacity (PFC) declines with increased age [41–45]. PFC is defined as "the ability to perform the physical tasks of daily life and the ease with which these tasks can be performed"[6]. Several researchers have investigated performance of aging elite athletes to more completely understand PFC changes with increased age. Aging elite athletes generally have fewer variables found than the aging general population including fewer/lesser changes in body composition, lesser changes in physical activity participation, and fewer comorbidities/degenerative diseases [6].

Donato and his coauthors [6] investigated the performance of 640 elite masters swimmers between 1988 and 1999 from the US Masters Swimming (USMS) Championships. The athletes studied placed in the top 10 in their age group in the 50 m or 1500 m during the 12-year study period [6]. A follow-up study was performed by Rubin et al. [46], and these authors performed a retrospective study collecting data from the USMS and International Masters Swimming Hall of Fame (IMSHOF) records. The inclusion criteria for subjects in Rubin's study include a minimum age of 25 years, participation in at least 16 years of masters swimming (competition spanning at least 4–5 year age groups), and IMSHOF recognition (Table 17.7) [6, 46].

Table 17.7 Age-related changes in the masters swimmer [6, 46]

Swimming performance [6, 46]	Declines progressively with age until ~70 years
	After 70 years, the decline becomes quadratic
	Strength and power declines
	Water resistance and drag increases
Event duration [6]	Long-duration event performance more affected by age than short duration
Females versus Males [6, 46]	Female swimmers show greater decline in performance
	Female swimmers demonstrate decreased muscular strength and power especially in the upper extremities
General [6]	Age-related decline is variable based on numerous factors including:
	Variability in training volume
	Variability in training intensity
	Athlete motivation
	Comorbidities
	General body fatigue in response to exercise

Common Injuries

Shoulder

The most common area prone to injury in a swimmer is the shoulder where 40–91 % swimmers have reported shoulder pain in their lifetime [13]. The shoulder's primary use is to aid the arm's ability to generate propulsion forces necessary to pull the body forward in the water. Males and females have similar injury risk and injury patterns, which appears to begin with muscle fatigue scapular dyskinesia, which has been found during practice even in healthy, pain-free swimmers [47]. During a swim practice quartered into breaks, scapular dyskinesia increased from 37 %, to 68 %, to 74 %, and eventually to 82 % by the end of practice in healthy swimmers [47]. Once scapular dyskinesia presented it never disappeared for the remainder of practice, suggesting vulnerability over time with high levels of repetition and training [47].

Tate et al. [48] studied risk factors associated with shoulder pain/disability across the lifespan of competitive swimmers in 2012. They found swimmers less than 12 years have shoulder pain, while older swimmers have shoulder pain and disability [48]. Hours swum per week were positively correlated with shoulder pain and disability, while participation in other sports, besides

water polo, was found to reduce the risk of injury [48]. Additionally, for younger swimmers, it appears that shoulder flexibility, weakness of the middle trapezius and shoulder internal rotators, and tightness of the latissimus dorsi predispose them to shoulder pain [48]. On the contrary, older swimmers present with pectoralis minor muscle tightness and core muscle weakness which predispose them to pain and disability [48].

Wolf et al. [30] and Walker et al. [49] highlight injury patterns and risk factors for the shoulder. They found that injuries that occur during swim practice were due to stroke technique errors and the use of hand paddles. Other risk factors were (a) strength and conditioning errors, (b) being freshmen in college, and (c) being female. Scapular dyskinesia, rotator cuff strength imbalances, glenohumeral laxity, and external rotation (ER) range of motion (ROM) <93° and ≥100° were risk factors that should be assessed and addressed to protect from injury to reinjury.

The risk for injury increases as the dynamic stabilizers fatigue and the static structures become overused which leads to the possibility of increased laxity over time [13]. An example of this during freestyle is at stroke entry, when the forward flexion and internal rotation of the glenohumeral joint during the recovery phase meets the hydrodynamic force of the hand hitting the water, forcing the hand to elevate the arm into an impingement position if not stabilized [13]. This impingement position was estimated from video analysis to be 24.8 % of the stroke time during freestyle [22]. Consider that a high-level swimmer trains for ~20–30 hours per week which can add up to ~500,000 strokes per arm; an untreated shoulder that experiences continued impingement can experience a spectrum of injuries including laxity, tendonitis, lesions, defects, and loose bodies [50].

Common clinical findings in the injured swimmers shoulder include [23]:

- Supraspinatus and subscapularis tendinopathy
- Subacromial impingement and thickening of the supraspinatus, infraspinatus, and teres minor
- Subacromial bursitis with lesions of the acromial joint (ACJ) that can lead to osteoarthritis (OA)
- Superior shoulder labral tear from anterior to posterior (SLAP)
- Bankart and long head of the biceps tendon lesions

Impingement is primarily caused by altered kinematics rather than subacromial pathological changes when [13, 51]:

(1) Anteroinferior acromion impinges the bursal surface of the rotator cuff.
(2) Anterosuperior glenoid and labrum impinge the rotator cuff and/or the bicep tendon.

This has been supported by Sein et al. [51] whose MRI images found only three out of 52 swimmers presented with acromion pathology. Additionally, he found that positive MRI findings were seen in healthy swimmers [51].

Glenohumeral joint rotation changes in unilateral overhead athletes have been shown to occur in the dominant shoulder when compared to the nondominant [52–54]. The competitive swimmer, however, is a bilateral upper extremity athlete, utilizing both dominant and nondominant arms. Humeral adaptations in bilateral upper extremity athletes depend on the muscle demands and technique of each swimmer. Research by

Potts et al. found a disparity in shoulder strength exists in swimmers due to the preferred breathing style, demonstrating bilateral breathers are better balanced than unilateral breathers [55]. Whiteley at el. [54] reported in elite swimmers significantly greater humeral retrotorsion (6.4°>ER) of the dominant versus nondominant arm in adolescent swimmers [56]; however, this is almost half the difference found in unilateral upper extremity athletes (11.9°>ER) [56].

Additional research by Riemann et al. supported this pattern of greater external rotation in the dominant arm found in all sexes across the age groups in youth, high school, and master programs [50]. These authors studied active range of motion (AROM) in 144 swimmers aged 12–61 years without recent history (<6 months) of shoulder pain or injury, with at least one year of competitive swimming experience, and practice frequency of ≥ 3× weekly were involved in the study. These swimmers demonstrated adaptive changes in the total arc of shoulder ROM with and without scapular stabilization in both the dominant and nondominant arms; commonly, the dominant arm will have greater ER AROM, while the nondominant arm will have greater IR AROM [50]. The rationale that may explain this finding is that, for example, a right-hand-dominant swimmer more frequently prefers to breathe right even when they report being bilateral breathers, which correlates to a need for more stability and more propulsive forces created underwater with the nondominant left arm [50]. However, the authors admit that more research needs to be done to investigate breathing pattern preferences and compare dominant and nondominant upper extremity strength and ROM values as this was not directly studied by the group.

Poor mechanics while swimming can be documented with both breathing and nonbreathing strokes. Abnormal mechanics also appear to be heightened in the presence of pain. One example of technique change is an increase in body rotation on the breathing side of the painful shoulder [57]. Musculoskeletal limitations in ROM could be a possible cause as a study by Thomas et al. found musculoskeletal limitations in ROM present after 12 weeks of swim practice [58]. These changes include decreased internal rotation and scapular protraction at 45° of elevation which can impact stroke performance [58]. Heinlein et al., Scovazzo et al., and Cools et al. each discuss variations in muscle activation for freestyle found from previous research, including an altered activation in the anterior and middle deltoid, upper trapezius, rhomboid, and serratus anterior which affect scapular upward rotation and protraction [59–61]. Similar studies highlight butterfly mechanical changes with noticeable altered upper trapezius, serratus anterior, supraspinatus, and teres minor activation, resulting in downward rotation of scapula [11, 59]. Further, previous research in breaststroke demonstrated altered muscle activation from latissimus dorsi, upper trapezius, subscapularis, and supraspinatus, resulting in the same decrease in scapular upward rotation that predisposes the shoulder to dyskinesia and impingement [17, 59].

Additional changes have been found in swimmers with painful shoulder during functional tasks, including greater activation of the sternocleidomastoid, upper trapezius, and anterior scalene on the involved side [62]. A study by Figueiredo et al. found muscles prone to fatigue in the last laps of 200 freestyle include flexor carpi radialis, biceps brachii, triceps brachii, pectoralis major, upper trapezius, rectus femoris, and biceps femoris [63]. A follow-up study in 2013 by Figueiredo found a kinematic change occurs in stroke mechanics at the onset of fatigue for the above muscles. He noted increased muscle activity and activation duration during the pull-through phase with the onset of muscle fatigue. Unfortunately, the increased muscle activation did not generate higher propulsion forces, causing a decrease in velocity in the last 50 of a 200 m swim [64].

This same phenomenon is most likely occurring during practice with similar injury risk and injury patterns, which appear to begin with muscle fatigue and compensation leading to scapular dyskinesia and other altered mechanics [47, 58]. Common corrective exercises and recommendations for injury prevention and rehabilitation will be discussed later.

Knee

Knee pain is the second most reported location injured among swimmers with 34–86 % incidence among swimmers [13]. The greatest incidence of knee pain is among breaststrokers, and the primary cause is the biomechanics of the breaststroke kick which generates high valgus loads during the adduction phase [13]. Evidence of repetitive stress to the medial compartment in breaststrokers includes synovitis, MCL strains, thickening of the medial plica, and pes anserine tendinitis or bursitis [65–67].

One study found a higher incident of knee pain when hip abduction angles were either less than 37° or greater than 42° [68]. Altered kicking kinematics have been seen in swimmers with medial patellar facet pain, as additional stress is accumulated when the swimmer increases hip abduction and flexion with increase in knee flexion [69]. These swimmers with MCL pain showed high velocity at the hips and knees, with the tibia increasing external rotation as the knees extended and the ankle plantar flexed [67].

The flutter kick used during backstroke and freestyle can also place repetitive stress thru the knee via patellofemoral overload [66]. This type of anterior knee pain may also be the result of improper starts and turns that place forceful muscle contractions through the knees in mini-squat position [66]. Additional considerations should be considered regarding tracking abnormalities, patellar instability, subluxations, impaired strength, endurance, and flexibility that may predispose a swimmer's knee to injury [13].

Swimmers may have abnormalities in stroke technique, training error, and dryland dysfunctional movements that take years to become symptomatic at the knee [13]. This statement is supported by a study in asymptomatic elite swimmers, 14–15 years of age, with abnormal MRI findings in 69.2 % compared to 31.1 % in age-matched controls [70]. The areas of MRI abnormalities include edema to the infrapatellar fat pad (53.8 %), bone marrow (26.9 %), prefemoral fat pad (19 %), and joint effusion (15.3 %) [70]. It is unknown whether or not these findings correspond to benign acute changes from training or if the stress findings become chronic damage, defect, or instability; additional research is warranted.

Spine

Similar to other swimming overuse injuries, muscle strength, endurance, and flexibility each have a role in back pain. Outside of myofascial strains that can result from the twisting motion with flip turns and body roll errors [23], it appears that degenerative disk changes at multiple levels are more common in swimmers than control [71]. Research has demonstrated little sex differences in low back pain; however training intensity, duration, and distance of the competitive swimmers appear to increase disk degeneration in elite swimmers (68%) compared to recreational swimmers (29%), in those ~20 years of age [72]. Another underlying cause could also be related to the aqueous training environment, which can lead to decreased bone mineral density as compared to athletes who compete on land [73].

The streamline position, used for starts and turns, may predispose the back to repeated stress. A study by Kobayashi et al. found the streamline position, while swimming increased lumbar lordosis, with a strong positive correlation to a streamline position on land [74]. This extended position can lead to repetitive loading of the posterior structures placing them at risk for spondylolysis and spondylolisthesis [13]. Similarly, the undulation motion that occurs at these hips and spine during butterfly and breaststroke can exaggerate lumbar lordosis [13]. Additional stressors to the lumbar spine can occur at practice with the utilization of fins, kick boards, and pull buoys, as each has been found to produce excessive hyperextension of the lumbar spine [75].

The number of training hours in adolescence may predispose swimmers to increased thoracic and lumbar spine injury without a balanced program. A study by Wojtys et al. found that lumbar lordosis and thoracic kyphosis angles increase in swimmers between 8 and 18 years of age in both sexes, compared to the smaller angles found in the age-matched youth who lacked sport participation [76]. During this time of development and growth in the age group swimmer, the bones have not ossified/hardened to protect against repeated stress [77]. If the training hours surpass the endurance of often weak abdominal muscles, then the hip flexors can increase lordosis and lead to other common back injuries in swimmers including: acute disk herniation, apophyseal fracture, strains, sprains, contusions, spondylolysis, and spondylolisthesis [77].

Altered activation patterns in the lumbo-pelvic musculature may predispose these athletes to overuse injuries to the vertebral joints, muscles, and ligaments [78]. It is imperative to assess and teach proper control of the lumbar spine at rest and against sport-specific demands to protect the swimmers' back during swimming tasks. An increase in lumbar lordosis is related to a decrease in internal oblique and transverse abdominal activation during the streamline position [74]. Further information regarding how to improve core control will be discussed later in the rehabilitation section of this chapter.

Hip

Similarly, control of the lumbo-pelvic musculature may also predispose a swimmer to injuries to the hip joint, ligaments, and musculature. Most common injuries include the hip flexor and the adductor magnus and brevis [66]. These adductor injuries can occur during the wide breaststroke kick that causes the breaststroker knee [23]. Chronic hip pain, femoral acetabulum impingement, structural instability, labral tears, and chondral lesions are all risks from repetitive hip internal rotation (IR) motions of the lower extremity (LE) that occur during the breaststroke kicking motion [79]. Impaired stability and movement patterns during a swimmer hip-driven kick should be assessed as research reports the presence of muscle weakness in those with chronic hip pain [79].

The muscles found to be weak and lacking neuromuscular control are those responsible for hip external rotation, internal rotation, and abduction [56, 79]. Utilizing fins and a kick board at practice can increase lumbar lordosis and apply additional stress to the hip structures [10]. Common corrective exercises and recommendations for injury prevention and rehabilitation will be discussed in further detail in the rehabilitation section of this chapter.

Ankle

The ankle is used in many ways to create underwater propulsion forces. Backstroke, freestyle, and butterfly share a similar kicking kinematics with a kick driven from the hips that transfer high forces against hydrodynamic resistance down the kinematic chain to a plantar-flexed foot. Additionally, these three strokes may all use an underwater, dolphin kick action to produce velocity from a start or turn into their breakout strokes.

Scientific evidence is lacking regarding effects of ankle flexibility in swimming, even though many swimming programs emphasize ankle plantar flexion stretches into their routine. A recent study by Willems et al. found muscle strength of plantar flexors, and internal rotators were predictors of power and performance during the dolphin kick in competitive swimmers [80]. They did not find a relationship between plantar flexion and internal rotation ROM on performance; however, the authors wanted to investigate the changes in mechanics in a swimmer with inadequate ankle plantar flexion ROM. By taping the tested ankle to temporarily increase joint stiffness, the authors altered kicking kinematics at the knee, increasing flexion and decreasing extension propulsion forces [80]. Kicking with a plantar-flexed ankle appears to be a skill learned through experience, as novice swimmers have demonstrated a dysfunctional kick with less plantar flexion, which was theorized as a reproduction of walking in the water [81]. With increased exposure, novice swimmers have been found to effectively achieve optimal plantar flexion ROM as evidenced by the performance of functional

kick movement patterns learned with increased experience [81, 82].

Ankle hypermobility and chronic instability may cause problems for those athletes who fatigue in their dynamic stabilizers or lack proper neuromuscular control to prevent repeated lateral ankle sprains. If untreated, chronic instability can develop into osteoarthritis as research had found ligamentous stabilizers could lengthen, tear, and allow the fibula to displace laterally and widen the ankle joint, which allows for excessive talar rotation [83]. This can lead to rear foot eversion movement that negatively impedes ground reaction forces and performance seen during a swim start [82].

Fin use has been associated with ankle injuries, as the foot requires more energy and torque depending on the type of fin used, and has been found to affect the body position during the kick [10, 80]. Using a swimmers' fin has been found to have a kinematic change that increase the kick frequency, amplitude, and depth of the kicking feet [80]. This may predispose the swimmer to injury as the increasing amplitude and speed creates a bigger wake and drag to overcome. Elipot et al. discovered higher-level swimmers have an improved coordination and less drag during their underwater undulation, as they are able to keep joint angles smaller than lower-level swimmers [84]. These higher-level swimmers move with a synergistic action between the ankle and hip and an independent knee action [84].

The extra stress applied through the ankle to the tibia during a swimmer's kick may predispose an athlete to repeated stress leading to medial tibial stress syndrome. This supports previous research that found swimmers have lower bone mineral density than athletes who compete in a weight-bearing sport [73]. Mudd et al. found the spine, pelvic, and lower legs to site-specific area prone less bone mineral in swimmers [73]. And a study by Palmer et al. found that swimmers who are symptomatic with medial tibial stress syndrome had a lower bone mineral density than non-symptomatic swimmers [85] which places them at higher risk for stress fractures in the lower extremities.

Swimming Injury Conclusion

Regardless of the injury, treatment should begin with relative rest, ice, and NSAIDS during the acute phase to reduce inflammation. Conservative rehabilitation should focus on the technique correction of muscle imbalances found during evaluation and during swim stoke. Corticosteroid injections have been suggested if pain is consistent and hinders rehabilitation [23]. The final option, if 3–6 months of conservative treatment was unsuccessful, is surgery. However, the research on overhead athletes with arthroscopy and subacromial decompressions includes few swimmers and suggests poor results with a 56 % return rate to swimming at prior level of function [23]. The return rate for posteroinferior capsular shift has been found to be 70 %, with a low recurrence rate of multidirectional instability [23].

Unique Pulmonary Considerations in Swimmers

Thoracic Outlet and Paget-Schroetter Syndrome

The cervical spine is also an area prone to injury in overhead athletes. Most injuries appear to be muscle strains, sprains, or contusions [86]. However, other conditions have been found in swimmers including thoracic outlet syndrome and Paget-Schroetter Syndrome, which is a medical emergency with a thrombosis of the subclavian vein [87, 88]. This effort thrombosis occurs from strenuous and repetitive activity of the upper extremities during swimming which presents similarly to thoracic outlet syndrome; exceptions include arms swelling with distention and dilation of visible veins across the shoulder and upper arm (Urschel's sign) [88]. Evidence supports that anatomical abnormalities of the thoracic outlet are involved in the pathogenesis of these thrombosis, including the cervical rib, congenital bands, hypertrophy of scalene tendons, and abnormal insertion of costoclavicular ligaments. Doppler ultrasonography is the preferred initial test, with contrast venography being the cold standard for diagnosis [88].

Swimming-Induced Pulmonary Edema

Swimming-induced pulmonary edema (SIPE) is not widely described in literature as it is difficult to capture as it is transient in nature. A diagnosis of SIPE is made when a swimmer reports shortness of breath accompanied with coughing in the absence of water aspiration [89]. Severity is categorized as "mild" when the swimmer is able to complete the swimming trial despite onset of symptoms and "severe" when the swimmer stops the swim due to symptoms. Miller and his coauthors surveyed athletes belonging to the US triathlon organization to assess prevalence and risk factors for SIPE. Based on their findings, SIPE may be present in 1.4 % of the population; only four of 31 cases occurred in the absence of these risk factors [90]. See Table 17.8 for SIPE risk factors.

Shupak et al. followed 35 males aged 18–19 years who were undergoing military training for open water swimming. None of the subjects had a history of pulmonary conditions, and none were habitual smokers ("some" smoked 2–3 cigarettes daily for 1–2 years). All swimmers completed five open water swim trials. Trials 1, 2, 3, and 5 were 2.4 km and trial 4 was 3.6 km. The water temperature was between 16 and 18 °C (61–64 °F), and all swimmers wore 6 mm thick neoprene diving jackets, swam supine, and utilized fins. During the duration of the study, 29 incidents of SIPE in 21 individuals (60 % incidence) were documented [89].

Shupak et al. propose that SIPE is induced by stress failure of the pulmonary capillaries. The failure of the pulmonary capillaries could be caused by the increased pulmonary blood flow and pressure which allows for the higher molecular weight protein edema fluid and red blood cells to leak into the interstitium and alveolar space [89]. The incidence of activity-induced pulmonary edema is higher in aquatic environments as compared with dryland environments. This is likely because immersion increases cardiac preload and pulmonary arterial pressure [89]. Additionally, cold water also increases risk for SIPE as cold water decreases core body temperature, which causes the body to shift the blood

Table 17.8 Risk factors for swimming-induced pulmonary edema (SIPE) [89–91]

1	Swimming in cold water
2	Oral fluid overload before a swimming event
3	History of hypertension
4	Participation in triathlon competition length of half-ironman distance or greater (1.2+ miles of swimming)
5	Female sex
6	Use of fish-oil supplements

Table 17.9 Swimming-induced pulmonary edema (SIPE) treatment guidelines [91]

On scene	Provide nebulized albuterol and supplemental oxygen (O_2)
	Continue O_2 until saturation of $\geq 95\%$ maintained (often 1–5 days)
Prevent hypothermia	Remove cold clothing
	Increase body warmth with towels and blankets
Continued care	Continue supplemental O_2 and beta 2-agonist for alveolar clearance and symptom improvement

from peripheral to more central (thoracic) blood vessels [92–95]. Cold water immersion also increases cardiac pre- and afterloads [96, 97].

Presentation in the emergency department is varied due to transportation times. Electrocardiography may show minor changes; some cases may present with positive troponin levels and transient left ventricular dysfunction [92, 98]. Pulmonary function tests may reveal rales, wheezes, and/or abnormal chest X-rays. Based on observation of three patients with SIPE, it was found that the gravity-dependent areas of the pulmonary vasculature were at higher risk to demonstrate abnormal lung sounds and chest X-ray results [91]. Other signs of SIPE presentation include dyspnea, cough (with our without hemoptysis), tachypnea, and confusion (Table 17.8) [89–91].

The above cardiopulmonary dysfunctions are not common in the swimming athlete but should be recognizable to health-care providers within differential diagnosis considerations to improve athlete outcomes and expedite return to prior level of swimming function as safely and efficiently as possible (Table 17.9) [91].

Rehabilitation

Rehabilitation of injured swimmers depends on many factors including past medical history, comorbidities, medications, allergies, and the timing of a conservative versus surgical rehabilitation on the return to sport for a competitive season. Many of the principles applied in the conservative and surgical rehabilitation program

are the same; however, protection of anatomic repair and any concomitant pathologies must be considered on an individual bases [99]. Regardless of the mechanism of injury, treatment starts with diminishing pain and inflammation and protecting the healing tissue while preventing the negative effects of immobilization and nonuse [99].

The following are recommendations and considerations regarding the rehabilitation of swimmers. Treatment should begin with setting the foundation of proper movement patterns, discouraging faulty movements early and throughout the return to sport.

Swimming is a unique sport in which ground reaction forces are rarely used. In the water, the trunk becomes the location of proximal stability to drive movement and propulsion from the upper and lower extremities. Regardless of injury, core stability and strengthening must be a significant focus of the rehabilitation. The end goal must be sport-specific control and endurance utilizing the upper legs, pelvis, trunk, and shoulders together.

Breathing

Breathing is an unconscious core muscle activation pattern that has been found to become disordered in athletes with dysfunctional movement patterns [100]. The normal and most efficient breathing pattern is termed "diaphragmatic breathing," and it involves the use of the diaphragm muscle to synchronize motion along the rib cage and abdomen [100]. One common dysfunctional breathing pattern is called "thoracic breathing," which involves the upper chest muscles expanding the upper rib cage and not utilizing movement from the lower rib cage and abdomen [100]. Studies have found a connection between the muscle compensation that occurs with thoracic breathing and neck pain, scapular dyskinesia, trigger point formation, and respiratory alkalosis [100]. Objectively, these dysfunctional movements have been researched utilizing a Functional Movement Screen [100]:

- 75 % of those who do not pass (score ≤ 14/21) demonstrated thoracic breathing.
- 66.6 % of those who passed (score ≥ 15/21) were diaphragmatic breathers.

Therefore, swimmers that demonstrate thoracic breathing may have more abnormal functional movement patterns and should be further evaluated for these in and out of the water.

Inspiratory muscle training has been shown to improve performance in both trained athletes and untrained individuals [101, 102]. A study by Wilson et al. found combining a standard warm-up with an inspiratory device improved performance in 100 m freestyle by 0.62 s [103]. It has been demonstrated that improved inspiratory volume and forced expiratory volume in 1 s can occur after 12 weeks of respiratory training [104]. Additional research has demonstrated that swimmers with 6 weeks of respiratory training have been able to improve 100 m and 200 m times but not 400 m [105] times; additional research is needed to understand training effects on distance events.

Breath Control/Pulmonary Function

Different strategies can be employed to improve breathing economy to gain a competitive edge with swimming. A training strategy utilized to improve swimming performance is apnea training. It has been documented that apnea training has several metabolic responses including increased lung volume [106] and decreased ventilatory responses to submaximal exercise/less dyspnea during exercise [107]. Lemaître and coauthors conducted a study of four male swimmers with no previous apnea training that performed a 3-month apnea training which consisted of performing 30 s apnea bouts (precipitated by a deep but not maximal breath to avoid Valsalva and Muller maneuvers) followed by 30 s of breathing room air while performing steady-state cycling at 30 % maximal oxygen uptake for 1 h as described in previous research [108, 109]. The test/ retest was performance based upon time to complete the 50 m freestyle spirnt without a breath. All four swimmers presented after 3 months with a significant increase in minimum arterial oxygen saturation (SaO_2min), maximal oxygen update (VO_2peak), and respiratory compensation point (RCP). Swimmers reported decreased perceived dyspnea, demonstrated delayed fatigue, increased stroke length (which has been reported to improve swimming performance), and greater propulsive continuity after apnea training. [107]. It must be noted that underwater apnea training to promote improved performance has been advised against in more recent years due to the more public awareness of accidental drownings.

Boyd and his coauthors have issued a public service announcement warning swimmers to avoid "dangerous underwater breath-holding behaviors" (DUBBSs) [110]. Hypoxic blackouts occur as a drop in partial pressure of oxygen in arterial blood gas occurs which results in hypoxia and then loss of consciousness underwater. Hyperventilation before swimming decreases carbon dioxide stores in the body, which delays the automatic response to come to the surface to breathe [110–112]. Four of 16 DUBB cases in New York between 1988 and 2011 resulted in deaths. Each of the four fatalities occurred in males who were known to be "expert" swimmers, and each performed hyperventilation activities before practicing underwater lap swimming [110]. 15 of the 16 drownings occurred in a pool facility, 14 of 15 of these had a lifeguard on duty with lifeguard rescue attempt, and more than half of the 16 incidents occurred with the drowning victim being accompanied by at least one other swimmer [110]. Due to the high and life-threatening risks associated with this type of training, the costs outweigh any benefits proposed and therefore it should be avoided.

An alternative to apnea training is a respiratory muscle warm-up. As mentioned earlier, Wilson et al. studied 15 elite swimmers (nine male, six female) to assess if an inspiratory muscle exercise (IME)-specific warm-up would improve swim performance as measured with a 100 m freestyle sprint [103]. Each swimmer had their own POWERbreathe device setup according to a percentage of their maximum inspiratory muscle pressure for the test. The swimmers were assigned to one of the four warm-up protocols. Protocol 1 included a swim-only warm-up. Protocol 2 included a IME warm-up with 2×30 reps of 40 % maximal inspiratory muscle pressure (40 % to prevent fatigue). Protocol 3 included the same swim warm-up as protocol 1 and included a sham IME warm-up (2×30 reps of 15 % maximal inspiratory muscle pressure). Lastly, protocol 4 included the same swim warm-up as protocol 1 followed by the IME warm-up described in protocol 2. The athletes performed their assigned warm-ups $1\times$ weekly for 4 weeks [103]. At retest, the results are as follows from fastest 100 m time to slowest: swim and IME warm-up, swim and sham IME warm-up, swim-only warm-up, and IME-only warm-up. The swim and IME warm-up was statistically faster than the swim-only warm-up and the IME-only warm-up but not statistically faster than the swim warm-up and sham IME warm-up. Follow-up investigation is needed, but these initial results demonstrate that the IME warm-up can be a safe and simple addition to swim training and improves performance [103].

Spine

Cervical

Endurance of the deep cervical spine muscles and pelvic and lumbar stabilizers are important in rehabilitation nontraumatic spine injuries. It is important to rule out red flags at the cervical and lumbar spine when warranted to determine if an appropriate referral or emergent care is needed. A recent literature review highlights how nonspecific neck pain in athletes maybe the result of minor sprains and strains during athletics [86]. It

appears these injuries result from deficits in cervical or upper thoracic mobility as well as cervical and upper thoracic muscle recruitment, strength, and endurance that effect repositioning acuity, postural stability, and oculomotor control [86]. This is supported by other researches found in overhead athletes, supporting thoracic ROM asymmetries and deficits are found even in healthy controls between the dominant and non-dominant arms [113].

Research also highlights the importance of stretching exercises for the scalenes, upper trapezius, levator scapulae, and pectoralis minor in athletes with neck pain [86, 114]. Tightness of these muscles can lead to axillary artery occlusion or thoracic outlet syndrome and compression of the subclavian artery, vein, or brachial plexus and/or axillary artery, with neurovascular symptoms of arm fatigue, pain, tenderness, and cyanosis [87, 114]. If an increase in thoracic kyphosis or anterior scapular tilt is present, then thoracic extension and pectoralis minor stretching have been recommended [86]. Nerve glides maybe needed for those athletes who have radicular symptoms down the upper extremity [86]. Other interventions include cervical retraction exercises to reduce forward-head position with improvement in deep neck musculature; a sample program is provided below (Appendix A) [86].

Lumbar

Treatment options for athletes with low back pain must be based upon sound clinical judgment to diagnose the appropriate care for a spondylolysis, spondylolisthesis, pars interarticularis stress fractures, avulsion fractures, and vertebral end plate fractures common in the young swimmer's back [115]. The purpose of this section will be to discuss interventions for trunk coordination, strengthening, and endurance exercises recommended in the clinical practice guidelines from the orthopedic section of the American Physical Therapy Association for low back pain [116]. It is recommended to begin these interventions for athletes with subacute and chronic low back pain with movement coordination impairments [116].

It was also recommended that manual therapy interventions should be utilized to reduce pain and disability in patients with mobility deficits at the spine and hip [116]. These manual techniques will be discussed in the hip section.

Trunk stability progression is a very important component of swim training. The more stable the core, the more efficient the swimmer. It is recommended to start strengthening and rehabilitation programs with abdominal bracing to improve effectiveness of trunk stability programs. Start with isolation of transverse abdominis and internal oblique muscles and move to larger, more surface-level muscles. Once isolation activation of these core muscles has been appropriately established, the athlete should progress then to more functional and swim-specific movements [117]. In order to encourage appropriate carryover to functional activities and swimming, training should utilize all three planes of motion with the strengthening program [117]. Trunk stability training is especially important for pediatric swimmers. During developmental ages, mechanical stroke technique is not commonly mastered yet, and movement inefficiencies can be prevalent. Allen et al. studied youth swimmers and found that trunk stabilization exercises over a 6-week period (utilized parallel roman chair dynamic back extension, prone and lateral plank, dynamic and static curl-up) are effective in a pediatric swimmer population with swim performance and injury prevention [118]. It can be extrapolated that strengthening and core activation exercises should be an important component of dryland training for swimmers of all ages.

Bilven et al. [119] discuss that an initial core stability program should include neutral spine awareness and proper postural muscle recruitment. In time, the athlete must gain proprioceptive, kinesthetic awareness and the ability to control the lumbar spine during return to sport progression. This is important because previous studies have found that altered neuromuscular control is a risk factor in patients with LBP [120]. Thus, it is recommended to begin with the local trunk stabilizers, training them without compensation, utilizing abdominal hallowing, bracing, and diaphragmatic breathing [119]. The follow-ing compilation of exercises for core stability is the focus of early neuromuscular progression from Bilven et al. [119], Kachingwe et al. [121], and Ellsworth et al. [122] (Appendix B).

Hip

It has been well documented that core muscle endurance and hip strength influence the risk for lower extremity injuries [119, 123, 124]. Research suggests that neuromuscular control of the core and hip musculature also play an important role in injury prevention [125, 126].

In swimmers, available research is limited regarding hip control and strength. However, a recent article by Semciw et al. compared the gluteus minimus and medius strength in swimmers versus nonswimmers. Their findings suggest there is an unloading effect from training in the water that affects muscle timing on land, not muscle size [56]. This gives insight into a key component to consider when treating an injured swimmer on land; dysfunctional movement patterns that are common in land athletes might be heightened/more pronounced in aquatic athletes. Thus, control deficits should be considered when screening for proper progression of dryland training or return to swimming rehabilitation.

One common soft-tissue hip injury resulting from pelvic instability and muscle imbalances is nonspecific groin pain/athletic pubalgia [124]. It is important for appropriate evaluation and diagnosis as many pathologies may cause referral pain to the groin that mimics these hip adductor and abdominal muscle injuries [122, 124]. According to Kachingwe et al., there are five signs indicative of athletic pubalgia (Table 17.10) [121, 122].

With these diagnoses, rehabilitation begins with pain and edema management, progressing within the physiology of soft-tissue healing [121, 122]. The acute phase goals (weeks 0–6) for nonoperative management of athletic pubalgia/sports hernia are based upon Ellsworths et al.'s [122] invited clinical commentary and should be used to guide the appropriate progression with individualized considerations for protection, rest, ice, and com-

Table 17.10 Signs and symptoms indicating athletic pubalgia [121, 122]

1. Subjective complaint of deep groin/lower abdominal pain
2. Pain increases with exertion: dryland, sprinting, resisted swimming, and kicking
3. Palpable tenderness over the pubic ramus at the insertion of the rectus abdominis and/or conjoined tendon
4. Pain with resisted hip abduction at 0°, 45°, 90° of hip flexion
5. Pain with resisted abdominal curl-up

pression as needed. Please refer to Appendix B for additional suggested progression details.

Additional considerations for manual and therapeutic exercise are based upon the core progression utilized prior to dynamic exercise in a case series by Kachingwe et al. that suggest conservative management is a viable option for return to higher-level sport [121]. Their nonoperative protocol guides the management of each athlete individually through an algorithm that considers the time of season as well as a suggestion to refer for surgery if <80 % improvement were not seen within 4–6 weeks [121]. Kachingwe et al. reported successful swimmers who returned to sport with the use of conservative treatments including soft-tissue and joint mobilization/manipulation, neuromuscular reeducation, manual stretching, and therapeutic exercise [72, 121]. The manual techniques and progression used are described in Fig. 17.9. Notice a suggested time frame for return to swim program may begin once the swimmer is able to reach phase 3 of the initial core exercise progression [121].

Knee

Similar mobilizations have been found to provide an immediate positive response to knee pain with activity for subjects with a side-to-side difference in hip internal rotation range of motion greater than 14° [127]. Research suggests that this patellofemoral pain is related to proximal hip dysfunctional movement patterns that cause stress to the patella from tracking errors and increased

mechanical load [128]. Conservative management has been supported by a recent systematic review, and meta-analysis by Lack et al. highlighting robust research supporting proximal rehabilitation combined with quadriceps strengthening produces a better result for both the short and the long term [128]. Other therapeutic aid considerations should include patella taping, orthotics, core control, and functional movement retraining [128].

Ankle

Swimmers primarily use the ankle passively as a propulsion surface to transfer forces created from the hip and knee musculature and joint actions while swimming in a plantar-flexed position [81, 129]. The opposite extremes of ROM must be considered at the ankle during closed kinetic chain activities when the ankle is dorsiflexed during dryland training, starts, and turns [129]. Rehab may be able to improve the closed kinematic chain activities in swimming based upon the literature available for land-based sports; however, additional information is needed for open chain considerations for swimmers.

Instead of the top-down approach from the core and hip, swimmers may benefit from an ankle rehabilitation program that focuses on a ground-up approach [130]. The extrinsic muscles of the foot should be considered part of the rehabilitation plan, but it is suggested to start with the intrinsic core of the foot for normal lower extremity function, including dynamic neuromuscular control [131]. Building the foundation of the foot has been associated with improving plantar fasciitis symptoms, posterior tibial tendon dysfunction, medial tibial stress syndrome, and chronic lower leg pain [131]. Learning to utilize the intrinsic muscles first has been suggested as important as learning the abdominal hallowing maneuver to address LE pain and dysfunction [131]. The ability to maintain and progress proper foot doming without extrinsic muscles is important throughout the progression from static to dynamic exercise for swimmers [131]. If a swimmer is able sense sitting subtalar neutral, with the

MOBILIZATION TECHNIQUES

Technique	Description of Technique	Illustration
Posterior ilium rotation mobilization	• Patient side lying, facing therapist, hip and knee at 60°-90° • Bottom hand makes contact over ischial tuberosity; top hand makes contact over ASIS • Force: 2 parallel forces with both hands to impart a "torque" or posterior rotation to the innominate • Can step in between patient's lower extremities and have patient perform isometric hip extension × 10 s, while therapist rests between mobilizations • After mobilization session done, do 2 sets of hold-relax (2-s hold, moderate contraction into ipsilateral hip extension, contralateral hip flexion, then adduction "setting")	
Anterior ilium rotation mobilization	• Patient prone • Therapist stands on contralateral side of ilium to be mobilized. Can have patient drop ipsilateral lower extremity off plinth • Bottom hand grasps anterior distal thigh (knee flexed or extended), bringing hip into extension • Contact with ulnar aspect of heel of hand over posterior ilium (pisiform by PSIS) • Force: Anterior-superior force over posterior ilium imparting a "torque" to induce anterior rotation of the innominate • Can have patient perform isometric hip flexion × 10 s, while therapist rests between mobilization sets • After mobilization session done, do 2 sets of hold-relax (2-s hold, moderate contraction into ipsilateral hip flexion, contralateral hip extension, then adduction "setting"	
Sacroiliac regional thrust manipulation technique	• Position the patient supine with ilium to be mobilized on opposite side of table • Passively side bend patient toward side to be treated • Therapist hooks cephalad elbow (ie, right elbow) inside patient's right elbow by threading arm through patient's clasped hand and stabilizing dorsum of hand against the patient's ribcage • Therapist places heel of caudal hand at the ASIS • While maintaining side-bent position, flex the patient's lumbar spine, while simultaneously rotating the individual towards you until the ASIS raises up off the table about 2.5 cm • Ask the patient to take a deep breath and, upon exhalation, take the available motion and perform a quick thrust at the ASIS in a posterior/inferior direction • After mobilization completed, have patient perform isometric adduction with your fist between patient's knees to "set" pubic symphysis	
Hip anterior glide mobilization	• Position patient prone • Stabilizing hand grasps anterior, distal femur, positioning hip in neutral, knee 90° • Mobilize hand contacts posterior, proximal femur • Exert anterior force	
Hip posterior glide mobilization	• Stand on opposite side of involved hip • Place cephalad hand underneath ischium (or can use wedge) to stabilize • Position hip in 90° flexion, 10° adduction • Caudal hand contacts patella, exerting posterior force through long axis of femur • Can use sternum for more contact/pressure	
Lumbar central PA mobilization	• Contact spinous process with pisiform/hypothenar eminence of cephalad (mobilizing) hand or can use thumb-dummy thumb technique directly over spinous process • Apply direct PA pressure with forearms directly in line with force	

Abbreviations: ASIS, anterior superior iliac spine; PSIS, posterior superior iliac spine; PA, posterior-to-anterior.

Fig. 17.9 Lumbar, sacral, and hip mobilizations [121]

calcaneus and the metatarsal head on the ground [131], then progression is suggested statically in standing on both legs and eventually to one before dynamic functional movements are progressed on stable and unstable surfaces [131].

Shoulder

Promoting dynamic stability in the shoulder while restoring pain-free ROM is a goal that starts immediately in rehabilitation [99, 114].

Research regarding overhead-throwing athletes highlights the importance of controlling the micro-instability at the shoulder to reduce risk of rotator cuff tendonitis, internal impingement, and labral lesions [114]. Reinold and Curtis [114] report principles of treating the overhead athlete with shoulder instability include (a) maintaining range of motion, (b) improving strength of the glenohumeral and scapulothoracic musculature, (c) emphasizing dynamic stabilization and neuromuscular control, and, finally, (d) integrating local and global stabilizers [114].

It is suggested to start with posture, correcting for the rounded shoulders and forward-head posture commonly seen in swimmers [114]. This posture has been associated with [114]:

- Weakness of the scapular retractors, deep neck flexors, lower trapezius, and serratus anterior
- Tightness of the pectoralis minor, upper trapezius, and levator scapula

Depending on the individual needs of each swimming injury, treatment of the shoulder often begins with the correction of the above dysfunction in strength and ROM.

It has been reported that overhead athletes can develop glenohumeral internal rotation deficits (GIRD) due to soft-tissue-acquired posterior shoulder tightness. To prevent ROM deficits that can cause injury and/or stroke asymmetry, stretching of the shoulder involving shoulder horizontal adduction with scapular stabilization should be integrated as a part of regular dryland swim training [132]. Additional benefits from instrument-assisted soft-tissue mobilization (IASTM) will be discussed in "Mobility" section.

In addition to ROM maintenance, promoting correct muscle activation while improving scapular proprioception has been promoted when rehabilitating overheard athletes [133–135]. The six scapular retraction exercises in Fig. 17.10 have been found to help retrain scapular muscles

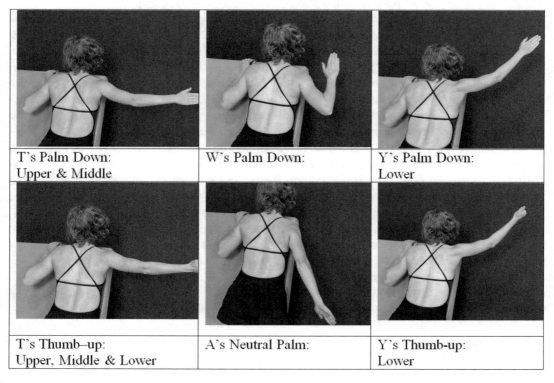

| T's Palm Down: Upper & Middle | W's Palm Down: | Y's Palm Down: Lower |
| T's Thumb–up: Upper, Middle & Lower | A's Neutral Palm: | Y's Thumb-up: Lower |

Fig. 17.10 Scapular exercises and trapezius activation [86]

responsible for scapular external rotation, upward rotation, and posterior tilt [135]. These exercises should be considered part of the swimmer rehabilitation program to gain necessary scapular muscle activation to reduce injury risk common to overhead athletes. Teaching the proper form early for endurance and enforcing scapular control with each dynamic movement progression back to the pool are critical (Fig. 17.10) [86].

Additional muscles that require strengthening in the shoulder include the middle and lower trapezius, the pectoralis muscle group, and the triceps. Moeller et al. [136] studied muscle activation patterns in common upper extremity exercises. Based on electromyography (EMG), Moeller et al. recommend using ER with scapular squeeze, to target middle and lower trapezius [136]. It was found that the bow and arrow exercise demonstrates higher upper trapezius activation despite cueing to increase mid- and low-trap muscle use and therefore can be less beneficial than the others with targeted scapular stabilizer strengthening [136]. An additional finding by that group included that individuals with and without shoulder injuries had the same scapular muscle activation ratios during these exercises. If the latissimus dorsi is the targeted muscle group, Anderson et al. [137] found that positioning with a wider grip while performing the lat pull-down exercise was most effective. Furthermore, in this wider grip position, there is less bicep co-activation with this hand position, which improves isolation of the muscle [137].

Strength training is an important component of dryland training in swimmers. However, proprioception is important in swimmers as it relates to body awareness. It has been reported that decreased proprioception in the shoulder joint correlates to shoulder joint instability. Salles et al. [138] found that after 8 weeks of training, the best results for proprioceptive improvement occurred with constant intensity and lower volume with exercises [138]. Progression consisted of isometric strength throughout a pain-free arc of motion prior to neuromuscular progression control of the glenohumeral and scapulothoracic joint [114]. Neuromuscular training progresses from rhythmic stabilization to reactive neuro-

muscular control drills, closed kinetic chain exercises, and plyometric exercises [114]. Proper muscle activation without compensation is an early goal to decrease scapular dyskinesia in overhead athletes (Appendix C) [99, 114, 133].

Frequently, swimmers demonstrate increased mobility of shoulder and scapular structures, and winging is a common presentation. Winging signifies imbalance between the pectoralis major and the serratus anterior muscles; this imbalance can be a source of abnormal shoulder mechanics with swimming. Subjects with winging demonstrate increased pectoralis major activation versus subjects without winging in all push-up plus exercise conditions (hands on the wall, quadruped, and standard flat plank) [139]. Park et al. found that increased weight-bearing increases serratus anterior activation and therefore recommends that once the athlete can tolerate increased weight-bearing through the upper extremity, the swimmer should be strengthened in standard push-up plus position to increase serratus anterior activation and decrease pectoralis major activation (Fig. 17.11) [139].

The use of TRX straps has become increasingly popular with dryland training for swimmers as it allows for the creation of an unstable surface. As an additional benefit, it was found that the suspension aspect of the upper extremity (UE) strength training increases muscle activation of all studied muscles (deltoids, pectoralis major, trapezius, and triceps) as the prone push-up motion was tested [140]. This is relevant to swim training as the triceps and pectoralis muscles are used largely for forward propulsion in swimming. Suspension training has also been found to increase the work of the rectus abdominis and external oblique [141] and should be incorporated as part of dryland strengthening program to enhance performance and decrease low back injury risk.

However, it should be noted that while TRX/suspended bands allow for activation of many target muscle groups simultaneously, this type of strengthening does not increase activation of one particular muscle group versus stable conditions. For rehabilitation purposes, if the goal is to focus on one particular muscle or muscle

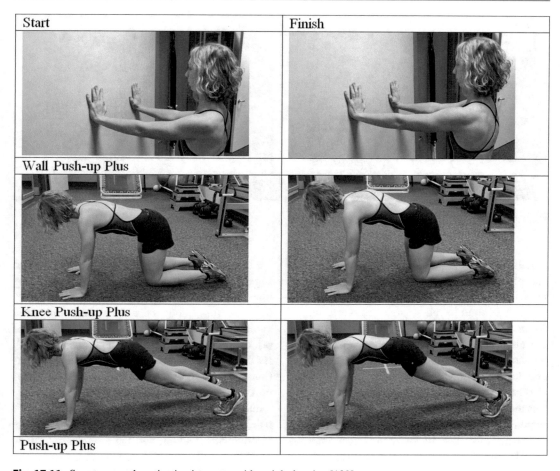

Fig. 17.11 Serratus muscle activation increases with weight-bearing [139]

group, closed kinetic chain strengthening is best [142]. Suspension training is helpful in addition to closed kinetic chain strengthening, and it is recommended that the swimming athlete should rotate between them (Fig. 17.12) [142].

Mobility

A literature review of myofascial origin of shoulder pain discovered that both active and latent myofascial trigger points are a mechanism of pain and sensitivity in those with shoulder pain [143]. Palpation is a useful tool to diagnose myofascial pain in those with nontraumatic shoulder pain, and the most prevalent trigger point locations were in the infraspinatus, upper trapezius, and levator scapulae muscles [143]. The presence of myofascial pain's effects on shoulder function includes reduced muscle strength, accelerated muscle fatigue, and simultaneous overloading of active motor units [143]. Techniques used to improve soft-tissue mobility may include instrument-assisted soft-tissue mobilization.

A study within overhead athletes found that the use of instrument-assisted soft-tissue mobilization (IASTM) to the posterior musculature demonstrated an increase in functional glenohumeral adduction ROM [144]. Other instruments such as foam rollers have been studied and found

Start	Finish

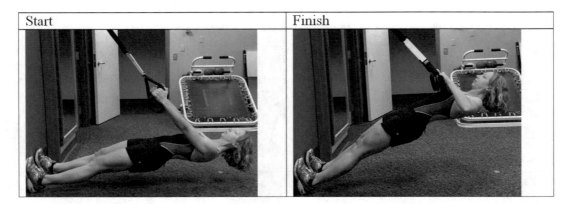

Fig. 17.12 Suspension training with TRX bands [142]

to reduce muscle soreness while improving active and passive ROM, as well as, performance with increased muscle activation. Foam roller use has also been found to reduce delayed onset muscle soreness after 10 min of treatment to the affected muscles [145]. In addition, the research found a tendency toward crossover effect to a contralateral limb [145]. Hip limitations in ROM have also been found to improve in athletes who have less than 90° of hamstring ROM, when utilizing a foam roller to assist the static stretches [146].

Foam roller use in swimmers can improve muscle length and performance. One study found improvement in maximum voluntary isometric contraction (MVIC) with foam roll use and static stretching combined as compared to either intervention alone [147]. However, because the improvement effects last only ~10 min [147], multiple applications may be needed throughout meets and practice to maintain unrestricted athletic performance.

Elastic Therapeutic Taping

A 2015 systematic review and meta-analysis reported elastic therapeutic taping (ETT) to be a treatment option that can reduce pain and disability from chronic musculoskeletal pain (>4 weeks) including shoulder impingement, myofascial pain, patellofemoral pain syndrome, plantar fasciitis, and mechanical neck and low back pain [148], which are common in swimmers. However,

the existing evidence does not support ETT to be superior to other treatment approaches including home exercises, joint manipulations, rigid taping, dry needling, and mechanical traction; used alone, the tape does not improve strength, proprioception, and functional performance [148]. ETT used in combination with other interventions may be more effective as two studies support both skilled exercise and ETT significantly reduced pain and disability in athletes with neck pain and shoulder impingement [149, 150]. The mechanism of action and the application details of ETT are still not well understood regarding the amount of tension or duration for most effective response although a preliminary study found the effect size of pain was lower when the tension was higher and the tape was applied longer [148].

Return to Sport Considerations

Swimmers are encouraged to continue dryland strengthening and physical therapy as needed while progressing through the return to swimming stages at the health-care provider's discretion. Return to swimming criteria as outlined by Hamman [34] includes (Table 17.11) the following.

A useful return to sport screening tool, in addition to range of motion and strength testing, is the utilization of the upper quarter and lower quarter Y-balance test (YBT-UQ/ YBT-LQ). Because swimming requires upper body strength, core strength, shoulder mobility, and shoulder

Table 17.11 Return to swimming criteria [34]

1	Ability to complete cardiovascular activities on land (physical education classes in school, running, recess participation, etc.)
2	Pain-free activities of daily living
3	Pain-free and normalized range of motion (including scapulohumeral rhythm if shoulder injury involved)
4	Strength within 90% of uninvolved side
5	Appropriate functional testing scores as performed by health-care provider [including functional movement screening (FMS), hop testing, Y-balance testing for the upper and lower extremities as needed]

stability, a functional test to quantify these variables can be helpful to assist with movement assessment and injury prevention. As previously discussed, female swimmers are at higher risk of upper quarter injuries as compared to their male counterparts at all levels [29, 30, 151]. Intrinsic risk factors for shoulder injury include shoulder joint laxity, decreased scapular and core muscle strength and endurance, and muscular imbalance between the shoulder joint and scapulothoracic joints [152].

Butler and his coauthors propose the use of the YBT-UQ test as an injury screen test because it is reliable and can be easily and cost-efficiently conducted to assess unilateral upper quarter dynamic function as it tests the swimmers' upper extremity (UE) strength, core strength, shoulder mobility, and shoulder stability [152–155]. It is important to note that no sex or bilateral differences exist in the YBT-UQ in the general population [152, 154, 155].

Butler et al. studied 43 male and 54 female National Collegiate Athletic Association Division I collegiate swimmers before the start of their season for testing, and all swimmers were pain-free at the time of participation. The authors found that while the swimmers demonstrated symmetrical performances between upper extremities for the three reaches tested (medial, inferolateral, and superolateral), males scored significantly higher with medial, inferolateral, and composite reaches [152]. Medial and inferolateral reaches require the largest amount of trunk mobility in the stabi-

lized posture, which may explain the lower scores in females. The authors suggest that improving core and shoulder strength/stability would improve performance with the YBT-UQ through strength and conditioning programs, female shoulder injury risk may decrease, and swim performance may improve [152].

YBT-LQ injury screens in land-based athletes found <95% limb asymmetry correlated with 6.5× increased risk for a lower extremity injury [156, 157]. A study by Ambegaonkar et al. used a related screen called the Star Excursion Balance Test (SEBT) and found an association between collegiate female athletes who demonstrated higher SEBT scores also had increased hip flexor, hip extensor, and hip abductor strength [123]. Therefore, it is suggested that coaches include lower extremity strengthening and stability training to decrease lower extremity injury risk.

Return to Swimming Protocol

There exist a large percentage of injuries, especially to the shoulder, of the swimming athlete during his/her career. These injuries are often caused by strength asymmetries, improper stroke technique, swim practice duration, and high yardage. Dryland rehabilitation can assist with the correction of the typical "swimmer posture" including forward-head and forward-shoulder posturing, scapular stabilization, shoulder and scapular neurological rehabilitation, and core strengthening [10]. However, dryland training does not appropriately activate the muscles in the same way that swimming does. Therefore the importance of return to swimming protocols (RTSP) increases. Spigelman et al. created a list of drills to aid the swimmer's stroke mechanical improvement [10]. Additionally, Hamman created a two-phase RTSP for the pediatric swimmer, and Spigelman et al. created an RTSP for the adult swimmer (Figs. 17.13 and 17.14) [10]. Both programs were created to address progression of yardage safely and create a guideline to assist clinicians communicate effectively with coaches and swimmers regarding appropriate return to sport advancement (Fig. 17.15) [34].

Table 2. *Swimming Drills. Drills used by swimmers to focus on technique during various phases of the stroke cycle.*

Drill	Guidelines to Perform Correctly	Focus of Drill	Phase of Stroke Cycle
Fingertip drag	The swimmer's face remains facing the bottom of the pool while the torso rotates on an imaginary long axis. As the swimmer begins the recovery portion of the arm stroke, he drags the fingers tips along the water surface during recovery.	Promotes a bent elbow recovery and symmetrical body roll	Recovery
Shoulder, Head, Enter	The swimmer performs freestyle, focusing on a high elbow that is flexed and recovers high out of the water. During the recovery, the swimmer taps the axillary's region, the head and then reaches in front of the body at the position of 1:00 on a clock to grab the water for hand entry.	Promotes high elbow recovery, symmetrical body roll, and proper hand entry	Recovery/Hand Entry
6/6	The swimmer is positioned on his side with the arm closest to the bottom of the pool over the head (ear against bicep). The swimmer performs 6 kicks on one side, takes three long freestyle stroke cycles focusing on a high elbow recovery, and 6 kicks on the opposite side.	Promotes symmetrical body roll	Recovery/Hand Entry/Early Pull Through
Left arm, right arm, both arm	Swimmer performs three strokes on the left side focusing on placing the hand in the water at 11 and 1 o'clock, and keeping a steady rhythmic kick (6-beat). The swimmer repeats the same motion on the right side.	Promotes proper hand entry, bent elbow recovery, symmetrical body roll	Hand Entry/Early Pull Through
Flutter kick without a kick board on side	Swimmer maintains tight core, arm closest to the bottom of the pool is extended next to the ear, and the swimmer should try to maintain this straight body position.	Core body strength	Early Pull Through/Late Pull Through
Catch up	Swimmer exaggerates the recovery and catch phase of the freestyle stroke. The left arm catches up to the right arm. The 6 beat kick should be focused on.	Promotes proper hand entry	Hand Entry
Fist	Swimmer makes a fist while performing the pull through phase of the stroke. Focus is on the rotation of the torso and the high elbow during the early pull phase of the stroke.	Helps to appreciate the sensation of the forearm while pulling the water. This is also known as appreciating the "feel the water" with the hand and forearm as a unit	Early Pull Through/Late Pull Through
4 strokes of backstroke/4 strokes of freestyle	Swimmer does four cycles of backstroke and four cycles of freestyle. Exaggeration can be placed on the roll of the body when switching from back to front. The hips/torso should drive the body rotation.	Promotes high elbow pull through	Early Pull Through/Late Pull Through
Distance per Stroke (DPS):	Swim freestyle trying to extend the arms and maximize stroke length. Swim freestyle, roll the body and extend the arms with each pull. As the body is extended, focus on rotating the hips from side to side and extending the arm. Try to reduce strokes with each 25 swam. This is best if performed in sets of 25's.	Helps to "feel the water" with the hand and forearm.	Early Pull Through/Late Pull Through
Sculling	Can be performed prone or supine. Slight motion of the hand and forearms back and forth just under the surface of the water to propel the swimmer forward. This is best if performed in sets of 25's.	Helps to appreciate the sensation of the forearm while pulling the water. This is also known as appreciating the "feel the water" with the hand and forearm as a unit	Hand Entry/Early Pull Through

Fig. 17.13 Drills for return to swimming progression [10]

Table 3. *Key Points of the Return to Swimming Protocol (RTSP). Overview of the RTSP including the major components of a swimming workout and criteria for progression.*

	Phase I			Phase II – Join Team	
	Week One 1000-1500	Week Two 1500-2200	Week Three 2200-3000	Week Four 2800-3900	Week Five 3500-4700+
Warm Up	(300-400)	(600-700)	(700-900)	(900-1100)	(1000-1200)
Drills	Stroke Technique using drills (300-500)	Stroke Technique using drills (400-600)	Stroke Technique using drills Incorporate drills in the beginning and end of practice (600-700)	Incorporate drills in the beginning and at the end of practice (700-900)	A drill set should be incorporated at the end of the workout (800-1000)
Kick	With fins or zoomers, but no kick board Kick on side or back Arms can be at side or streamlined position if pain free (400-600)	With fins or zoomers but no kick board Kick on side or back Arms can be at side or streamlined position if pain free (500-900)	With fins or zoomers, but no kick board Kick on side or back Arms can be at side or streamlined position if pain free (700-900)	With fins or zoomers Kick board if comfortable Kick on side or back Arms can be at side or streamlined position if pain free (700-900)	Kick with board if pain free Or Kick in streamlined position, on side or supine with arms at sides Fins and zoomers are optional (700-900)
Intervals	None	None	1 set on interval at 70% effort 1 set on interval about 10 slower than regular practice pace (200-500)	Gradually increase number of sets with interval work Maintain correct stroke technique (500-1000)	Start on interval 5-10 sec slower than pre-injury pace, progress to pre-injury interval gradually Maintain correct stroke technique (800-1300)
Pull Set	None	None	None	None	Start pull set conservatively (200-300) Increase pulling yardage by 300 as tolerated DO NOT USE PADDLES! Stop immediately if pain or discomfort is felt.
Rest between repetitions	20-30 seconds for all	10-20 seconds for all	10-15 seconds between repetitions Interval 5-10 seconds rest Longer swims should have longer rest periods	10-15 sections between repetitions Interval 5-10 seconds rest Longer swims should have longer rest periods	5-15 sections between repetitions Interval 3-10 seconds rest Longer swims should have longer rest periods
Criteria to Progress	1.Pain free 2. Proper stroke technique during drills per coaches assessment a. Bent elbow recovery b. 4-6 beat kick c. Symmetrical body roll	1.Pain free 2.Proper stroke technique during drills per coaches assessment a. Bent elbow recovery b. 4-6 beat kick c. Symmetrical body roll	1.Pain free during and after practice 2. Ability to maintain good stroke technique at end of practice. 3. No shoulder pain during interval work	Join Team 1.Pain free during and after practice 2. Ability to maintain good stroke technique 3. No pain or discomfort during interval work	1.Completely pain free 2. Maintain stroke technique 3. Complete pull work pain free 4. No pain or discomfort during interval work
All distance is represented in yards.					

Fig. 17.14 Return to swimming protocol for adults [10]

Hamman offers a clinical commentary with regard to a return to swimming guideline specific to the pediatric swimmer. He provides three phases for return to swimming for the nonoperative swimmer after injury. Hamman emphasizes not only progressive return to normal practice distance but also swimmer's exertion level progresses [34]. The phases were not created to be used in a linear fashion, so pre-organization of individualized swimmer needs and circumstances will dictate where to begin and end for the athlete's full return to sport (Table 17.12) [34].

APPENDIX A

Return to Swim Protocol

Dry land and home exercise program to be performed as instructed by your physical therapist.
How pain influences protocol:

- -Pain during warm up that continues throughout practice or goes away then returns: take 2 days off, drop 1 level or stay at lowest level for full week
- -Pain during warm up that goes away: Stay at level
- -Pain the day after lifting or dryland (not muscle soreness): 1 day off, do not advance to next level
- -No soreness for 1 week: progress to next level

Phase I: No Organized Practice (If Swimmer has been deactivated from swimming for 6 weeks or greater)
Perform each stage 3 times with at least 1 full day off between sessions. Freestyle stroke only throughout Phase I

Stage I (do not complete whole practice in less than 30 minutes):
-2x200 warm up; 30 seconds rest
-4x100; 20 seconds rest
-4x50; 15 seconds rest
-6x50 kick in streamline (if arm, shoulder, or neck injured) or pull (if low back or leg injured) down, swim back; 15 seconds rest
-2x100 cool down; 20 seconds rest

Stage II (do not complete whole practice in less than 45 minutes):
-400 warm up; 30 seconds rest
-4x100; 20 seconds rest
-4x50 kick (if arm, shoulder, or neck injured) or pull (if low back or leg injured) down, swim back; 15 seconds rest
-2x200 active recovery; 20 seconds rest
-4x100; 10 seconds rest
-4x50 kick (if arm, shoulder, or neck injured) or pull (if low back or leg injured) down, swim back; 10 seconds rest
-2x100 cool down; 20 seconds rest

Stage III (do not complete whole practice in less than 60 minutes):
-400 warm up; 30 seconds rest
-4x100; 20 seconds rest
-4x50 kick (if arm, shoulder, or neck injured) or pull (if low back or leg injured) down, swim back; 15 seconds rest
-2x200 active recovery; 20 seconds rest
-4x100; 10 seconds rest
-4x50 kick (if arm, shoulder, or neck injured) or pull (if low back or leg injured) down, swim back; 10 seconds rest
-2x200 active recovery; 20 seconds rest
-4x100; 10 seconds rest
-4x50 kick (if arm, shoulder, or neck injured) or pull (if low back or leg injured) down, swim back; 10 seconds rest
-2x100 cool down; 20 seconds rest

The International Journal of Sports Physical Therapy | Volume 9, Number 3 | June 2014 Page 391

Fig. 17.15 Pediatric return to swimming protocol [34] parts—A and B

Phase II: Organized Practice (if completed Phase I or has been deactivated less than 6 weeks)

	Stage I	Stage II	Stage III	Stage IV	Stage V
Practice Yardage	60% Total Distance	70% Total Distance	80% Total Distance	90% Total Distance	Full Participation
Short Course Pace	100 pace time divided by 4, then add 2 seconds	100 pace time divided by 4, then add 1.5 seconds	100 pace time divided by 4, then add 1 second	100 pace time divided by 4, then add 0.5 second	Full Participation
Long Course Pace	100 pace time divided by 4, then add 4 seconds	100 pace time divided by 4, then add 3 seconds	100 pace time divided by 4, then add 2 seconds	100 pace time divided by 4, then add 1 second	Full Participation

Example Stage I Short Course 100 pace of 1:20:
      25 no faster than 0:22
      50 no faster than 0:44
      100 no faster than 1:28
      200 no faster than 2:56
Example Stage I Practice
      10,000 yard total practice
      2,000 yard warm up + 2,000 yard cool down+ 2,000 yard remaining distance = 6,000 yards or 60% of 10,000 yards
Must perform full warm up and cool down each practice and may not go faster than pace time
May perform all stroke beginning at Stage II
No pull buoys or paddles (for upper extremity and neck injuries) and no kickboard or fins (for low back or lower extremity injuries) until Stage III
Progress to next stage after 1 full week without symptoms
If symptoms occur return to previous stage

Phase III (Double Practices)
Complete Phase II Stage V prior to beginning Phase III. When starting doubles, repeat Phase II for secondary practice while fully participating with primary practice

Fig. 17.15 (continued)

Table 17.12 Return to swimming criteria [34]

Phase 1: reintroduction to water. Focus is on normalizing stroke mechanics	a. Used if the swimmer has been removed from sport for greater than or equal to 6 weeks due to injury
	b. No participation in formalized practice to prohibit competition and refocus on stroke technique
	c. Only freestyle performed as it comprises more than half of their training volume regardless of stroke specialization
	d. Rest involved body part:
	i. Neck, upper extremity injuries: swimmers are to perform on their back in a streamline position and kick
	ii. Low back, lower extremity injuries: swimmers use the pull buoy
Phase 2: emphasis on technique restoration	a. Used if the swimmer has been removed from sport for less than 6 weeks or has already completed phase 1
	b. Return to organized swim practice with team
	c. Yardage and pacing restrictions outlined for safe progression to prior level of function
Phase 3: multiple practices in 1 day	a. Dictates to follow practice guidelines normally during first practice of day
	b. Restricts second practice of day to follow the guidelines outlined in phase 2
	c. During second practice, allow for relative rest of involved body part(s): (until phase 2, stage 3)
	i. Neck, upper extremity injuries: no pull buoy or paddle use
	ii. Low back, lower extremity injuries: no use of kickboard or fins

Training Considerations

Equipment Considerations

Research is still needed to fully understand the appropriate use and progression to swimming equipment. What is currently supported includes the utilization of in-water resistance training as it can improve maximal swimming force, power, and velocity; assisted elastic-band swimming was found to enhance technical skills including decreasing stroke rate while decreasing stroke depth [158, 159]. Wanivenhaus et al. discuss the therapeutic use of fins to decrease upper body stress while swimming as well as a pull buoy to reduce drag and stress on the shoulder [13].

The evidence, however, is lacking to support the use of a swim bench for rehabilitation [153]. Barbosa et al. raise concern for the selection of paddle size by age group or for rehabilitation as their results showed an increase in paddle size had a significant effect on increasing peak force, average force, minimum force, time to peak force, stroke duration, rate of force development, and impulse [160]. This increased muscular intensity and duration must be considered for a swimmer on an individual assessment. Additional stressors from equipment include those to the lumbar spine that occur during practice with the utilization of fins, kick boards, and pull buoys, as they have been found to produce excessive hyperextension of the lumbar spine [160]. Fins have also been associated with ankle injuries as the foot requires more energy and torque which has been found to affect the body position during the kick [10, 80].

Spigelman et al. highlight additional use and considerations of equipment here (Fig. 17.16) [10].

Table 1. *Swimming Tools. Tools commonly used by competitive swimmers. Tools should be used with caution depending on swimmer's injury.*

Tool	Name	Use/Indications	Contraindications
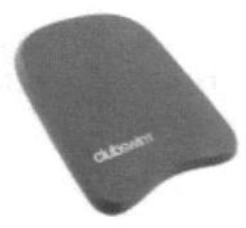	Kickboard	Used to focus on kicking only; Most commonly used with arms extended in front of the body; creates lumbar lordosis	Shoulder injuries; spondylolysis
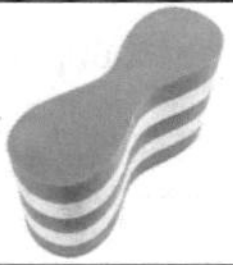	Pull buoy	Used to focus on arm stroke only; Placed between upper legs to prevent kicking while providing buoyancy to the lower body	Shoulder tendinitis/tendinosis; elbow or forearm pain
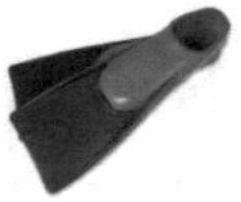	Fins	Used to increase leg length and surface area of the feet; increase propulsion of stroke	Acute ankle injuries; knee pain
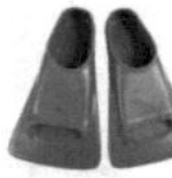	Zoomers	Used to increase leg strength; increase surface area of the feet, but are shorter than fins and allow for rapid leg motions to increase forward propulsion	Acute ankle injuries; knee pain
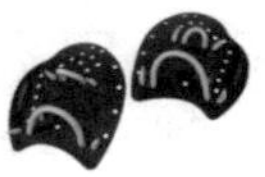	Paddles	Worn on hands; come in variety of sizes; increase surface area of the hand; slow down pull when worn, but build strength while pulling	Shoulder injury or pain; improper stroke technique

Fig. 17.16 Swimming equipment—uses and contraindications [10]

Coach/Trainer Resistance Training Expertise

Communication with coaches, PE teachers, and strength-training coaches is critical in the assessment of benefits versus barriers to swimmer health. If the athlete is not appropriately educated on appropriate resistance training and safe mechanics, they sustain injuries and unsafe training regimens for themselves. McGladrey et al. [161] investigated coach and teacher awareness of safe resistance training practices to assess knowledge of the instructors. McGladrey and his group evaluated 287 strength coaches and PE teachers and 140 university PE teacher education students and gave them a 90-question examination covering safety, training regimen, and prescription, as well as mechanics. It was found that coaches who instructed athletes in resistance training had a pass rate of 9.5 %, the university PE education students had a pass rate of 16 %, coaches, and those that had a resistance training certification (CSCS, USAW) passed at 50 % [161]. Subjects demonstrated the lowest scores occurred in the "safety knowledge" section which is concerning. Knowledge of safe practices and mechanics as well as communication with other care providers are crucial to the safety of athletes.

When training, there are several factors the instructor/therapist/coach and the swimmer should consider. First, once an injury or risk of injury has been accurately identified, it is important that the swimmer focus on the activation of individual muscles instead of movement itself in order to best increase/improve activation of targeted muscles with rehabilitation [136]. Athletes often use commonly practiced motor activation patterns, which may usurp the activation of the desired muscle groups—thus perpetuating the muscle imbalance cycle.

Efficacy of Dryland Strength Training

Dryland training has historically been utilized to improve swimming performance and prevent injuries. In a study by Gatta et al., swimmers per-

formed either dryland training in addition to swim practice or performed additional swimming drills before swim practice for 6 weeks [162]. It was found that power increased in the dryland strength-training group and not the swim training group after 6 weeks of preseason training in 20 male masters swimmers [162]. Therefore, it is recommended to use high-intensity, lower-repetition dryland training to increase power and performance in swimmers.

Another group studied the effects of eccentric strengthening. During rehabilitation, restoration of function is a top priority, and the focus is commonly the involved/injured side. However, Lepley and his coauthors found that eccentrically strengthening the uninjured side carries over to the injured side and therefore should be used in addition to focused strengthening of the injured side. The resultant effects can be useful both for injury prevention and rehabilitation strategies for swim training [163].

Efficacy of Swim Training Regimen

The perfect prescription of training volume, intensity, and frequency to result in optimal exercise performance has yet to be discovered in sport. In swimming, historically, high-volume training has been the routine with athletes swimming anywhere from 4000 to 10,000 yards per high school or club swim practice for competitive events that range in completion time between 20 s and 15 min (50 yards through 1500 m). However, recent studies have experimented with bouts of high-intensity, low-volume training finding success with swimmer competitive performance [164–167]. And due to the high level of overuse injuries in swimmers, especially of the shoulder complex, lower volume may be beneficial to injury prevention in swimmers which makes investigation into this topic even more important.

In a study by Faude et al. [166], ten high-level teenage swimmers altered their normal training routine to perform two different four-week training periods, both followed by one identical taper week. The athletes continued to be coached by their home coach, but during the high-volume training trial, their total training volume increased 30 % above normal. During the swimmers' high-intensity training, the training volume decreased 40 % below their normal level. After 4 weeks of training, both the high-volume and high-intensity trials increased the individual anaerobic threshold to higher than pre-training values. Additionally, the high-intensity group increased their maximal blood lactate concentration. Swimmer 100m and 400m performance times were not significantly different between groups before and after the 4-week training trials [166]. Overall, this study found no significant differences in performance and heart rate with maximal and submaximal swim speeds. Lastly, there was no difference between trials in subject "Profile of Mood States" (POMS) questionnaire which assesses possible overtraining by measuring changes in vigor, fatigue, depression, and anger [166].

These results are in agreement with those found by Kilen et al. [165]. Kilen and his coauthors studied 41 elite swimmers (average age = 20 years) and assigned them to a control group or high-intensity training group. The high-intensity group (HIT) reduced their training volume to 50 % of their normal volume and increased the intensity to 50 % more than normal. After 12 weeks of training, these authors found no significant difference between the high-intensity training and the control groups with regard to swimming performance, swim-specific VO_2max, body composition, blood metabolic markers, and swimming economy. However, it was found that VO_2max normalized to body weight decreased in the high-intensity group only and did not change in the control group [165].

It has been found in other studies that younger swimmers (average age = 10) demonstrated improved swimming performance with high-intensity training [168]. This could signify that the age of the participant has a different effect on training results. It is also possible that there exists an upper limit to how much exposure to high-intensity, low-volume training is present as the elite swimmers in the Kilen study had performed high-intensity and low-volume training as part of

their normal regimen for several years [165]. Pugliese studied the high-intensity training effect on ten male masters swimmers (average age = 32 years) [167]. Pugliese et al. put his swimmers through both a high-volume, low-intensity training regimen for 6 weeks and then a high-intensity, low-volume training regimen for the next 6 weeks [167]. These swimmers responded with improved peak oxygen consumption and improvements in the 400 and 2000 m swim performance after the high-volume, low-intensity training. After the subsequent high-intensity, low-volume training, these same swimmers did not demonstrate changes in their peak oxygen consumption nor changes in their 400 and 2000 m time from their post high-volume, low-intensity training. They did, however, improve their individual anaerobic threshold and their 100 m swim performance [167].

In a similar study, Laursen et al. split groups of cyclists/triathletes into three different groups for three different kinds of high-intensity, low-volume training [164]:

- Group 1 completed eight intervals at VO_2peak power output for a duration equal to time to exhaustion as calculated from a progressive exercise test with a recovery ratio of 1:2.
- Group 2 completed eight intervals at VO_2peak power output for a duration equal to time to exhaustion as calculated from a progressive exercise test with a recovery time as long as needed to allow the body to return to 65 % of max heart rate.
- Group 3 completed 12×30 s bouts of 175 % peak power outlet with a 4.5 min recovery in between bouts.
- The control group did not alter their normal training regimen.

Their results demonstrated that groups 1 and 2 demonstrated the biggest improvement in endurance performance (40 km time trial), peak power output, and VO_2peak. Laursen et al. [164] report that time to exhaustion intervals could be more rigorous than other study protocols. Additionally, effort adjustments in protocol training were made after reassessments as were performed to monitor cyclist progress throughout the trial. These effort adjustments also increased the rigor of the training.

It is important to note that while the above studies do not demonstrate improved performance with high-intensity, low-volume training, subjects did not note a decrease in performance which means that both methods, as understood so far, produce similar results. Perhaps high-intensity, low-volume training can reduce the risk of overuse injuries by reducing training time and allowing longer recovery time between training sessions. Current training programs incorporate variations of intensity, volume, and frequency in their routine, but the exact proportions required to produce the best and safest performance has yet to be determined. Laursen et al. [169] recommend a mixture of both high-volume, low-intensity and high-intensity, low-volume regimens into a highly trained athletes' plan. Laursen et al. [169] also suggest that because the metabolic adaptations occur with both training strategies overlap significantly, but the molecular events are different, both should be incorporated. Laursen et al. suggest a ratio of approximately 75 % high-volume, low-intensity training, and 10–15 % of the training regimen should be high-intensity, low-volume training [169].

Training Effort and Communication with Coaches

Communication between athletes and coaches is very important to ensure the status of goal achievement, training plan compliance, and athlete safety. Barroso published two articles regarding communication between swimmers and coaches. Barroso et al. [170, 171] defined communication during one training workout as "session rating of perceived exertion" (SRPE). The authors studied 160 swimmers of different age categories (11–12-year-olds, 13–14-year-olds, and 15–16-year-olds) and different competitive swimming experience and nine coaches. The coaches rated the SRPE before the training session as falling within these three categories: easy (SRPE < 3), moderate (SRPE 3–5), and

difficult (SRPE > 5). The SRPE was indicated by the swimmers 30 min after the end of the session. Barroso et al. [170] found that increased age and competitive swimming experience improved coach and athlete SRPE agreement. It was found that younger swimmers (ages 11–14) rated training intensity differently from coaches in all three categories. The 15–16-year-old swimmers demonstrated agreement with the easy and moderate SRPE but differed in the SRPE difficult category [170].

Additionally, in a follow-up study, Barroso et al. [171] investigated SRPE and how training volume and intensity may affect agreement between swimmers and coaches. Using the three SRPE categories defined above, coaches recorded the desired SRPE levels before the session and swimmers recorded their response 30 min after the training concluded. Thirteen moderately trained swimmers (average 21 years ± 1.1 year) were given different swim volumes (10×100 m, 20×100 m, 10×200 m, and 5×400 m) at the same relative intensity. Athlete and coach SRPE differed in 10×200 m and 5×400 m. Therefore SRPE is affected by intensity, volume, and distance. It is recommended that coaches ensure thorough communication with swimmers especially with increased volume, longer distance, and higher intensity to ensure desired training effort is applied by the athletes and to prevent injuries [170, 171].

Altitude Training

One training type that can be feasibly difficult due to opportunity, cost, and traveling logistics is altitude training. Altitude dosing has been established as living high enough (>2000 m), spending enough hours at that height daily (>14–16 h/day), for a duration of >19–20 days to create the hypoxic erythropoietic effect. This equates to approximately 300–400 h of exposure [172, 173]. It has been documented that an increase in hemoglobin mass of 1 % per 100 h of exposure can occur in endurance athletes [174, 175]. However, increased hemoglobin mass changes are highly variable, and even the

Table 17.13 Notable training considerations at altitude

Increased dehydration [172]	*Definition:* increased and unanticipated fluid loss through the upper respiratory system due to the low humidity of the higher altitudes and the body's need to compensate to maintain a moisturized airway
	Monitor urine color/osmolality
	Monitor pre- and post-training water weight loss (dehydration is a loss of greater than 2% body mass after training)
	Monitor headaches
Quality of sleep [172]	At moderate altitude (2000–3500 m)
	Sleep disturbances only occur in approximately 25% of athletes
	Usually resolves within 2–3 nights of sleeping at the same altitude as the athlete acclimatizes
	At high altitudes (over 3500 m)
	40–50% of athletes will have disordered breathing with sleep
	These athletes may need to follow the rest high, train low, sleep low paradigm to avoid the disordered breathing
Compromised immune system [172]	Higher risk of upper respiratory tract infection due to the decreased humidity of the air
	Potential sleep disturbances can decrease resting/recovery quality
	It is recommended to ease into normal training routine in order to progress workload and decrease the stress of the altitude change on the athlete's body
Food intake changes [178, 179]	Carbohydrates are used more in hypoxic environments and therefore increase consumption of carbs pre-training decreases oxygen desaturation
	Carbohydrates have been found to improve quality of interval training at altitude

hypoxic erythropoietic effect dose ranges from "no change" to "increased by 15%" after 3–4 weeks at altitude [172, 173, 176, 177]. It is recommended to use caution when exercising above 3000 m due to general fatigue experienced by some athletes. These athletes' training intensity will decrease over time, and therefore they will miss several of the intended benefits of altitude training. Some individuals are sensitive to higher altitudes and the effects of hypoxia as it can create acute mountain sickness, decreased appetite, generalized muscle fatigue and even muscle wasting, increased ventilatory work, and protein synthesis inhibition—all which negate the beneficial effects of the altitude training concepts (Table 17.13) [172, 178, 179].

Injury Prevention

Video Analysis

Along with focused strengthening and stabilization techniques used inside and outside of the pool, poor or abnormal stroke biomechanics are risk factors for developing pain and pathology [22, 180]. Video swim stroke analysis can be a useful tool to provide the swimmer with technique feedback to address current abnormal movement patterns and also reduce future injury risk. Refer to the "Common Stroke Technique Errors" section at the beginning of this chapter for common biomechanical stroke errors that can be improvable with use of video analysis.

Feedback

The ability to communicate between coaches and swimmers is inhibited by the aquatic environment. In other sports, coaches and clinicians can easily provide verbal simultaneous feedback to athletes to provide comments/critiques on mechanics and form. However, due to the nature of water, both swimmers hearing and vision are diminished which limits coaches' ability to communicate.

Zaton and Szczepan [181] studied the effectiveness of immediate verbal feedback (IVF) in swimmers. The goal was to modify stroke length in freestyle. The authors communicated with the swimmers in the experimental group, so the swimmer could hear feedback immediately while swimming. The control group received no feedback at all but understood the goal of the exercise was to lengthen the stroke to improve freestyle speed. Using two different methods to measure stroke length (the SIMI 2D movement analysis software) and the Hay method [182] which describes stroke length as the number of stroke cycles completed within a fixed distance. Between both measurements, the experimental group increased stroke rate between 5 and 7 % improving speed and efficiency, while the control group did not create significant change in performance [181].

The authors found that IVF had the ability to correct misperceptions of coach's information immediately to redirect the swimmer to more desirable swimming mechanics [183, 184] and also increased athlete interest in making these corrections [185].

A Proposed Injury Screen

Preseason injury screens use common clinical tools to assess injury risk with the goal of decreasing and preventing athlete injury in season. While swimming is a bilateral overhead sport where both arms are frequently (and ideally) performing symmetrical repetitive movements through symmetrical ranges of motion, range of motion and strength normative values in the pain-free athlete are not yet fully understood. For screening purposes, it can be expected that younger athletes will have greater ROM availability (even through high school age) especially in the composite IR and total arc ranges of motion [50]. And again, the dominant arm will likely have greater ER AROM, while the nondominant arm will have greater IR AROM [50]. The goals of these screens are to help identify individuals at higher risk for injury allowing targeted treatment to be appropriated to promote healthier, safer, and pain-free performance in sport.

A Proposed Dynamic Warm-Up

The Federation Internationale de Football Association (FIFA) has an injury prevention program created to help prevent soccer sports injury. Characteristics of the program include core stability, proprioception, dynamic stability, plyometrics, minimal equipment needed, and less than 15 min to complete. Barengo et al. performed a systematic review investigating the effectiveness of the use of the FIFA 11+ injury prevention program [186]. From the review, it was found that the FIFA 11+ injury prevention program reduces the injury incidence and improves athlete sport performance. It is recommended that a coach administer the program to ensure athlete "buy-in" and compliance. Additionally, the review concluded that increased compliance frequency improved injury prevention [186].

The authors of this textbook chapter propose a swim-specific version of the FIFA 11+ injury prevention program to decrease injury risk in swimmers (Appendices D, E, and F) [186, 187].

Appendix A: General Rehab—Neck Pain for Swimmers [86]

Goals	• Reduce pain
	• Reestablish proper flexibility, strength, and ROM
	• Adequately prepare the athlete for the demands of sport:
	• Proper muscle recruitment with oculomotor control
Treatment	• Begin with low-intensity exercise, below pain threshold
	• Progress to muscular endurance and strength
	• Minimize sternocleidomastoid and scalenes activation
	• Modalities PRN
Mobility	• Stretches for scalenes, upper trapezius, levator scapulae,
	• pectoralis minor, and pectoralis major
	• Thoracic extension self-mobilization using foam roller
Primary muscles	• Deep cervical flexors: longus capitis and colli, rectus capitis
	• Anterior and lateralis, hyoid muscles
	• Deep cervical extensors: semispinalis cervicis, multifidus,
	• Rectus capitis posterior major and minor
Criterion to progress to return to swimming program	• Pain-free activity
	• Full neck range of motion and strength
	• Sport-specific repositioning acuity, postural stability
	• Oculomotor control

Cervical stabilization program			
Exercise	1	2	3
Chin nods and cervical rotation	1 × fatigue	1–2 × fatigue	1–5 × fatigue
Cervical stretch and thoracic spine mobilization	1 × fatigue	1–2 × fatigue	1–5 × fatigue
Balance and oculomotor exercises	1 × fatigue	1–2 × fatigue	1–5 × fatigue
Cervical and thoracic muscle endurance		1–2 × fatigue	1–5 × fatigue
Cervical and thoracic muscle strength			1–5 × fatigue
Aerobic	Walk 10–20 min	Swim 20 min without starts	Swim 20–45 min with starts

Appendix B: General Rehab—Trunk Program (Lumbar and Hip) [119, 121, 122]

Goals	• Reduce pain
	• Reestablish proper flexibility, strength, and ROM
	• Adequately prepare the athlete for the demands of sport
	• Dynamic lumbo-pelvic stability and neuromuscular control
Treatment	• Begin with abdominal bracing and neutral spine awareness
	• Progress proper recruitment with dynamic movements
	• Modalities PRN
Mobility	• Full functional ROM of lumbar spine, pelvis, and hips
	• Therapeutic mobilization techniques as medically
	• necessary
Primary muscles	• Gluteus maximus and medius, longissimus thoracic, lumbar
	• multifidus, external and internal obliques, transverse
	• abdominis, rectus abdominis, and hamstrings
Criterion to progress to return to swimming program	• Pain-free activity
	• Full lumbar, pelvis, and hip range of motion and strength
	• Sport-specific awareness to self-correct neutral spine and hip control with dynamic movements

Trunk stabilization program

Exercise	1	2	3
Dead bug	Support, arms overhead, marching, 3×30 s	Unsupported, arms overhead, one leg extended, 3×1 min	Unsupported, arms alternate with legs extended, 3×2 min
Partial sit-ups	Forward, hands on the chest, 1×10	Forward hands on the chest, 3×10	3×10 forward, 3×10 left, and 3×10 right
Bridging	Slow reps, double leg, 2×10	Slow reps, double leg with weight, 2×20	Single leg, one leg extended 3×20
Bird-dog	Alternate the arm/leg with gluteal set, 1×10	Alternating the arm/leg 2×10 hold 5 s	On ball, alternating the arm/leg 2×10 hold 5 s
Quadruped	Alternating arms and legs, 1×10 hold 5 s	Alternating the arm and leg, 2×10 hold 5 s	Alternating the arm and leg, 3×10 hold 5 s
Wall squats	Less than 90° 1×10	At 90° 1×10 hold 20 s	At 90° 1×10 hold 30 s
Aerobic	Water walk 10 min	Water run 10 min	20–30 min swim

Appendix C: General Rehab—Shoulder Program [99, 114, 133]

Goals	• Reduce pain and inflammation
	• Reestablish proper flexibility, strength, and ROM
	• Adequately prepare for the demands of sport
	• Posterior strength and dynamic neuromuscular endurance
Treatment	• Begin with abdominal bracing and neutral spine activation
	• Progress proper recruitment with dynamic movements
	• Modalities PRN
Mobility	• Full, pain-free total arc of motion, horizontal ADD
	• scapulothoracic posture, and a lumbar neutral streamline
	• Self-mobilization and stretch: latissimus dorsi, pectoralis
	• minor and major, trapezius, thoracic extension and rotation
Primary muscles	• Rotator cuff muscles, with a focus on ER,
	• Serratus anterior, lower and middle trap
Criterion to progress to return to swimming program	• Pain-free activity
	• Full thoracic and shoulder motion and strength
	• Sport-specific dynamic stability and endurance

Trunk stabilization program

Exercise	1	2	3
Rotator cuff strengthening	Submaximal, mutli-angle isometrics, pain-free ranges	Begin in supine and progress to standing with tubing/manual rotator cuff program	Continue to advance rotator cuff program resistance/weight
Scapular strengthening	Isometric, pain-free scapular retraction, depression, and protraction	Begin in prone and progress to standing with tubing/manual rotator cuff program	Continue to advance rotator cuff program resistance/weight
Dynamic and rhythmic stabilization exercises	IR and ER with arm in scapular plane, 30° of abduction, and supine multidirectional elevated to 90–100°	Supine multidirectional rhythmic stabilization, elevated to 90–100°	Multidirectional stabilization 45–120° of elevation with and without protraction
Closed kinetic chain exercises	Quadruped weight shifts, multidirections, and push-up plus	Plank variations, dynamic, rhythmic stabilization, and push-up plus	Two-hand drills with suspension training
Bilateral UE plyometrics		Begin with side-to-side and chest pass	Progress, overhead throws, and slams
Unilateral UE plyometrics			Deceleration throws and throw with bounce back
Aerobic	Stationary bike, 20 min	Bike 30 min and upper body ergometer, 5 × 1 min alternating direction	Bike 30 min and upper body ergometer, 5 × 2 min alternating direction

Appendix D: Part 1—Dynamic Shoulder, Spine, Hip, Knee, and Ankle Warm-Up (All 2 × 15 Reps) [186, 187]

Diaphragmatic breathing		
	Supine	Standing
Shoulder ER to IR		
	Start	Finish
Scapular squeezes		
	Start	Finish
90/90 abduction to adduction		
	Start	Finish

90/90 ER to IR		
	Start	Finish
Scapular squeezes to streamline		
	Start	Finish
Hip IN and OUTs		
	Start	Finish
Dynamic ankle and knee		
	Start	Finish

Appendix E: Part 2—Strength/Plyometric/Balance/Reaction Time Progression [186]

Plank progression			
	TrA activation hold, 2×20–30 s	Alt LE lift for 2 s holds, 2×40–60 s	Alt LE lift for 20–30 s, 2×20–30 s
Side plank progression			
	Side plank hold, 2×20–30 s	With hip ABD reps for time, 2×20–30 s	With hip ABD reps for time, 2×20–30 s
Eccentric hamstring drop progression			
	Slowly lower, 1×3–5 reps	Slowly lower, 1×7–10 reps	Slowly lower, 1×12–15reps
T, A, and W's progression			
	All three prone, 2×15 reps	All three prone with perturbations, 2×30 s each side	All in quadruped with perturbations, 2×30 s each side

(continued)

Exercise			
Turkish get-up progression (see figure # for mechanics)	No weight 2×3–5 repetitions on each side	Water bottle in hand 2×3–5 on each side	5 s partner perturbations at each phase, 2×3–5
Reaction jump progression (take your mark, go!)	Reaction starts squat jump with 5 s holds, 2×5	Split squat jump with 5 s holds 1×5 on each side	Relay start squat jump, double leg step with 5 s hold, 2×5

Appendix F: Part 3—Aquatic Swimming-Specific Drills [186, 187]

Out of water, streamline with core hallowing 2 × 20 s on, 10 s off		
In water streamline from: block × 1 and wall × 1 2 × max distance with easy swim		
Prone sculling, catch 2 × 25 yards		
Prone sculling, mid-pull 2 × 25 yards		
Supine sculling, finish 2 × 25 yards		
Six-kick stroke with 180° rotation 2 × 25 yards		

| Corkscrew swimming, alternating direction by 25

2 × 25 yards | | |
| Speed work × 1 fast between walls and flags and ×1 fast between flags

2 × 25 yards | | |

References

1. Swimming. Encyclopedia Britannica. Encyclopedia Britannica Online. http://www.britannica.com/sports/swimming-sport. Accessed 21 June 2015.
2. FINA Sports—Swimming. www.FINA.org. Accessed 11 June 2015.
3. NCAA. 2014 NCAA men's swimming and diving championships results and records. NCAA online. http://www.ncaa.org/championships/statistics/2014-ncaa-mens-swimming-and-diving-championships-results-and-records. Accessed 11 June 2015.
4. NCAA. 2014 NCAA women's swimming and diving championships results and records. NCAA online. http://www.ncaa.org/championships/statistics/2014-ncaa-womens-swimming-and-diving-championships-results-and-records. Accessed 11 June 2015.
5. Barbosa TM, Bragada JA, Reis VM, Marinho DA, Carvalho C, Silva AJ. Energetics and biomechanics as determining factors of swimming performance: updating the state of the art. J Sci Med Sport. 2010;13(2):262–9.
6. Donato AJ, Tench K, Glueck DH, Seals DR, Eskurza I, Tanaka H. Declines in physiological functional capacity with age: a longitudinal study in peak swimming performance. J Appl Physiol (1985). 2003;94(2):764–9.
7. Psycharakis SG, McCabe C. Shoulder and hip roll differences between breathing and non-breathing conditions in front crawl swimming. J Biomech. 2011;44(9):1752–6.
8. Counsilman JE. Science of swimming. Englewood Cliffs: Prentice-Hall; 1968.
9. Weldon III EJ, Richardson AB. Upper extremity overuse injuries in swimming: a discussion of swimmer's shoulder. Clin Sports Med. 2001;20:423–38.
10. Spigelman T, Sciascia A, Uhl T. Return to swimming protocol for competitive swimmers: a post-operative case study and fundamentals. Int J Sports Phys Ther. 2014;9(5):712–25.
11. Pink M, Jobe FW, Perry J, Browne A, Scovazzo ML, Kerrigan J. The painful shoulder during the butterfly stroke: an electromyographic and cinematographic analysis of twelve muscles. Clin Orthop Relat Res. 1991;288:60–72.
12. Pink MM, Edelman GT, Mark R, Rodeo RA. Applied mechanics of swimming. In: Manske RC, Magee DJ, Quillen WS, Zachazewski JE, editors. Athletic and sport issues in musculoskeletal rehabilitation. 1st ed. Saint Louis: Saunders; 2011. p. 331–49.
13. Wanivenhaus F, Fox AJ, Chaudhury S, Rodeo SA. Epidemiology of injuries and prevention strategies in competitive swimmers. Sports Health. 2012;4:246–51.
14. Hara R, Muraoka I. Open water swimming performance. In: Kanosue K, Nagami T, Tsuchiya J, editors. Sports performance. Chapter 24th ed. Japan: Springer; 2015. p. 313–22.
15. Riewald S. The biomechanics of swimming. Independent Study Course 23.1.6. Orthopaedic Management of the Runner, Cyclist, and Swimmer: APTA. Orthopedica Section. 2013. p. 1–39.
16. Andrews C, Bakewell J, Scurr JC. Comparison of advanced and intermediate 200-m backstroke swimmers' dominant and non-dominant shoulder entry angles across various swimming speeds. J Sports Sci. 2011;29(7):743–8.
17. Ruwe PA, Pink M, Jobe FW, Perry J, Scovazzo ML. The normal and the painful shoulders during the breaststroke. Electromyographic and cinematographic analysis of twelve muscles. Am J Sports Med. 1994;22(6):789–96.

18. Nakashima M, Hasegawa T, Kamiya S, Takagi H. Musculoskeletal simulation of the breaststroke. JBSE. 2013;8(2):152–63.

19. Alberty M, Potdevin F, Dekerle J, Pelayo P, Gorce P, Sidney M. Changes in swimming technique during time to exhaustion at freely chosen and controlled stroke rates. J Sports Sci. 2008;26(11):1191–200.

20. Pink MM, Tibone J. The painful shoulder in the swimming athlete. Orthop Clin North Am. 2000;31(2):247–61.

21. Virag B, Hibberd EE, Oyama S, Padua DA, Myers JB. Prevalence of freestyle biomechanical errors in elite competitive swimmers. Sports Health. 2014; 6(3):218–24.

22. Yanai T, Hay J. Shoulder impingement in front-crawl swimming: II. Analysis of stroking technique. Med Sci Sports Exerc. 2000;32(1):30–40.

23. Gaunt T, Maffulli N. Soothing suffering swimmers: a systematic review of the epidemiology, diagnosis, treatment and rehabilitation of musculoskeletal injuries in competitive swimmers. Br Med Bull. 2012;103(1):45–88.

24. Junge A, Engebretsen L, Mountjoy ML, Alonso JM, Renström PA, Aubry MJ, Dvorak J. Sports injuries during the summer Olympic games 2008. Am J Sports Med. 2009;37:2165–72.

25. Engebretsen L, Soligard T, Steffen K, Alonso JM, Aubry M, Budgett R, Dvorak J, Jegathesan M, Meeuwisse WH, Mountjoy M, Palmer-Green D, Vanhegan I, Renström PA. Sports injuries and illnesses during the London Summer Olympic Games 2012. Br J Sports Med. 2013;47:407–14.

26. Mountjoy M, Junge A, Benjamen S, Boyd K, Diop M, Gerrard D, van den Hoogenband CR, Marks S, Martinez-Ruiz E, Miller J, Nanousis K, Shahpar FM, Veloso J, van Mechelen W, Verhagen E. Competing with injuries: injuries prior to and during the 15th FINA World Championships 2013 (Aquatics). Br J Sports Med. 2015;49:37–43.

27. Mountjoy M, Junge A, Alonso JM, Engebretsen L, Dragan I, Gerrard D, Kouidri M, Luebs E, Shahpar FM, Dvorak J. Sports injuries and illnesses in the 2009 FINA World Championships (Aquatics). Br J Sports Med. 2010;44:522–7.

28. Kerr ZY, Baugh CM, Hibberd EE, Snook EM, Hayden R, Dompier TP. Epidemiology of National Collegiate Athletic Association men's and women's swimming and diving injuries from 2009/2010 to 2013/2014. Br J Sports Med. 2015;49(7):465–71.

29. McFarland EG, Wasik M. Injuries in female collegiate swimmers due to swimming and cross training. Clin J Sport Med. 1996;6:178–82.

30. Wolf BR, Ebinger AE, Lawler MP, Britton CL. Injury patterns in division I collegiate swimming. Am J Sports Med. 2009;37:2037–42.

31. Evershed J, Burkett B, Mellifont R. Musculoskeletal screening to detect asymmetry in swimming. Phys Ther Sport. 2014;15(1):33–8.

32. Hellard P, Dekerle J, Avalos M, Caudal N, Knopp M, Hausswirth C. Kinematic measures and stroke rate variability in elite female 200-m swimmers in the four swimming techniques: Athens 2004 Olympic semi-finalists and French National 2004 Championship semi-finalists. J Sports Sci. 2008;26(1):35–46.

33. Pacholak S, Hochstein S, Rudert A, Brücker C. Unsteady flow phenomena in human undulatory swimming: a numerical approach. Sports Biomech. 2014;13(2):176–94.

34. Hamman S. Considerations and return to swim protocol for the pediatric swimmer after non-operative injury. Int J Sports Phys Ther. 2014;9(3):388–95.

35. Lätt E, Jürimäe J, Mäestu J, Purge P, Rämson R, Haljaste K, Keskinen KL, Rodriguez FA, Jürimäe T. Physiological, biomechanical and anthropometrical predictors of sprint swimming performance in adolescent swimmers. J Sports Sci Med. 2010; 9(3):398–404.

36. Ratel S, Poujade B. Comparative analysis of the energy cost during front crawl swimming in children and adults. Eur J Appl Physiol. 2009;105(4):543–9.

37. Poujade B, Hautier CA, Rouard A. Determinants of the energy cost of front-crawl swimming in children. Eur J Appl Physiol. 2002;87(1):1–6.

38. Van Praagh E. Developmental aspects of anaerobic function. In: Armstrong N, Kirby B, Welsman JR, editors. Children and exercise XIX. London: E & FN Spon; 1997. p. 267–90.

39. Jurimae J, Haljaste K, Clcchella A, Latt E, Purge P, Lepplk A, Jurimae T. Analysis of swimming performance from physical, physiological, and biomechanical parameters in young swimmers. Pediatr Exerc Sci. 2007;19:70–81.

40. Dormehl SJ, Osborough CD. Effect of age, sex and race distance on front crawl stroke parameters in sub-elite adolescent swimmers during competition. Pediatr Exerc Sci. 2015;27(3):334–44.

41. Buskirk ER, Hodgson JL. Age and aerobic power: the rate of change in men and women. Fed Proc. 1987;46(5):1824–9.

42. Joyner MJ. Physiological limiting factors and distance running: influence of gender and age on record performances. Exerc Sport Sci Rev. 1993;21:103–33.

43. Martin JC, Farrar RP, Wagner BM, Spirduso WW. Maximal power across the lifespan. J Gerontol A Biol Sci Med Sci. 2000;55(6):M311–6.

44. Rogers MA, Evans WJ. Changes in skeletal muscle with aging: effects of exercise training. Exerc Sport Sci Rev. 1993;21:65–102.

45. Tanaka H, Seals DR. Age and gender interactions in physiological functional capacity: insight from swimming performance. J Appl Physiol (1985). 1997;82(3):846–51.

46. Rubin RT, Lin S, Curtis A, Auerbach D, Win C. Declines in swimming performance with age: a longitudinal study of Masters swimming champions. Open Access J Sports Med. 2013;4:63–70.

47. Madsen PH, Bak K, Jensen S, Welter U. Training induces scapular dyskinesis in pain-free competitive swimmers: a reliability and observational study. Clin J Sport Med. 2011;21(2):109–13.

48. Tate A, Turner GN, Knab SE, Jorgensen C, Strittmatter A, Michener LA. Risk factors associated with shoulder pain and disability across the lifespan of competitive swimmers. J Athl Train. 2012;47(2):149–58.

49. Walker H, Gabbe B, Wajswelner H, Blanch P, Bennell K. Shoulder pain in swimmers: a 12-month prospective cohort study of incidence and risk factors. Phys Ther Sport. 2012;13:243–9.

50. Riemann BL, Witt J, Davies GJ. Glenohumeral joint rotation range of motion in competitive swimmers. J Sports Sci. 2011;29(11):1191–9.

51. Sein ML, Walton J, Linklater J, et al. Shoulder pain in elite swimmers: primary due to swim-volume-induced supraspinatus tendinopathy. Br J Sports Med. 2010;44:105–13.

52. Kibler WB, Chandler TJ, Livingston BP, Roetert EP. Shoulder range of motion in elite tennis players. Effect of age and years of tournament play. Am J Sports Med. 1996;24(3):279–85.

53. Ellenbecker TS, Roetert EP, Bailie DS, Davies GJ, Brown SW. Glenohumeral joint total rotation range of motion in elite tennis players and baseball pitchers. Med Sci Sports Exerc. 2002;34(12):2052–6.

54. Whiteley RJ, Ginn KA, Nicholson LL, Adams RD. Sports participation and humeral torsion. J Orthop Sports Phys Ther. 2009;39(4):256–63.

55. Potts AD, Charlton JE, Smith HM. Bilateral arm power imbalance in swim bench exercise to exhaustion. J Sports Sci. 2002;20(12):975–9.

56. Semciw AI, Green RA, Pizzari T. Gluteal muscle function and size in swimmers. J Sci Med Sport. 2015;pii: S1440-2440(15)00129-2.

57. Payton CJ, Bartlett RM, Baltzopoulos V, Coombs R. Upper extremity kinematics and body roll during preferred-side breathing and breath-holding front crawl swimming. J Sports Sci. 1999;17:689–96.

58. Thomas S. Glenohumeral rotation and scapular position adaptations after a single high school female sports season. J Athl Train. 2009;44(3):230–7.

59. Heinlein SA, Cosgarea AJ. Biomechanical considerations in the competitive swimmer's shoulder. Sports Health. 2010;2(6):519–25.

60. Scovazzo ML, Browne A, Pink M, Jobe FW, Kerrigan J. The painful shoulder during freestyle swimming: an electromyographic cinematographic analysis of twelve muscles. Am J Sports Med. 1991;19:577–82.

61. Cools AM, Witvrouw EE, Declercq GA, Danneels LA, Cambier DC. Scapular muscle recruitment patterns: trapezius muscle latency with and without impingement symptoms. Am J Sports Med. 2003;31(4):542–9.

62. Hidalgo-Lozano A, Calderón-Soto C, Domingo-Camara A, Fernández-de-Las-Peñas C, Madeleine P, Arroyo-Morales M. Elite swimmers with unilateral shoulder pain demonstrate altered pattern of cervical muscle activation during a functional upper-limb task. J Orthop Sports Phys Ther. 2012;42(6):552–8.

63. Figueiredo P, Sousa A, Goncalves P, Pereira SM, Soares S, Vilas-Boas JP, Fernandes RJ. Biophysical analysis of the 200 m front crawl swimming: a case study. In: Kjendlie PL, Sallman RK, Cabri J, editors. Biomechanics and medicine in swimming XI. Oslo: Norwegian School of Sports Sciences; 2010. p. 79–81.

64. Figueiredo P, Sanders R, Gorski T, Vilas-Boas JP, Fernandes RJ. Kinematic and electromyographic changes during 200 m front crawl at race pace. Int J Sports Med. 2013;34(1):49–55.

65. Rovere GDNA. Frequency, associated factors, and treatment of breaststroker's knee in competitive swimmers. Am J Sports Med. 1985;13(2):99–104.

66. Rodeo SA. Knee pain in competitive swimming. Clin Sports Med. 1999;18(2):379–87.

67. Keskinen K, Eriksson E, Komi P. Breaststroke swimmer's knee: a biomechanical and arthroscopic study. Am J Sports Med. 1980;8(4):228–31.

68. Vizsolyi P, Taunton J, Robertson G. Breaststroker's knee: an analysis of epidemiological and biomechanical factors. Am J Sports Med. 1987;15(1):63–71.

69. Stulberg SD, Shulman K, Stuart S, Culp P. Breaststroker's knee: pathology, etiology, and treatment. Am J Sports Med. 1980;8(3):164–71.

70. Soder RB, Mizerkowski MD, Petkowicz R, Baldisserotto M. MRI of the knee in asymptomatic adolescent swimmers: a controlled study. Br J Sports Med. 2012;46(4):268–72.

71. Hangai M, Kaneoka K, Hinotsu S, Shimizu K, Okubo Y, Miyakawa S, Mukai N, Sakane M, Ochiai N. Lumbar intervertebral disk degeneration in athletes. Am J Sports Med. 2009;37(1):149–55.

72. Kaneoka K, Shimizu K, Hangai M, et al. Lumbar intervertebral disk degeneration in elite competitive swimmers: a case control study. Am J Sports Med. 2007;35(8):1341–5.

73. Mudd LM, Fornetti W, Pivarnik JM. Bone mineral density in collegiate female athletes: comparisons among sports. J Athl Train. 2007;42(3):403–8.

74. Kobayashi K, Kaneoka K, Takagi H, Sengoki Y, Takemura M. Lumbar alignment and trunk muscle activity during the underwater streamline position in collegiate swimmers. J Swim Res. 2015;23(1): 33–43.

75. Nyska M, Constantini N, Cale-Benzoor M, Back Z, Kahn G, Mann G. Spondylolysis as a cause of low back pain in swimmers. Int J Sports Med. 2000;21(5):375–9.

76. Wojtys EM, Ashton-Miller JA, Huston LJ, Moga PJ. The association between athletic training time and the sagittal curvature of the immature spine. Am J Sports Med. 2000;28(4):490–8.

77. Haus BM, Micheli L. Back pain in the pediatric and adolescent athlete. Clin Sports Med. 2012;31(3): 423–40.

78. Emami M, Arab AM, Ghamkhar L. The activity pattern of the lumbo-pelvic muscles during prone hip extension in athletes with and without hamstring strain injury. Int J Sports Med. 2014;9(3):312–9.

79. Harris-Hayes M, Mueller MJ, Sahrmann SA, Bloom NJ, Steger-May K, Clohisy JC, Salsich GB. Persons with chronic hip joint pain exhibit reduced hip

muscle strength. J Orthop Sports Phys Ther. 2014; 44(11):890–8.

80. Willems TM, Cornelis JA, De Deurwaerder LE, Roelandt F, De Mits S. The effect of ankle muscle strength and flexibility on dolphin kick performance in competitive swimmers. Hum Mov Sci. 2014;36: 167–76.

81. Sanders RH. Kinematics, coordination, variability, and biological noise in the prone flutter kick at different levels of a "learn-to-swim" programme. J Sports Sci. 2007;25(2):213–27.

82. McCullough AS, Kraemer WJ, Volek JS, Solomon-Hill Jr GF, Hatfield DL, Vingren JL, Ho JY, Fragala MS, Thomas GA, Häkkinen K, Maresh CM. Factors affecting flutter kicking speed in women who are competitive and recreational swimmers. J Strength Cond Res. 2009;23(7):2130–6.

83. Kobayashi T, Suzuki E, Yamazaki N, Suzukawa M, Akaike A, Shimizu K, Gamada K. Fibular malalignment in individuals with chronic ankle instability. J Orthop Sports Phys Ther. 2014;44(11):872–8.

84. Elipot M, Houel N, Hellard P, Dietrich G, editors. Motor coordination during the underwater undulatory swimming phase of the start for high level swimmers. The XIth international symposium for biomechanics and medicine in swimming in Oslo, June 16–19, 2010.

85. Palmer KL, Clasey JL, Hosey RG, Mattacola CG. Bone mineral density of the distal tibia in swimmers with and without medial tibial stress syndrome following dry-land, weight-bearing training. Athl Train Sports Health Care. 2013;5(4):160–7.

86. Durall CJ. Therapeutic exercise for athletes with nonspecific neck pain: a current concepts review. Sports Health. 2012;4(4):293–301.

87. Nitz AJ, Nitz JA. Vascular thoracic outlet in a competitive swimmer: a case report. Int J Sports Phys Ther. 2013;8(1):74–9.

88. Alla VM, Natarajan N, Kaushik M, Warrier R, Nair CK. Paget-Schroetter syndrome: review of pathogenesis and treatment of effort thrombosis. West J Emerg Med. 2010;11(4):358–62.

89. Shupak A, Weiler-Ravell D, Adir Y, Daskalovic YI, Ramon Y, Kerem D. Pulmonary oedema induced by strenuous swimming: a field study. Respir Physiol. 2000;121:25–31.

90. Miller III CC, Calder-Becker K, Modave F. Swimming-induced pulmonary edema in triathletes. Am J Emerg Med. 2010;28(8):941–6.

91. Lund KL, Mahon RT, Tanen DA, Bakhda S. Swimming-induced pulmonary edema. Ann Emerg Med. 2003;41(2):251–6.

92. Beinart R, Matetzky S, Arad T, Hod H. Cold water-induced pulmonary edema. Am J Med. 2007;120(9):e3.

93. Arieli R, Kerem D, Gonen A, Goldenberg I, Shoshani O, Daskalovic YI, Shupak A. Thermal status of wet-suited divers using closed circuit O2 apparatus in sea water of 17–18.5 degrees C. Eur J Appl Physiol Occup Physiol. 1997;76(1):69–74.

94. Wolff AH, Coleshaw SR, Newstead CG, Keatinge WR. Heat exchanges in wet suits. J Appl Physiol. 1985;58(3):770–7.

95. Kurss DI, Lundgren CEG, Pasche AJ. Effect of water temperature on vital capacity in head-out immersion. In: Bachrach AJ, Matzen MM, editors. Underwater physiology VII. Proceedings of the seventh symposium on underwater physiology. Bethesda, MD: Undersea Medical Society Inc; 1981. p. 297–301.

96. Keatinge WR, McIlroy MB, Goldfien A. Cardiovascular responses to ice-cold showers. J Appl Physiol. 1964;19:1145–50.

97. Wilmshurst PT, Nuri M, Crowther A, Webb-Peploe MM. Cold-induced pulmonary oedema in scuba divers and swimmers and subsequent development of hypertension. Lancet. 1989;1(8629):62–5.

98. Koehle MS, Lepawsky M, McKenzie DC. Pulmonary oedema of immersion. Sports Med. 2005;35(3):183–90.

99. Wilk KE, Macrina LC, Cain EL, Dugas JR, Andrews JR. The recognition and treatment of superior labral (SLAP) lesions in the overhead athlete. Int J Sports Phys Ther. 2013;8(5):579–600.

100. Bradley H, Esformes J. Breathing pattern disorders and functional movement. Int J Sports Phys Ther. 2014;9(1):28–39.

101. Sheel AW. Respiratory muscle training in healthy individuals: physiological rationale and implications for exercise performance. Sports Med. 2002;32:567–81.

102. Edwards AM, Wells C, Butterly R. Concurrent inspiratory muscle and cardiovascular training differentially improves both perceptions of effort and 5000 m running performance compared with cardiovascular training alone. Br J Sports Med. 2008; 42:823–7.

103. Wilson EE, McKeever TM, Lobb C, Sherriff T, Gupta L, Hearson G, Martin N, Lindley MR, Shaw DE. Respiratory muscle specific warm-up and elite swimming performance. Br J Sports Med. 2014;48(9):789–91.

104. Wells GD, Plyley M, Thomas S, Goodman L, Duffin J. Effects of concurrent inspiratory and expiratory muscle training on respiratory and exercise performance in competitive swimmers. Eur J Appl Physiol. 2005;94:527–40.

105. Kilding AE, Brown S, McConnell AK. Inspiratory muscle training improves 100 and 200 m swimming performance. Eur J Appl Physiol. 2010;108: 505–11.

106. Schagatay E, van Kampen M, Emanuelsson S, Holm B. Effects of physical and apnea training on apneic time and the diving response in humans. Eur J Appl Physiol. 2000;82(3):161–9.

107. Lemaître F, Seifert L, Polin D, Juge J, Tourny-Chollet C, Chollet D. Apnea training effects on swimming coordination. J Strength Cond Res. 2009; 23(6):1909–14.

108. Joulia F, Steinberg JG, Faucher M, Jamin T, Ulmer C, Kipson N, Jammes Y. Breath-hold training of

humans reduces oxidative stress and blood acidosis after static and dynamic apnea. Respir Physiol Neurobiol. 2003;137(1):19–27.

109. Joulia F, Steinberg JG, Wolff F, Gavarry O, Jammes Y. Reduced oxidative stress and blood lactic acidosis in trained breath-hold human divers. Respir Physiol Neurobiol. 2002;133(1–2):121–30.

110. Boyd C, Levy A, McProud T, Huang L, Raneses E, Olson C, Centers for Disease Control and Prevention (CDC). Fatal and nonfatal drowning outcomes related to dangerous underwater breath-holding behaviors—New York State, 1988–2011. MMWR Morb Mortal Wkly Rep. 2015;64(19):518–21.

111. Lanphier EH. Breath-hold and ascent blackout. Presented at: the physiology of breath-hold diving, Undersea and Hyperbaric Medical Society Workshop, Buffalo, NY, October 28–29, 1985.

112. Barlow HB, MacIntosh F. Shallow water black-out. Royal Naval Physiological Laboratory Report R N P 44/125 UPS 48(a).

113. Laudner K, Lynall R, Williams JG, Wong R, Onuki T, Meister K. Thoracolumbar range of motion in baseball pitchers and position players. Int J Sports Phys Ther. 2013;8.

114. Reinold MM, Curtis AS. Microinstability of the shoulder in the overhead athlete. Int J Sports Phys Ther. 2013;8(5):601–16.

115. Petering RC, Webb C. Treatment options for low back pain in athletes. Sports Health. 2011;3(6):550–5.

116. Delitto A, George SZ, Van Dillen LR, Whitman JM, Sowa G, Shekelle P, Denninger TR, Godges JJ, Orthopaedic Section of the American Physical Therapy Association. Low back pain. J Orthop Sports Phys Ther. 2012;42(4):A1–57.

117. Maeo S, Takahashi T, Takai Y, Kanehisa H. Trunk muscle activities during abdominal bracing: comparison among muscles and exercises. J Sports Sci Med. 2013;12(3):467–74.

118. Allen BA, Hannon JC, Burns RD, Williams SM. Effect of a core conditioning intervention on tests of trunk muscular endurance in school-aged children. J Strength Cond Res. 2014;28(7):2063–70.

119. Huxel Bliven KC, Anderson BE. Core stability training for injury prevention. Sports Health. 2013;5(6):514–22.

120. Akuthota V, Standaert CJ, Chimes GP. Core strengthening. Arch Phys Med Rehabil. 2004;85(3) Suppl 1:S86–92.

121. Kachingwe AF, Grech S. Proposed algorithm for the management of athletes with athletic pubalgia (sports hernia): a case series. J Orthop Sports Phys Ther. 2008;38(12):768–81.

122. Ellsworth AA, Zoland MP, Tyler TF. Athletic pubalgia and associated rehabilitation. Int J Sports Phys Ther. 2014;9(6):774.

123. Ambegaonkar JP, Mettinger LM, Caswell SV, Burtt A, Cortes N. Relationships between core endurance, hip strength, and balance in collegiate female athletes. Int J Sports Phys Ther. 2014;9(5):604.

124. Tyler T, Silvers HJ, Gerhardt MB, Nicholas SJ. Groin injuries in sports medicine. Sports Health. 2010;2(3):231–6.

125. Leeturn DT, Ireland ML, Willson JD, Ballantyne BT, Davis IM. Core stability measures as risk factors for lower extremity injury in athletes. Med Sci Sports Exerc. 2004;36(6):926–34.

126. Lawrence 3rd RK, Kernozek TW, Miller EJ, Torry MR, Reuteman P. Influences of hip external rotation strength on knee mechanics during single-leg drop landings in females. Clin Biomech. 2008;23(6):806–13.

127. Iverson CA, Sutlive TG, Crowell MS, Morrell RL, Perkins MW, Garber MB, Moore JH, Wainner RS. Lumbopelvic manipulation for the treatment of patients with patellofemoral pain syndrome: development of a clinical prediction rule. J Orthop Sports Phys Ther. 2008;38(6):297–312.

128. Lack S, Barton C, Sohan O, Crossley K, Morrissey D. Proximal muscle rehabilitation is effective for patellofemoral pain: a systematic review with meta-analysis. Br J Sports Med. 2015;49(21):1365–76.

129. Hutchinson AC. Performance implications of rear foot movement in the swimming kick star. University of Western Ontario—Electronic Thesis and Dissertation Repository Paper 2279 2014.

130. Baltich J, Emery CA, Stefanyshyn D, Nigg BM. The effects of isolated ankle strengthening and functional balance training on strength, running mechanics, postural control and injury prevention in novice runners: design of a randomized controlled trial. J Sports Sci. 2014;15(1):407.

131. McKeon PO, Hertel J, Bramble D, Davis I. The foot core system: a new paradigm for understanding intrinsic foot muscle function. Br J Sports Med. 2015;49(5):290.

132. Salamh PA, Kolber MJ, Hanney WJ. Effect of scapular stabilization during horizontal adduction stretching on passive internal rotation and posterior shoulder tightness in young women volleyball athletes: a randomized controlled trial. Arch Phys Med Rehabil. 2015;96(2):349–56.

133. De Mey K, Danneels LA, Cagnie B, Huyghe L, Seyns E, Cools AM. Conscious correction of scapular orientation in overhead athletes performing selected shoulder rehabilitation exercises: the effect on trapezius muscle activation measured by surface electromyography. J Orthop Sports Phys Ther. 2013;43(1):3–10.

134. Mottram SL, Woledge RC, Morrissey D. Motion analysis study of a scapular orientation exercise and subjects' ability to learn the exercise. Man Ther. 2009;14:13–8.

135. Oyama S, Myers JB, Wassinger CA, Lephart SM. Three-dimensional scapular and clavicular kinematics and scapular muscle activity during retraction exercises. J Orthop Sports Phys Ther. 2010;40:169–79.

136. Moeller CR, Huxel Bliven KC, Valier AR. Scapular muscle-activation ratios in patients with shoulder

injuries during functional shoulder exercises. J Athl Train. 2014;49(3):345–55.

137. Andersen V, Fimland MS, Wiik E, Skoglund A, Saeterbakken AH. Effects of grip width on muscle strength and activation in the lat pull-down. J Strength Cond Res. 2014;28(4):1135–42.

138. Salles JI, Velasques B, Cossich V, Nicoliche E, Ribeiro P, Amaral MV, Motta G. Effect of strength training on shoulder proprioception. J Athl Train. 2015;50(3):277–80.

139. Park KM, Cynn HS, Kwon OY, Yi CH, Yoon TL, Lee JH. Comparison of pectoralis major and serratus anterior muscle activities during different push-up plus exercises in subjects with and without scapular winging. J Strength Cond Res. 2014;28(9):2546–51.

140. Borreani S, Calatayud J, Colado JC, Tella V, Moya-Nájera D, Martin F, Rogers ME. Shoulder muscle activation during stable and suspended push-ups at different heights in healthy subjects. Phys Ther Sport. 2014;pi:S1466-853C.

141. Byrne JM, Bishop NS, Caines AM, Crane KA, Feaver AM, Pearcey GE. Effect of using a suspension training system on muscle activation during the performance of a front plank exercise. J Strength Cond Res. 2014;28(11):3049–55.

142. De Mey K, Danneels L, Cagnie B, Borms D, T'Jonck Z, Van Damme E, Cools AM. Shoulder muscle activation levels during four closed kinetic chain exercises with and without Redcord slings. J Strength Cond Res. 2014;28(6):1626–35.

143. Sergienko S, Kalichman L. Myofascial origin of shoulder pain: a literature review. J Bodyw Mov Ther. 2015;19(1):91–101.

144. Laudner K, Compton BD, McLoda TA, Walters CM. Acute effects of instrument assisted soft tissue mobilization for improving posterior shoulder range of motion in collegiate baseball players. Int J Sports Phys Ther. 2014;9.

145. Jay K, Sundstrup E, Søndergaard SD, et al. Specific and crossover effects of massage for muscle soreness: randomized controlled trial. Int J Sports Phys Ther. 2014;9(1):82–91.

146. Mohr AR, Long BC, Goad CL. Effect of foam rolling and static stretching on passive hip-flexion range of motion. J Sport Rehabil. 2014;23(4):296–9.

147. Škarabot J, Beardsley C, Štirn I. Comparing the effects of self-myofascial release with static stretching on ankle range-of-motion in adolescent athletes. Int J Sports Phys Ther. 2015;10(2):203–12.

148. Lim EC, Tay MG. Kinesio taping in musculoskeletal pain and disability that lasts for more than 4 weeks: is it time to peel off the tape and throw it out with the sweat? A systematic review with meta-analysis focused on pain and also methods of tape application. Br J Sports Med. 2015;49(24):1558–66.

149. Simsek HH, Balki S, Kekik SS, et al. Does Kinesio taping in addition to exercise therapy improve outcomes in subacromial impingement? A randomized, double-blinded, controlled clinical trial. Acta Orthop Traumatol Turc. 2013;47:104–10.

150. Dawood RS, Kattabei OM, Nasef SA, et al. Effectiveness of Kinesio taping versus cervical traction on mechanical neck pain dysfunction. Int J Ther Rehabil Res. 2014;2:1–5.

151. Sallis RE, Jones K, Sunshine S, Smith G, Simon L. Comparing sports injuries in men and women. Int J Sports Med. 2001;22(6):420–3.

152. Butler R, Arms J, Reiman M, Plisky P, Kiesel K, Taylor D, Queen R. Sex differences in dynamic closed kinetic chain upper quarter function in collegiate swimmers. J Athl Train. 2014;49(4):442–6.

153. Aspenes ST, Karlsen T. Exercise-training intervention studies in competitive swimming. Sports Med. 2012;42(6):527–43.

154. Gorman PP, Butler RJ, Plisky PJ, Kiesel KB. Upper quarter y balance test: reliability and performance comparison between gender in active adults. J Strength Cond Res. 2012;26(11):3043–8.

155. Roush JR, Kitamura J, Waits MC. Reference values for the closed kinetic chain upper extremity stability test (CKCUEST) for collegiate baseball players. N Am J Sports Phys Ther. 2007;2(3):159–63.

156. Vrbanić TS, Ravlić-Gulan J, Gulan G, Matovinović D. Balance index score as a predictive factor for lower sports results or anterior cruciate ligament knee injuries in Croatian female athletes–preliminary study. Coll Antropol. 2007;31(1):253–8.

157. Plisky PJ, et al. Star excursion balance test as a predictor of lower extremity injury in high school basketball players. J Orthop Sports Phys Ther. 2006;36(12):911–9.

158. Girold S, Maurin D, Dugué B, Chatard JC, Millet G. Effects of dry-land vs. resisted-and assisted-sprint exercises on swimming sprint performances. J Strength Cond Res. 2007;21(2):599–605.

159. Gourgoulis V, Antoniou P, Aggeloussis N, Mavridis G, Kasimatis P, Vezos N, Boli A, Mavromatis G. Kinematic characteristics of the stroke and orientation of the hand during front crawl resisted swimming. J Sports Sci. 2010;28(11):1165–73.

160. Barbosa AC, Castro Fde S, Dopsaj M, Cunha SA, Andries Jr O. Acute responses of biomechanical parameters to different sizes of hand paddles in front-crawl stroke. J Sports Sci. 2013;31(9):1015–23.

161. McGladrey BW, Hannon JC, Faigenbaum AD, Shultz BB, Shaw JM. High school physical educators' and sport coaches' knowledge of resistance training principles and methods. J Strength Cond Res. 2014;28(5):1433–42.

162. Gatta G, Leban B, Paderi M, Padulo J, Migliaccio GM, Pau M. The development of swimming power. Muscles Ligaments Tendons J. 2014;4(4):438–45.

163. Lepley LK, Palmieri-Smith RM. Cross-education strength and activation after eccentric exercise. J Athl Train. 2014;49(5):582–9.

164. Laursen PB, Jenkins DG. The scientific basis for high-intensity interval training: optimising training programmes and maximising performance in highly trained endurance athletes. Sports Med. 2002;32(1):53–73.

165. Kilen A, Larsson TH, Jørgensen M, Johansen L, Jørgensen S, Nordsborg NB. Effects of 12 weeks high-intensity & reduced-volume training in elite athletes. PLoS One. 2014;9(4), e95025.

166. Faude O, Meyer T, Scharhag J, Weins F, Urhausen A, Kindermann W. Volume vs. intensity in the training of competitive swimmers. Int J Sports Med. 2008;29(11):906–12.

167. Pugliese L, Porcelli S, Bonato M, Pavei G, La Torre A, Maggioni MA, Bellistri G, Marzorati M. Effects of manipulating volume and intensity training in masters swimmers. Int J Sports Physiol Perform. 2015;10(7):907–12.

168. Sperlich B, Zinner C, Heilemann I, Kjendlie PL, Holmberg HC, Mester J. High-intensity interval training improves VO(2peak), maximal lactate accumulation, time trial and competition performance in 9-11-year-old swimmers. Eur J Appl Physiol. 2010;110(5):1029–36.

169. Laursen PB. Training for intense exercise performance: high-intensity or high-volume training? Scand J Med Sci Sports. 2010;20 Suppl 2:1–10.

170. Barroso R, Cardoso RK, do Carmo EC, Tricoli V. Perceived exertion in coaches and young swimmers with different training experience. Int J Sports Physiol Perform. 2014;9(2):212–6.

171. Barroso R, Salgueiro DF, do Carmo EC, Nakamura FY. Training volume and repetition distance affect session rating of perceived exertion and internal load in swimmers. Int J Sports Physiol Perform. 2015;10(7):848–52.

172. Girard O, Amann M, Aughey R, Billaut F, Bishop DJ, Bourdon P, Buchheit M, Chapman R, D'Hooghe M, Garvican-Lewis LA, Gore CJ, Millet GP, Roach GD, Sargent C, Saunders PU, Schmidt W, Schumacher YO. Position statement—altitude training for improving team-sport players' performance: current knowledge and unresolved issues. Br J Sports Med. 2013;47(Suppl):i8–16.

173. Robertson EY, Aughey RJ, Anson JM, Hopkins WG, Pyne DB. Effects of simulated and real altitude exposure in elite swimmers. J Strength Cond Res. 2010;24(2):487–93.

174. Garvican-Lewis LA, Clark SA, Polglaze T, McFadden G, Gore CJ. Ten days of simulated live high:train low altitude training increases Hbmass in elite water polo players. Br J Sports Med. 2013;47 Suppl 1:i70–3.

175. Clark SA, Quod MJ, Clark MA, Martin DT, Saunders PU, Gore CJ. Time course of haemoglobin mass during 21 days live high:train low simulated altitude. Eur J Appl Physiol. 2009;106(3):399–406.

176. Friedmann B, Frese F, Menold E, Kauper F, Jost J, Bärtsch P. Individual variation in the erythropoietic response to altitude training in elite junior swimmers. Br J Sports Med. 2005;39(3):148–53.

177. Wachsmuth NB, Völzke C, Prommer N, Schmidt-Trucksäss A, Frese F, Spahl O, Eastwood A, Stray-Gundersen J, Schmidt W. The effects of classic altitude training on hemoglobin mass in swimmers. Eur J Appl Physiol. 2013;113(5):1199–211.

178. Charlot K, Pichon A, Richalet JP, Chapelot D. Effects of a high-carbohydrate versus high-protein meal on acute responses to hypoxia at rest and exercise. Eur J Appl Physiol. 2013;113(3):691–702.

179. Bishop DJ, Thomas C, Moore-Morris T, Tonkonogi M, Sahlin K, Mercier J. Sodium bicarbonate ingestion prior to training improves mitochondrial adaptations in rats. Am J Physiol Endocrinol Metab. 2010;299(2):E225–33.

180. O'Donnell CJ, Bowen J, Fossati J. Identifying and managing shoulder pain in competitive swimmers: how to minimize training flaws and other risks. Phys Sportsmed. 2005;33(9):27–35.

181. Zaton K, Szczepan S. The impact of immediate verbal feedback on the improvement of swimming technique. J Hum Kinet. 2014;41:143–54.

182. Hay JG, Guimaraes ACS, Grimston SKA. Quantitative look at swimming biomechanics. In: Hay JG, editor. Starting, stroking & turning. A compilation of research on the biomechanics of swimming. Iowa: The University of Iowa; 1983.

183. Lee T, Swinnen S, Serrien J. Cognitive effort and motor learning. Quest. 1994;46:328–44.

184. Schmidt RA, Lee TD. Motor control and learning: a behavioural emphasis. Human Kinetics: Champaign; 1999.

185. Yerg BJ. The impact of selected presage and process behaviors on the refinement of a motor skill. J Teach Phys Educ. 1990;3:38–46.

186. Barengo NC, Meneses-Echavez JF, Ramierez-Velez R, Cohen DD, Tovar G, Bautista JE. The impact of the FIFA11+ training program on injury prevention in football players: a systematic review. Int J Environ Res Public Health. 2014;11:11986–2000.

187. Edelman GT. An active shoulder warm-up for the competitive swimmer. 2009. http://www.udel.edu/PT/PT%20Clinical%20Services/journalclub/sojc/09_10/Nov09/Active%20Warmup%20George.pdf. Accessed Feb 24, 2015.

Mental Skills for Endurance Sports

18

Jennifer E. Carter and Stephen Graef

Introduction

Ask athletes the percentage of sport performance that is mental, and they will often give estimates around seventy-five percent. Next, ask what percentage of their *training* is mental. Zero is the common response. While sport psychologists do not advocate for athletes to substitute a 50-mile bike ride with a 3 h imagery session, we do recommend supplementing physical training with mental training. Sport psychologists assist athletes with mental health and mental skills training in order to improve their sport performance. In this chapter, we focus on mental skills training for endurance sports.

Mental skills training can "…enhance athletes' chances of performing at their highest level under very demanding, stressful, and sometimes even hostile conditions" [1]. Imagine a cross-country skier battling icy wind, a cyclist trying to avoid a crash while flying down a steep decline, or a runner trudging through mile 20 of a marathon. Endurance sports often present such stressful, demanding conditions, and athletes who are mentally prepared will be the ones to thrive.

Mental skills training has positive effects on endurance sport performance, according to one literature review [2]. In particular, goal setting, imagery, and self-talk show consistent effectiveness for endurance sport performance. More research is needed to learn how and for whom these mental skills work.

Mental training interventions occur individually or in packages. Individually, mental skills include motivation, goal setting, arousal or energy management, self-talk, focus, imagery, routines, mindfulness, and team building. While sport psychologists commonly teach several mental skills in combination, more research is needed to determine if mental training packages add more improvement than individual skills. Packages including goal setting, energy management, imagery, and self-talk have improved triathlon performance [3] and 1600 m running performance [4].

Get ready to psyche up for endurance sports! Because it takes inordinate discipline to excel as an endurance athlete, we start with a discussion about motivation. Then we dive into specific mental skills to train your mind as well as your body. We finish the chapter with a discussion of finding balance in exercise. Here is the order of topics in this chapter:

- Motivation
- Goal setting
- Energy management
- Self-talk
- Focus

J.E. Carter (✉) • S. Graef
Sports Medicine, Ohio State University Sports
Medicine Center and Athletic Department,
Pavilion, Third Floor, 2050 Kenny Road, Columbus,
OH 43221, USA
e-mail: carter.270@osu.edu; graef.7@osu.edu

© Springer International Publishing Switzerland 2016
T.L. Miller (ed.), *Endurance Sports Medicine*, DOI 10.1007/978-3-319-32982-6_18

- Imagery
- Performance routines
- Mindfulness
- Exercise balance

Motivation

Motivation is likely one of the most important psychological constructs in sport, especially within endurance sport. The ongoing energy required for endurance athletes to persist in repetitive high-quality, grueling training sessions, even in the face of adversity and other life demands, exemplifies motivation as a foundational requirement for high performance and achievement. As such, it is no surprise that trainers, coaches, organizations, and athletes alike all have vested interest in understanding, developing, and maintaining motivation.

Research has consistently shown that motivation is a crucial factor in human behavior because it influences the initiation, direction, intensity, and persistence of specific goal-directed behavior [5]. Self-determination theory [5] focuses on the strength of athletes' motivation to perform particular behaviors and has been increasingly applied to sport [6]. SDT focuses on the factors that influence athletes' decisions to perform and persist in sport. One such factor is the goals or motives that athletes cite for engaging in their sport [6]. Specifically, a distinction is made between *intrinsic* (i.e., establishing meaningful relationships, feeling a sense of community, gaining knowledge, finding stimulation, and achieving personal growth) and *extrinsic* goals or motives (i.e., winning, seeking fame, obtaining an appealing appearance, and achieving financial success) [5].

Within self-determination theory [5], goal type has implications for personal and relational functioning. Intrinsic goals focus on developing personal interests, values, and potential and are inherently satisfying to pursue [6]. According to SDT, the pursuit of intrinsic goals will lead to both sustained engagement in the behavior as well as more positive psychological outcomes (e.g., well-being, self-esteem) [7]. In contrast, extrinsic goals are more outwardly oriented, directed toward *external* indicators of worth, leading to the less inherent satisfaction and human development [7]. While the desire to win to prove something to others can be motivating, athletes must be careful in their utilization of extrinsic motives for they may undermine the development of intrinsic motivation. Relying solely on extrinsic motives might limit the ability for endurance athletes to sustain training requirements for the long haul and decrease their enjoyment of the process.

Some strategies for increasing intrinsic motivation include building on past success, preparation, positive reinforcement, variety in training, and athlete contribution to training [8]. Successful experiences increase perceived intrinsic ability and strengthen personal competence. For example, athletes experience success by setting small goals and reaching them. Adequate preparation is also essential for endurance athletes. Slowly progressing through a training protocol will be more motivating than going for a long distance without sufficient training. Rewards that are contingent with performance can be beneficial. For example, Bill has been gunning for a particular pace on a training run, and once he reaches it, he rewards himself with his favorite meal.

Verbal and nonverbal praise from athletes and coaches can provide positive feedback that helps increase motivation. Further, motivational self-talk has also been shown to improve performance in whole body endurance activity [2]. Mixing up the training process by varying drill sequences or activity days can keep training stimulating and more motivating. Finally, allowing athletes to have a say in training, and other related decisions, can increase autonomy and intrinsic motivation. Understanding the need for increasing and maintaining higher motivation levels is critical for athletic success in endurance sport. Appropriately tapping into intrinsic and extrinsic motivation is essential to developing this performance fuel.

Goal Setting

A goal is a target, specific standard, or accomplishment that one strives to attain, usually within a specified period of time [9]. Goal setting and

has been shown to consistently facilitate sport performance [10]. Objective goals are those that are measureable, such as "I want to run a half-marathon in under two-hours" [11]. Subjective goals, on the other hand, are more general statements of intent, such as wanting to do well at the race [11].

Goals have commonly been further divided based on whether the intention of the goal is outcome, performance, or process driven [11]. An outcome goal usually focuses on the result of an event, such as wanting to win a race, gain entry into an event, or earn a medal. Performance goals focus on achieving objectives that are in comparison to one's own previous performance rather than the performance of competitors. For instance, wanting a personal record in a marathon or lowering one's swim time during a triathlon are examples of performance goals. Finally, process goals focus on executing concrete actions in order to perform well [11]. For instance, focusing on spearing the hand into the water during each swim stroke or pushing and pulling with each pedal revolution are pertinent process goals. When used systematically, goals help athletes plan, evaluate, and manage their behavior and thoughts [10].

In general, when compared to no goals or vague "do your best" goals, specific goal setting has been shown to enhance athletes' performance [9]. Outcome goals, though uncontrollable, are attractive and exciting—useful in enhancing the motivation needed for the physical and mental grind of training [9]. Performance goals offer more control and flexibility, thus allowing athletes the opportunity to raise and lower their goal difficulty to remain challenged and excited [9]. Athletes use process goals in immediate situations to enable focus on specific task demands in productive ways [9]. Considered collectively, setting outcome, performance, and process goals offers unique benefits to maximizing performance.

Within endurance sport, goal setting has been shown to improve performance. In particular, using goals helped high school runners improve their 2.3 km times and nonathletes cycle for longer durations during an incremental test [2]. Further, in a gymnasium sprint triathlon, outcome,

performance, and process goals all positively impacted race day performance [3]. These endurance sport data, combined with many years of goal setting research in other sport performance domains, yield clear and consistent results for goal setting as a performance-enhancing strategy.

There are guidelines which improve the effectiveness of goal setting [10]. Set specific goals in measurable and behavioral terms, which makes it easier to detect progress. Set moderately difficult but realistic goals to remain challenged enough to be motivated, instead of frustrated from repeated failure. Set short-range and long-range goals to stay focused on the path and experience small successes along the way. As noted above, outcome, performance, and process goals all offer benefits to enhancing performance when used appropriately. Set goals in both practice and competition to enhance performance. Set positive goals instead of negative goals, which allows athletes to focus on what they want to accomplish, not reminding themselves of what they do *not* want to accomplish. Identify targets for goal attainment to improve focus and promote a sense of urgency, such as completing a half marathon within 4 months. Finally, write goals down and frequently evaluate them to stay on the path toward success.

Energy Management

Too high or too low? Some athletes experience excessive anxious energy prior to competition, causing tense muscles and wasted energy. Others feel too flat or tired to perform well. Athletes have an optimal zone of energy (also known as arousal or emotion) in which they perform best, and mental training helps them find that ideal energy zone.

Following the tenet of "moderation in all things," it appears a moderate level of energy works well for most athletes [12, 13]. But due to the complexity of behavior, researchers have theorized more multifaceted relationships between energy and performance. Hanin proposes that individuals vary in the amount of energy they need to succeed in sport, depending on their personality and sport event [14]. For example, sensation-seeker Shannon swims faster in shorter events like the 200 freestyle when she has high energy, whereas anxiety-prone Sean rows best in the longer single sculls event when he's more relaxed.

Individual interpretation of energy level is also important, according to reversal theory [15]. Shannon views her fast heartbeat as excitement and a sign she's ready to swim fast. Sean, however, interprets the butterflies in his stomach as unpleasant anxiety—a feeling of dread. McGonigal found that stress can be good for us if we reframe a thumping heartbeat and butterflies flitting about in the stomach as a sign our bodies are preparing to rise to the challenge [16].

When athletes have too much energy or anxiety, relaxation strategies are often helpful [17]. A key skill is diaphragmatic breathing, also known as belly breathing. To practice diaphragmatic breathing:

– Place one hand on your chest and one hand on your belly (below belly button).
– Inhale through your nose, exhale through your mouth.
– When you inhale, keep the hand on your chest still, while pushing out the hand on your belly with air (the opposite of "sucking it in").
– Exhale completely…let your shoulders droop as you breathe out.
– The diaphragm is the muscle beneath your lungs…you'll feel that drop or push down as you inhale, which allows your lungs to expand down into your chest cavity.

Another calming breathing strategy is paced breathing which involves a shorter inhale and a longer exhale [18]. For example, breathe in to a count of two, and breathe out to a count of four. Paced breathing has been shown to reduce heart rate.

When athletes are too low in energy, they often feel tired and flat and may suffer a "let down" [19]. Strategies to increase energy include quick, shallow breaths and jumping up and down. According to Cuddy, holding the body in a "power pose" for 2 min decreases cortisol (stress)

Table 18.1 Energy management strategies

Too nervous? Chill out	Too flat? Pump up
Take diaphragmatic breaths, paced breaths	Take fast, shallow breaths
Repeat trigger word like "Just do my best"	Move your body. Jump up and down
Focus on the process, the controllables	Alternate contracting and relaxing muscles
Reexperience your best performance	Review your most important goal
Get perspective—it's just a sport!	Walk and talk quickly. Act as if you're energized
Listen to happy music, a comedy routine	Listen to pump up music
Talk to a friend about your stress	Repeat an affirmation "I've got great stamina"
Hold a power pose for 2 min	Hold a power pose for 2 min

and increases testosterone (feelings of energy and power) [20]. See Table 18.1 for more "chill out" and "pump up" strategies [17, 19–21].

Self-Talk

"Push harder." "I can't keep up." "Why the *hell* am I doing this?"

Sound familiar? Self-talk is what athletes say to themselves before, during, and after training and competition. Cognitive-behavioral theory, which challenges dysfunctional self-talk, is a cornerstone of mental training for sports.

Cognitive theories espouse that our reactions do not stem from the events that happen to us, but rather from how we *interpret* those events. For example, Amy and Sienna both swallow water during the swim of a triathlon. Amy thinks, "Oh, no! Why does this always happen to me? I suck at swimming. My race is ruined." In contrast, Sienna thinks, "Yuck. This happens to lots of swimmers. Breathe. One stroke at a time." Both Amy and Sienna experience the negative event of swallowing water, but Sienna reacts more effectively due to her evidence-based self-talk.

Cognitive-behavioral therapy teaches skills to challenge dysfunctional thoughts like overgeneralization [22]. Athletes who overgeneralize interpret one negative event as a never-ending pattern, making broad conclusions about themselves and others. While training for a tramping event in New Zealand, Daniel's old knee injury acts up, and he has to cut one practice short. If he thinks, "I'll never be ready for this event. I screw up everything," he is overgeneralizing. One abbreviated training session doesn't mean that he will be ill-prepared for the race, nor does it imply that he fails at *everything* in his life. Such negative thoughts can lead to feelings of anxiety, hopelessness, and irritability, which can then impair training and sport performance [1].

Another classic dysfunctional thinking style is "should" statements. When thoughts like "I should've known better" or "I should beat that athlete" pop up, athletes often become too tense or angry to perform well. Ellis advises us to stop "shoulding" all over ourselves [23]. Instead, use words like "prefer," or acknowledge the facts, such as "Just because I have a better ranking doesn't mean I should beat that athlete. Rankings are meaningless on any given day."

Do self-talk interventions improve sport performance? In a 2011 meta-analysis, Hatzigeorgiadis et al. reported a moderate positive effect size [24]. For instructional self-talk such as "Follow through," fine motor skills like golf putting benefit more than gross motor skills like running. Motivational self-talk ("Just keep swimming") may be more useful for gross motor skills used in endurance sports. Anticipation of positive consequences like "I'll feel wonderful crossing the finish line!" is a type of motivational self-talk helpful in endurance events [25].

Regarding endurance sports, studies find that self-talk interventions have improved performance in swimming [26] and marathon running [25]. Hamilton, Scott, and McDougall found that positive self-talk improved cycling performance, particularly when audio of positive messages reinforced the cyclists' self-talk [27]. The authors also found that negative self-talk slightly improved performance and explained that some athletes perceive negative statements like "You can't keep up this pace" as surprisingly motivating. This study highlights the unique responses of athletes to mental training interventions.

Self-talk interventions do not focus only on challenging negative self-talk but also on brief self-coaching instructions prior to performance. Intelligent athletes may tend to overthink, which can cause muscular tension, hesitation, poor focus, and mental fatigue. Decreased athletic performance may result. Their internal dialogue may sound something like this:

> I really want to PR today. Why does *that* athlete have to be in this race? So annoying. Are my water bottles full? Coach told me to get after the third mile. Ooh, I like that guy's bike. How does he afford that? I hope my quad doesn't cramp up. Crap, that work deadline's approaching. What if I don't finish? That'd be awful. Is it going to rain? Remember to pick up milk on the way home. C'mon, focus. PR, baby.

Such rambling self-talk impairs concentration. For increased focus, sport psychologists often teach "trigger words": words or phrases under the athlete's control, about the task at hand, that focus on one thing at a time [28]. Behind the blocks, swimmers might use trigger words like "Fast and loose," "Hop on the third one hundred," or "Do my best." In the above example, Sienna uses trigger words like "Breathe" and "One stroke at a time" to refocus after swallowing water during a swim.

Concentration

Concentration is the ability to focus attention on the task at hand without distraction from irrelevant external or internal stimuli. It is a learned skill of limiting reactions and distractions to unimportant information, which has a profound effect on athletic performance [1, 2]. When athletes concentrate well, they respond to changing performance demands, control emotion and performance state, and release muscular tension [29]. Attentional focus has been theorized to reside on two dimensions: width (broad or narrow) and direction (external or internal) [30]. A broad attentional focus allows a person to perceive several stimuli simultaneously, such as scanning the entire lake prior to the swim. Narrow attentional focus occurs when an athlete only focuses on one or two cues, like a competitor's tire when making a pass on the bike. An external attentional focus directs attention outward to an object, such as biking toward your specific transition spot. Finally, an internal attentional focus is directed inward to thoughts and feelings, like working through the heavy legs after a bike.

Another important quality of focus is whether athletes associate, i.e., focus on bodily sensations or performance-specific cues, or dissociate, i.e., focus on external stimuli as a means of distracting themselves. Early studies suggested that elite athletes gravitate toward associative strategies, and nonelite athletes favor dissociative strategies, but 35 years of subsequent research has resulted in equivocal findings regarding the best attentional focus for peak performance [31]. Brick et al. recommended future research breakdown associative strategies into active self-regulation and internal sensory monitoring and dissociative strategies into active distraction and involuntary distraction [31].

Additional support for the value of concentration comes from Moran [32]. He contends that a focused state of mind requires deliberate mental effort and intentionality. Although skilled athletes can divide their attention between two or more concurrent actions, they can focus consciously on only thought at a time. (Focusing on only one thing is also known as the *one-mindful* mindfulness skill.) During peak performance states, athletes' minds are so focused that there is no difference between what they are thinking and what they are doing. Athletes tend to lose their concentration when they pay attention to events and experiences that are in the future, in the past, out of their control, or otherwise irrelevant to the task. Excessive anxiety can also undermine optimal performance by leading performer's focus on inappropriate cues as well as focus too much on conscious, instead of automatic, control of movement. Considered collectively, concentration is a worthwhile mental skill that needs to be deliberately trained and sharpened.

Fortunately there are many supported strategies for improving concentration. Simulating competitive demands in practice can aid with concentration on event day [33]. Simulation offers the opportunity to learn how to cope effec-

tively with distractions and practice strategies for refocusing the mind. Self-talk, especially trigger words, can be used to trigger an identified response. Using nonjudgmental thinking about performance also helps athletes stay in the present moment and not be distracted by past or future performances. (See the section "Mindfulness" for more details.) Performance routines allow athletes to focus on what is under their control and reduce distractions that may come up on race day as well as ready the mind for reaching the zone. Plans for competitions also offer athletes a way to remain focused during the event by reminding themselves of strategies, goals, and techniques. Finally, another strategy to enhance concentration is to overlearn the skills required to perform. Cyclists focus better on race strategy if they aren't overly concerned about how to effectively engage the pedal stroke. A well-learned stroke will be automatic, thus allowing cyclists to focus on other elements necessary for great performance.

Imagery

Imagery is using all of the senses to create an experience in the mind [33]. Imagery, visualization, mental rehearsal, mental blueprint, and mental practice all refer to the process of recalling from memory pieces of information stored from experience and shaping these pieces into meaningful images [34]. It is an act of simulation that occurs internally within the mind. Anyone can use imagery, in any setting, to learn and practice skills and performance strategies, correct mistakes, prepare a mental focus for competition, automate preperformance routines, build and enhance mental skills, and aid in the recovery from injuries [33].

How does imagery work? When engaging in visualization, similar neural impulses occur in the brain and muscles, mimicking those actually fired when physically performing the action [34]. For example, picturing yourself biking up a tough hill will actually fire neurons in your brain and body that are responsible for making your quads and hamstrings move. Imagery also facilitates performance by helping athletes blueprint the movements or strategies necessary for success, so they become more automatic [34]. For instance, picturing a technically sound swimming stroke increases the likelihood of performing a perfect stroke. Athletes are also able to develop coping responses to potential stressful situations [34]. As such, a cyclist can image racing confidently on a rainy course. Finally, imagery allows athletes to create the optimal levels of energy and concentration required for their performance endeavor [34]. A marathoner who is nervous before a race might picture a beach scene to relax her mind and body.

Evidence supporting the use of imagery in endurance performance has been well-documented. For example, nonathletes using pre-performance imagery of skill execution and successful performance outcomes showed improvement in a 1.5-mile run [2]. In a small group of competitive youth swimmers, imagery training and listening to an imagery script improved performance in a 1000-yard practice set [2]. Another study of a small group of indoor gymnasium triathlon participants showed that imagery helped in the tolerance of pain, increased motivation and confidence, and improved race strategy [3]. These examples, as well as supplemental research involving participants in varying levels of ability and sport type, offer support for the use of mental imagery in enhancing performance.

To set up an effective imagery training program and maximize the potential overlap in neural activation between real and imaged behaviors, it has been suggested to use the PETTLEP model [35]. The PETTLEP model outlines seven elements (Physical, Environment, Task, Timing, Learning, Emotion, and Perspective) that amplify the relatedness between the imaged and actual performance [36]. For instance, the physical element suggests imaging in a similar physical environment (i.e., imaging the swim while standing in the pool or floating in the water). The timing element suggests imaging the performance in real time (note: obviously this may be difficult when imaging endurance sport, though picturing a swimming stroke or run cadence in real time would be ideal). Hence, deliberately engaging in

imagery in ways that best utilize and approximate the elements of the PETTLEP model would offer the greatest benefit [35]. Further, it is essential to assess which aspect of performance that will be imaged [33]. For instance, does the athlete need to focus on technique, dealing with a flat tire, or picturing strength while running up a hill? All require a different type of imagery. Another obvious key to imagery includes being able to control the image [33]. If athletes have difficulty creating the image they want, backtracking to individual behaviors and building off of what they can controllably image are appropriate.

Performance Routines

Throughout this chapter we have introduced mental skills to enhance athletic endurance performance. Though helpful in isolation, these mental skills can serve additional purpose when combined in unison before, during, and after competition. Such deliberate packaging of mental skills to ready the mind and body for a successful performance is known as performance routines. Performance routines are a sequence of task-relevant thoughts and actions systematically engaged in prior to performing a specific sport skill [37]. Though most commonly used in closed-sport situations such as golf putting or free throw shooting, routines also have a place in longer repetitive activities such as endurance sport. In this case, routines would be utilized the night before, the day of, or immediately before competition to prime the athlete for a ready state to perform. In addition, athletes may employ routines *after* performance to aid in their mental and physical recovery.

Performance routines can aid in building confidence, composure, and concentration. For instance, with confidence, every night before a race, a triathlete might eat the same dinner, take time visualizing herself feeling strong the entire race, double check her gear bag, and write positive self-talk statements in her journal. Doing this the night before each race builds confidence for a successful race. An athlete who is prone to performance anxiety or is participating in high-stake races might use performance routines to calm his nerves. He may begin race day with a deep breathing exercise prior to leaving for the race venue. He may sit quietly after his swim gear is on and his transition corral is organized. Picturing a calm mind and body throughout the race allows him to maintain composure up until the race begins. Finally, preperformance routines allow athletes to automate their behaviors leading up to race day and start. As such, they are able to focus solely on the race, rather than irrelevant information such as gear, navigating the venue, etc. All the potential stress and mental chatter has been silenced by developing a routine that effectively addresses these areas in an automated manner.

Routines have received substantial support in the empirical literature in a variety of sporting domains [29]. Although routines often occur before or between competitive performances, it is optimal to use them systematically during training so they are learned and easily transferable to competition. Developing appropriate and effective prerace routines may take some time. It is important to use mental skills and routine strategies in a way that fits with the individual. This is not a one size fits all approach. It is necessary to assess what athletes need on race day. What would they like from the routine—confidence, composure, concentration, or all three? What mental skills do the athletes tend to use the most and with the greatest amount of success? Include these skills in the routine. Developing a routine takes time and may require some trial and error. Stay patient and be flexible. Make sure that the components of the routine help enhance performance and not distract from it.

Mindfulness

Mindfulness is experiencing the moment without reacting to the moment [38]. Jon Kabat-Zinn described mindfulness as "the awareness that emerges through paying attention on purpose and nonjudgmentally to the unfolding of experience moment by moment" [39]. It is "affective, compassionate, and nonreactive." Mindfulness is at the heart of Buddha's teachings and has been incorporated in clinical treatments like dialectical behavior therapy [38].

Mindfulness develops an accepting relationship with one's inner experience, instead of trying to control thoughts and feelings like in traditional cognitive-behavioral approaches [40]. Cognitive models attempt to replace negative thoughts with evidence-based thoughts. In contrast, mindful approaches notice the thoughts without reacting to them. For example, athletes might think, "I'm a failure." Cognitive interventions encourage the athlete to challenge that belief with evidence like "I didn't pace the race well but that doesn't mean I'm a failure in all things—I did succeed by managing my nutrition effectively." Mindfulness training encourages responses like "I notice the thought 'I'm a failure'. I'm aware of a tightness in my chest; a feeling of insecurity."

Interest in mindfulness interventions in sport has increased recently [1]. Control isn't all it's cracked up to be, especially when attempts to control backfire. Strategies designed to suppress or replace negative thoughts may paradoxically increase those thoughts [41]. Gardner and Moore argue that traditional mental skills training has reduced negative mental states in some studies but has not translated into consistent improvement in sport performance [40]. Because some athletes struggle to achieve control over their cognitive processes via traditional skills training, acceptance approaches like mindfulness offer promise for the future.

Kabat-Zinn first applied mindfulness to endurance sport performance by studying mindfulness meditation and rowers [42]. More recently, soccer players who trained in mindfulness reported feeling calmer and less reactive to negative emotional states [43]. Thompson et al. found that mindfulness training improved runners' mile times and feelings of relaxation [44]. The mindfulness training was also associated with decreased anxiety and irrelevant thoughts. One unique study explored the usefulness of mindfulness for recovering from burnout in sport [45].

Mindfulness increases awareness of all things, including experiences of confidence and mastery, which may enhance feelings of flow. Peak athletic performance is known as being in the zone or in a state of "flow": the optimal zone where skill meets challenge [46]. Pineau et al. studied mindfulness in rowers and found an association between mindfulness, efficacy, and flow [47]. The authors theorized that mindfulness increased awareness of mastery experiences, thereby increasing feelings of efficacy and flow.

To practice mindfulness skills, endurance athletes might start with observing nonjudgmentally [38]. The *observe* skill involves noticing the present moment without reacting. Athletes may feel stuck in the past when they berate themselves for mistakes or stuck in the future when they worry about the outcome of a race. They can become more anchored in the present by observing with their five senses: "I see the red buoy. I hear the splash of water. I feel coolness on my skin. I notice my breathing is shallow." The *nonjudgmental* skill is noticing facts without evaluating them as good or bad. Athletes who judge themselves with thoughts like "I shouldn't get angry" can practice the nonjudgmental skill by listing five facts about the situation ("I *am* angry," "Everyone feels anger," "Anger is different from aggression," etc.) and/or asking what a supportive person in their life would say (e.g., "It's okay to be angry").

Balanced Exercise

Exercise has countless physical, mental, and emotional benefits, and endurance athletes know these benefits well. But many people do not exercise at all, and most don't get enough exercise [48]. There are fewer who get too *much* exercise [49]. Endurance athletes are more at risk for excessive exercise [50], thereby increasing their risk for developing eating disorders and physical injuries [51]. Finding the balance between too little and too much exercise is important for health [48].

Various terms for excessive exercise include compulsive exercise, obligatory exercise, exercise addiction, exercise dependence, and exercise abuse. To manage psychological distress, exercise joins food restriction, binge eating, substance use, gambling, and other addictive behaviors as a potential means to escape or numb painful emotion. Similar to other compulsive behaviors, excessive exercise provides short-term relief of negative emotional states but often adds to distress in the long run. It can be difficult to detect excessive exercise, particularly in competitive athletes. Think about athletes who run the extra mile or train multiple times a day—others often applaud their unparalleled discipline. For this reason, it may be a challenge to recognize exercise as an addictive, potentially harmful behavior.

How do athletes know if they are overexercising? Powers and Thompson recommend determining if exercise has a negative impact on physical, emotional, or psychological health as well as interfere with daily activities like school, work, or relationships [48]. Exercise is also problematic if it occurs at inappropriate times or settings or continues despite injury. Examples include the compulsion to take a long bike ride in lieu of attending to family needs. The American College of Sports Medicine recommends taking at least one day off exercise per week [52, 53].

The quality of exercise may be more important than the quantity [48]. Qualities to consider include motivation for exercise and level of control over exercise. What motivates athletes to exercise? If the motivation is solely to burn calories, punish themselves, give permission to eat, or compensate for calories eaten, exercise may represent an eating disorder symptom. More balanced motivations include health, training for a sport, stress reduction, fun, and mind-body connection. It's also helpful to gauge the level of control individuals feel over exercise. If exercise feels compulsive or obligatory, the athlete's health may be compromised. For instance, cyclists with uncontrollable urges to go on long bike rides experienced more internal conflict [54] (Table 18.2).

Individuals who are concerned about inadequate or excessive exercise will find *The Exercise Balance* by Pauline Powers and Ron Thompson to be a helpful resource.

Table 18.2 Signs of balanced and unbalanced exercise

Signs of balanced exercise	Signs of unbalanced exercise
Improved physical and mental health	Avoidance of all exercise
Supported by adequate nutrition	Exercising without fueling your body
Increased sensation and awareness of body	Obsession with weight and calories burned
Exercise as one of many coping skills for stress	Exercising to allow yourself to eat
Exercise what you like, not exercise what you dislike	Skipping work, class, or social plans for exercise
Balance of cardiovascular, strength, and flexibility exercise	Not taking a day off (even when sick or injured)
Being able to stop when injured	Exercising to compensate for calories eaten
Including leisure activities like hiking	Judging a day as good or bad depending on how much you exercise

Conclusion

The mind of an endurance athlete is a terrible thing to waste. Hopefully this chapter provides an informative introduction into the mental world of sport and how to make the most of what is between the ears to achieve greater performance. Much like the physical and technical training necessary to for endurance sport success, systematic training of mental skills can be difficult and requires tremendous self-discipline. We encourage you to identify the mental skills that interest you most (perhaps imagery, energy management, goal setting, and/or mindfulness) and practice these skills until they become part of you. Start small and have fun along the way!

References

1. Birrer D, Rothlin P, Morgan G. Mindfulness to enhance athletic performance: theoretical considerations and possible impact mechanisms. Mindfulness. 2012;3:235–46. doi:10.1007/s12671-012-0109-2.
2. McCormick A, Meijen C, Marcora S. Psychological determinants of whole-body endurance performance. SportsMed.2015;45:997–1015.doi:10.1007/s40279-015-0319-6.
3. Thelwell RC, Greenlees IA. Developing competitive endurance performance using mental skills training. Sport Psychol. 2003;17:318–37.
4. Patrick TD, Hrycaiko DW. Effects of a mental training package on an endurance performance. Sport Psychol. 1998;12:283–99.
5. Deci EL, Ryan RM. Overview of self-determination theory: a organismic-dialectical perspective. In: Deci EL, Ryan RM, editors. Handbook of self-determination research theory. Rochester: University of Rochester Press; 2002. p. 3–33.
6. Standage M. Motivation: self-determination theory and performance in sport. In: Murphy SM, editor. The Oxford handbook of sport and performance psychology. New York: Oxford University Press; 2012. p. 233–49.
7. Sebire SJ, Standage M, Vansteenkiste M. Goal content for exercise questionnaire. J Sport Exerc Psychol. 2008;30:353–77.
8. Weinberg RS, Motivation GD. Foundations of sport and exercise psychology. 4th ed. Champaign: Human Kinetics; 2007. p. 51–76.
9. Vealey R. Mental skills training in sport. In: Tenenbaum G, Eklund R, editors. Handbook of sport psychology. 3rd ed. Hoboken: Wiley; 2007. p. 287–309.
10. Gould D. Goal setting for peak performance. In: Williams J, editor. Applied sport psychology: personal growth to peak performance. 5th ed. Boston: Mcgraw Hill; 2006. p. 240–59.
11. Weinberg D, Gould D. Goal Setting. In: Foundations of sport and exercise psychology. 4th ed. Champaign: Human Kinetics; 2007. p. 345–64.
12. Landers DM, Arent SM. Physical activity and mental health. In: Singer R, Hausenblas H, Janelle C, editors. Handbook of sport psychology. 2nd ed. New York: Wiley; 2001. p. 740–65.
13. Yerkes RM, Dodson JD. The relation of strength of stimulus to rapidity of habit formation. J Comp Neurol Psychol. 1908;18:459–82.
14. Hanin YL. An individualized approach to emotion in sport. In: Hanin YL, editor. Emotions in sport. Champaign: Human Kinetics; 2000. p. 65–90.
15. Kerr J. Motivation and emotion in sport: reversal theory. East Sussex: Psychology Press; 1997.
16. McGonigal K. How to make stress your friend. 2013. [Video File] http://www.ted.com/talks/kelly_mcgonigal_how_to_make_stress_your_friend.
17. Pineschi G, Pietro AD. Anxiety management through psychophysiological techniques: relaxation and psyching-up in sport. J Sport Psychol Action. 2013;4:181–90.
18. Wehrenberg M, Prinz SM. The anxious brain. New York: Norton; 2007.
19. Loehr JE. The new toughness training for sports. New York: Dutton; 1995.
20. Cuddy A. Your body language shapes who you are. 2012. [Video File] http://www.ted.com/talks/amy_cuddy_your_body_language_shapes_who_you_are.
21. Balk YA, Adriaanse MA, de Ridder DT, Evers C. Coping under pressure: employing emotion regulation

strategies to enhance performance under pressure. J Sport Exerc Psychol. 2013;35:408–18.

22. Beck A. Cognitive therapy of depression. New York: Guilford Press; 1979.

23. Ellis A, Grieger R. Handbook of rational-emotive therapy. New York: Springer; 1977.

24. Hatzigeorgiadis A, Zourbanos N, Galanis E, Theodorakis Y. Self-talk and sports performance: a meta-analysis. Perspect Psychol Sci. 2011;6(4):348–56. doi:10.1177/1745691611413136.

25. Schüler J, Langens TA. Psychological crisis in a marathon and the buffering effects of self-verbalizations. J Appl Soc Psychol. 2007;37(10):2319–44.

26. Hatzigeorgiadis A, Zourbanos N, Galanis E, Theodorakis Y. Self-talk and competitive sports performance. J Appl Sport Psychol. 2014;26:82–95. doi:10.1080/10413200.2013.790095.

27. Hamilton RA, Scott D, MacDougall MP. Assessing the effectiveness of self-talk interventions on endurance performance. J App Sport Psychol. 2007;19:226–39. doi:10.1080/104132007012 30613.

28. Moran A. Concentration/attention. In: Hanrahan SJ, Andersen MB, editors. Routledge handbook of applied sport psychology. New York: Routledge; 2010. p. 500–9.

29. Weinberg R, Gould D. Concentration. In: Foundations of sport and exercise psychology. 4th ed. Champaign: Human Kinetics; 2007. p. 365–95.

30. Nideffer R, Sagal M. Concentration and attentional control training. In: Applied sport psychology: personal growth to peak performance. 5th ed. New York: McGraw-Hill; 2006. p. 382–403.

31. Brick N, MacIntyre T, Campbell M. Attentional focus in endurance activity: new paradigms and future directions. Int Rev Sport Exerc Psychol. 2014;7(1):106–34. doi:10.1080/1750984X.2014.885554.

32. Moran A. Concentration: Attention and Performance. In: The Oxford handbook of sport and performance psychology. New York: Oxford University Press; 2012. p. 117–30.

33. Weinberg RS, Gould D. Imagery. In: Foundations of sport and exercise psychology. 4th ed. Champaign: Human Kinetics; 2007. p. 295–319.

34. Vealey R, Greenleaf C. Seeing is believing: understanding and using imagery in sport. In: Williams J, editor. Applied sport psychology: personal growth to peak performance. 6th ed. New York: McGraw-Hill Higher Education; 2010. p. 306–48.

35. Williams S, Cumming J. The role of imagery in performance. In: Murphy S, editor. The Oxford handbook of sport and performance psychology. New York: Oxford University Press; 2012. p. 213–32.

36. Holmes PS, Collins DJ. The PETTLEP approach to motor imagery: a functional equivalence model for sport psychologists. J Appl Sport Psychol. 2001; 13:60–83.

37. Moran AP. The psychology of concentration in sport performers: a cognitive analysis. Hove: Psychology Press; 1996.

38. Linehan M. DBT skills training handouts and worksheets. New York: Guilford; 2015. p. 39.

39. Kabat-Zinn J. Mindfulness-based interventions in context: past, present, and future. Clin Psychol Sci Pract. 2003;10:144–56. doi:10.1093/clipsy/bpg016.

40. Gardner FL, Moore ZE. Mindfulness and acceptance models in sport psychology: a decade of basic and applied scientific advancements. Can Psychol. 2012;53(4):309–18. doi:10.1037/a0030220.

41. Beilock SL, Afremow JA, Rabe AL, Carr TH. "Don't miss!" The debilitating effects of suppressive imagery on golf putting performance. J Sport Exerc Psychol. 2001;23(3):200–21.

42. Kabat-Zinn J, Beall B, Rippe J. A systematic mental training program based on mindfulness meditation to optimize performance in collegiate and Olympic rowers. Paper presented at the World Congress in Sport Psychology, Copenhagen. 1985.

43. Baltzell A, Caraballo N, Chipman K, Hayden L. A qualitative study of the mindfulness meditation training for sport: division I female soccer players' experience. J Clin Sport Psychol. 2014;8:221–44. doi:10.1123/jcsp.2014-0030.

44. Thompson RW, Kaufman KA, DePetrillo LA, Glass CR, Arnkoff DB. One year follow-up of mindful sport performance enhancement (MSPE) with archers, golfers, and runners. J Clin Sport Psychol. 2011;5:99–116.

45. Jouper J, Gufstasson H. Mindful recovery: a case study of a burned-out elite shooter. Sport Psychol. 2013;27:92–102.

46. Jackson SA, Csikszentmihalyi M. Flow in sports. Champaign: Human Kinetics; 1999.

47. Pineau TR, Glass CR, Kaufman KA, Bernal DR. Self- and team-efficacy beliefs of rowers and their relation to mindfulness and flow. J Clin Sport Psychol. 2014;8:142–58. doi:10.1123/jcsp.2014-0019.

48. Powers P, Thompson RA. The exercise balance. Carlsbad: Gurze; 2008.

49. Mónok K, Berczik K, Urbán R, Szabo A, Griffiths MD, Farkas J, Magi A, Eisinger A, Tamás K, Kökönyei G, Kun B, Paksi B, Demetrovics Z. Psychometric properties and concurrent validity of two exercise addiction measures: a population wide study. Psychol Sport Exerc. 2012;13:739–46.

50. Thompson RA, Sherman RT. Eating disorders in sport. New York: Taylor & Francis; 2010.

51. Lichtenstein MB, Christiansen E, Elklit A, Bilenberg N, Støving RK. Exercise addiction: a study of eating disorder symptoms, quality of life, personality traits and attachment styles. Psychiatry Res. 2014;215:410–6.

52. American College of Sports Medicine. ACSM position stand: the recommended quantity and quality of exercise

for developing and maintaining cardiorespiratory and muscular fitness, and flexibility in healthy adults. Med Sci Sports Exerc. 1998;30:975–91.

53. Garber CE, Blissmer B, Deschenes MR, Franklin BA, Lamonte MJ, Lee I-M, et al. Quantity and quality of exercise for developing and maintaining cardiorespiratory, musculoskeletal, and neuromotor fitness in apparently healthy adults. Med Sci Sports Exerc. 2011;43(7):1334–59.

54. Stenseng F, Haugen T, Torstveit MK, Høigaard R. When it's "All About the Bike"—intrapersonal conflict in light of passion for cycling and exercise dependence. Sport Exerc Perform Psychol. 2015;4(2):127–39. doi:10.1037/spy0000028.

Optimizing Nutrition for Endurance Training

Jackie Buell

Endurance athletes should know that nutrition affects performance-specific characteristics like fatigue levels [1–4], the immune system [5], muscle breakdown versus maintenance or growth [6–8], and even coordination [9–11]. As endurance athletes become more serious about their desired body changes and performance goals, they often become more intentional about their training diet and seek advice related to their goals.

The fuel for aerobic metabolism (assuming a mixed diet that includes carbohydrate, protein, and fat) depends on the intensity and duration of exercise [12, 13]. Higher-intensity work uses higher carbohydrate (less fat), while lower intensities can rely more heavily on fat as the primary fuel. The longer an endurance event lasts, the less stored carbohydrate (glycogen) in the muscle and the higher the reliance on fat for energy. Environmental factors like extreme heat or stress will also increase the muscle's reliance on carbohydrate as fuel [4, 14, 15]. Reliance on carbohydrate uses the glycolytic pathways, while the utilization of fat trains the lipolytic or ketogenic pathways. In general, there is always some mixture of fat and carbohydrate oxidation occurring simultaneously. "Optimization" for the endurance athlete is finding the mixture of these fuels that allows for best performance while maintaining gastrointestinal comfort and muscle fueling [16]. It is important for endurance athletes to consider how to best train these two metabolic pathways and to use intentional nutrition to achieve desired results.

Important Nutrition Components and Current Recommendations

Approximate *energy balance* is a primary nutritional consideration for endurance athletes. It is difficult to improve performance when there is not enough energy in the diet, or at least the energy needs to be adequate to promote optimal changes desired from the training program. Athletes desiring to lose body fat likely need to adopt a slight energy deficit to achieve the goal, but not such a large deficit to induce metabolic consequences [17–19]. The other common goal of gaining lean mass or strength must be accompanied by a training diet high enough in calories and protein to promote muscle protein synthesis. Calorie balance is important to achieving the desired goals and should be intentional in endurance athletes.

Calorie balance can also be considered from an energy availability perspective [18]. From work relative to the female athlete triad paradigm, we understand that low energy availability contributes to decreased reproductive hormone status (and amenorrhea) as well as potential decreases in bone mass [20]. The triad has

J. Buell (✉)
Department of Medical Dietetics, Ohio State University, 306 K Atwell Hall, 453 West 10th Ave, Columbus, OH 43210, USA
e-mail: buell.7@osu.edu

© Springer International Publishing Switzerland 2016
T.L. Miller (ed.), *Endurance Sports Medicine*, DOI 10.1007/978-3-319-32982-6_19

recently been expanded to include (damage to) many other metabolic characteristics including immunological, gastrointestinal, cardiovascular, psychological, developmental, hematological, endocrine, and metabolic changes [19]. While this under-fueling and its ramifications have long been largely considered female issues, current literature is beginning to recognize the same poor fueling sequelae in male endurance athletes [21–24]. Eating enough to support training as well as the underlying basal metabolism is important to long-term health as well as short-term performance benefits.

Energy availability is a specific calculation to ensure fueling is adequate to support the underlying metabolism in addition to exercise [25].

$$EA = \frac{\left(\text{calorie in} - \text{calories spent in exercise}\right)}{\text{kg fat free mass}}$$

Optimal energy availability is considered to be an energy intake greater than 45 kcals/kg fat-free mass to allow for normal menstrual function [25], growth or gain of body mass, and normal body and brain function. Alternatively, intakes below 30 kcals/kg fat-free mass have been demonstrated to change menstrual function or have health implications, and this should be seen as an inadequate fueling plan for endurance athletes [26]. Training diets with 30–45 kcals/kg fat-free mass are minimal, but should allow for healthy weight loss or changes in body composition. It should be noted that the individual athlete's response to restriction level must be considered, as the threshold values are the result of research where group data were considered and may not be accurate for poor training responses for individuals. The bottom line for energy balance for the endurance athlete is that training volume must be included in decisions about how much energy to consume in the intentional training diet.

The Macro Mixture

Once the calorie level of a training diet is determined to help fuel the athlete, consideration is given to the macronutrient profile of the diet:

Table 19.1 Current position statement macronutrient recommendations

Macronutrient	ACSM/AND [29] statement	IOC statement [30]
Carbohydrate	6–10 g/kg/day	6–10 g/kg/day
Fat	20–35 % intake	
Protein	1.2–1.7 g/kg/day	1.2–1.6 g/kg/day

How much carbohydrate, fat, and protein does the endurance athlete need? Carbohydrates and fats are considered the primary fuels for endurance exercise [27]. There is some evidence that endurance athletes can use slightly more protein as an energy source compared with other athletes [28], but the protein recommendations are not typically considered from a fueling perspective. The current evidence-based guidelines for fueling an endurance athlete include a diet high in carbohydrate and moderate in fat and protein [29, 30]. There are two current position statements for athlete nutrition summarized in Table 19.1.

The traditional training diet follows these professional recommendations and focuses on carbohydrate as the primary fuel, which results in a well-trained glycolytic system that allows the athlete to teach the muscle to store muscle glycogen for use during endurance events [31, 32]. As muscle glycogen decreases with high intensity and/or longer duration, the muscle becomes more dependent on lipid oxidation and can presumably continue exercise at a lower intensity [33]. Consideration should be given to training both systems adequately within the periodization of an endurance program. In general, this is a personalized program and is not likely easy to determine from any cookie cutter recommendation.

Working with the spectrum of endurance athletes from the elite Olympic hopeful to the weekend marathon warrior requires consideration of the athlete's physique and performance goals and then personalization of the eating plan. The body's use of the energy systems to fuel exercise is the direct result of the energy sources (carbohydrate or fat) provided to the system [33]. If you want to train your system to be the highest in intensity, it must rely on carbohydrate thus provided with carbohydrate for fuel. If you do not care about intensity of exercise and wish to maximize your use of fat as fuel, it may require a distinctly different diet.

An evolving paradigm in endurance nutrition is the *keto-adapting* diet where the athlete forces the body to rely on fat for fuel by depriving the muscle of carbohydrate. Intuitively, this means undertraining the glycolytic pathways therefore a loss of "high gear" [34]. But if the athlete is not concerned about high gear or high intensity, this "keto" method of fueling likely taps into the body fat stores much more than the mixed or high-carbohydrate diet. Some athletes will want to try periods of keto-adapting to see if specific training of the fat-burning pathways improves how long they can run. Many carb-trained athletes rely on a high-carbohydrate intake during exercise, which causes a fair amount of gastrointestinal distress. Thus, the keto-fueling plan can also improve gastrointestinal comfort during running. Some ultra-endurance athletes are well-known "keto" athletes [35, 36] and maintain various (carbohydrate) habits around their training and race days. This method of fueling is largely understudied in athletes, and a few well-respected laboratories for elite athletes denigrate the method due to the loss of high gear [34, 37]. When working with adult endurance athletes who are as concerned about losing body fat as they are performing, this style of fueling may be able to help reach the desired outcomes. Unfortunately, most of the "evidence" is anecdotal at this point and does not seem well accepted in the dietetics community. This is an area where additional funding and research activities are needed. It is possible that the current sports nutrition literature is biased toward a carbohydrate-trained muscle, and more studies on true keto-adapting will help practitioners and athletes understand the potential differences in the fueling styles.

In addition to the overall strategy for macronutrient composition of the diet, there are fueling strategies to understand about each macronutrient. It might be best to categorize the carbohydrate as the jet fuel in the muscle, the protein as the building blocks for repair and growth, and the fat as the long-distance fuel that is needed for good hormonal health.

Since *carbohydrates* are utilized for the higher-intensity exercises, it is the focus of most training diets [30, 38, 39]. For health implications, complex carbohydrates are preferred over simple carbohydrates for the advantages of higher fiber and more nutrients (less processed, more nutrient dense). However, fueling around exercise might benefit from some of the metabolic handling characteristics of simple carbohydrates [40, 41]. Simple carbohydrates (when taken alone) will empty from the stomach more quickly, be absorbed by the intestine and into the blood system more quickly (higher glycemic index), will stimulate a higher insulin response (anabolic to muscle), and can support blood glucose more quickly than complex carbohydrates. Therefore the use of simple carbohydrates around exercise may help some endurance athletes. It has also been shown that using a mixture of simple carbohydrates can enhance absorption thus provide more rapid support to the working muscle [4, 40]. However, high simple carbohydrate loads cause gastric distress (bloating, gas, diarrhea) for some athletes [42]. These athletes might experiment with more complex carbohydrates to see if they tolerate the higher molecular weight.

The timing of carbohydrate intake around exercise is pretty standardized [30, 38, 39]. Carbohydrate or glycogen loading (consuming high-carbohydrate diet) for a few days prior to a big event is a popular fueling strategy for many athletes. In addition, if the athlete wishes to top off the glycogen stores in the muscle prior to exercise, a small carbohydrate-rich snack or drink may help accomplish the extra muscle fuel. It is important to remember that fluids or foods high in calories in the stomach will slow gastric emptying [43], so the preperformance snack should be intentional and commensurate with the athlete goals and timing before the event. If the athlete wishes the pre-event snack to enter the system more slowly, consuming a small amount of fat or more complex carbohydrates may help achieve this goal. An athlete who has fueled poorly over the course of the day who just wants to get some additional fuel to the muscle would be smart to rely solely on carbohydrate prior to exercise as it should reach the muscle sooner. Some athletes fear that consuming high carbohydrate just prior to endurance exercise will make them bonk (become hypoglycemic). There are athletes who would rebound to hypoglycemia, but insulin and epinephrine are part of a redundant hormonal system, and epinephrine should override the influence of insulin. Of course, if an athlete knows simple carbohydrate prior to exercise causes them as an individual to become hypoglycemic, they should certainly adopt another strategy. In general, 30–60 g of carbohydrate within the hour of endurance exercise is promoted to top off the glycogen stores [30, 38].

Carbohydrate consumption during exercise depends on numerous factors: overall fueling prior to exercise, duration and intensity of exercise, and individual tolerance and level of training. In general, the current recommendation is for athletes exercising longer than 60–90 min to consume small quantities of carbohydrate during endurance exercise to facilitate maintaining a high intensity. While most novice and average competitors can use 30–60 g of exogenous carbohydrate per hour, elite athletes may be able to assimilate as much as 90 g of carbohydrate per hour [44].

After exercise, there is a window of recovery where the muscle will replace glycogen at a faster pace [45]. There is also evidence that immediate protein consumption can promote muscle repair and synthesis [6, 8]. Given these two pieces of information, it is no surprise that current recovery snack practices ask the athlete to consume good carbohydrate with a small amount of good quality protein to promote muscle recovery [30, 38]. Additionally, carbohydrate intake is shown to help immune function and potentially avoid overtraining [5, 46]. Current generic guidelines would have an endurance athlete consume 40–60 g of carbohydrate along with ~20 g of good quality protein immediately after exercise to promote muscle recovery [38]. Athletes might consider that they exercise to get desired changes in the muscle, and the recovery snack is a priority to facilitate those changes.

Fat is important to the overall training diet as well as good health. Low-fat diets do not help fuel the muscle or endurance exercise. The intramuscular triglyceride (IMTG) stores are an important source of fueling for endurance exercise [33], so the endurance athlete needs to ensure a variety of fats within energy balance for the training diet. Of course, a keto-adapting athlete would rely on fats as the primary fuel within a carb-restricted diet.

A commonly asked dietary fat question is the consumption of omega-3 fatty acids to help control inflammation and promote cardiovascular or brain health [47–50]. Omega-3 fatty acids are found naturally in foods like fatty fish (salmon, mackerel), walnuts, flax, and chia seeds or their oils. The current dietary recommendation for all of us is to eat fatty fish such as salmon two times per week. Instead, many Americans choose to take fish oil capsules as a dietary supplement. Like all dietary supplements, the consumer should look for a brand that is third party verified, but the evidence to fully support this supplement for athletes is still equivocal.

Protein is not typically considered fuel for exercise, but nitrogen excretion studies on male runners demonstrate a small amount of protein can be used for fuel. The current trend in sports nutrition is to move the paradigm for protein intake from adequate to optimal. Therefore, endurance athletes are recommended to consume higher protein than nonathletic counterparts. The essential amino acids [8, 51], and leucine in particular [52], have been shown to stimulate muscle protein synthesis after exercise, so the use of good quality proteins in the recovery snack has become standard advice. Additionally, some counselors like their athletes to have a little leucine late in the evening to support the muscle in the overnight repair process.

The macronutrient comparison of a traditional endurance athlete diet with a keto-adapted athlete diet is provided for an example day in Table 19.2. The arbitrary choice to demonstrate this with about 2400 kcals would make this a reasonable example for a female endurance athlete running about 5–8 miles per day.

Table 19.2 Traditional and keto-adapted nutritional plans for endurance training

~2400 kcals each	Traditional	Keto-adapted
Pre-run	½ banana, one slice toast with jelly, and water	Water
Breakfast	One cup oatmeal with two TBSP raisins and one cup skim milk, one egg scrambled with 1 oz cheese	Two eggs scrambled with 1 oz cheese and 2 oz ham, with spinach, onions, mushrooms, olives sautéed in three tsp olive oil, water
Snack	One mozzarella cheese stick and small apple, with 1 oz pretzels	Celery with two TBSP peanut butter
Lunch	Turkey sandwich with three ounces meat on two slices whole grain bread with lettuce, tomato, and ¼ medium avocado with 8 oz skim milk to drink	One cup lettuce and greens with 4 oz grilled chicken, 1 oz feta cheese, half medium avocado with two TBSP regular salad dressing, and water to drink
Snack	¼ cup cottage cheese with ½ cup peaches, ½ cup carrots with one TBSP ranch dip, and water	Two Colby-Jack cheese sticks with ½ cup cut up cauliflower with two TBSP dip
Dinner	1.5 cup pasta with ½ cup tomato-based sauce with 3 oz meatballs, one cup dinner salad with one TBSP dressing, water	5 oz salmon steamed in one TBSP oil with garlic salt, 1.5 cups stir-fried vegetables with two TBSP almond slivers, water
Snack	One Greek yogurt with ½ cup granola	One cup almond milk as base for smoothie with 15–20 g protein, spinach greens, and two TBSP flax
Approximate nutrition	285 g carb, 130 g pro, 80 g fat	50 g carb, 150 g pro, 175 g fat

Both plans are high in protein. On the traditional plan, athletes may decrease some protein intake in exchange for more carbohydrate

Hydration

Hydration is often considered during and after exercise, but many athletes fail to think about hydrating throughout the day. Of course fluids are important to hydration, but so are the electrolyte nutrients like sodium, potassium, and chloride. While there are position statements favoring a scheduled drinking plan prior to, during, and after exercise [53], there is also a current push to simply drink when thirsty [54]. This is a catch 22 because the thirst mechanism lags behind the physiology: the feedback loop to the thirst center depends on dehydration to stimulate thirst. The "drink as thirsty" advocates are responding to case studies and prevention of hyponatremia. When endurance athletes lose a lot of sweat, they are losing water and salt. When they are replacing sweat with plain water (low in sodium), they are actually further diluting the serum sodium concentrations and this can cause symptoms of hyponatremia. It stands to reason that a good hydration plan should address the replacement of electrolytes along with enough fluids to stay hydrated.

It is best for endurance athletes to have a plan for fluids that includes electrolytes and carbohydrates during endurance competitions [30, 38, 55]. Of course, they should practice the race routine a number of times in long runs to be sure it will help, not hinder, the race. For heavy-salt-loss athletes, this includes an adequate amount of salt. Many endurance athletes use very high-sodium commercial products to this end. Overhydration or hyponatremia can result in the same race failure as dehydration.

Common Micronutrient Issues

The vitamins and minerals make up the micronutrients athletes need for good health and performance. Endurance athletes sometimes supplement blindly with the belief that extra nutrients can magically improve performance. The habitual diet is an important consideration when athletes are choosing dietary supplements.

Iron-deficiency anemia can be limiting to the endurance athlete's performance [56]. Once an athlete becomes anemic, it is hard to correct the anemia in a short period of time [57, 58]. It is best to avoid the anemia by having the ferritin, iron-binding capacity, and hemoglobin values in blood checked periodically. The detrimental effect of low hemoglobin is self-explanatory as it carries oxygen to the tissues. Ferritin has become the pre-anemia or iron-insufficiency marker of interest as some research has demonstrated that correcting a low ferritin can also improve performance [59]. The advances in the science behind athlete's iron status propose low-iron intake and absorption to influence muscle structure, function, and repair in ways that are likely to increase regular testing as practitioners catch up with the science [60].

Females are more susceptible than males to iron insufficiency due to heavy menstrual cycles, poor diet quality, and/or caloric restriction [61]. Meats are the best (most absorbable) dietary iron sources due to the heme iron. We can get iron from beans and green leafy vegetables, but it is best to educate the athlete that we absorb a smaller fraction of the iron from plant foods (nonheme iron). While the practice of blindly supplementing iron can be dangerous to athletes with a predisposition to hemochromatosis, it may be necessary to supplement athletes with low fer-ritin values. Iron supplements are notorious for causing GI issues like constipation or upset stom-ach, so low-level supplementation may be more comfortable than high-dose therapies. Athletes with absorptive issues such as Crohn's disease may benefit from intravenous infusions for better health as this is typically more than a perfor-mance issue for those athletes.

Calcium is another nutrient of concern, espe-cially for female athletes with a low body mass [58]. Body mass is strongly tied to bone mass in endurance athletes, so consuming enough cal-cium to permit good bone health deserves atten-tion. Athletes with multiple stress fractures, high mileage, and amenorrhea may benefit from know-ing their bone mass to encourage better overall diet consumption and potentially different exer-cise habits. Other nutrients known to affect bone mass include vitamins A, D, and K, magnesium, and phosphorus. Balancing a varied diet with exercise volume is important to skeletal health.

Many athletes have adopted the practice of having serum *vitamin D* measured periodically.

Vitamin D receptors are found in many tissues throughout the body including muscle and bone [62]. While it is common knowledge that vitamin D influences bone health, it is less known that vitamin D has important roles in muscle function and a plethora of other systems [63]. Another research suggests the immune system may also benefit from optimal vitamin D status [64]; thus blind supplementation of this nutrient is also common. Caution is warranted for high doses of vitamin D as it can be toxic if too high. The occa-sional checkup for serum vitamin D status may be important for performance for endurance athletes.

Most athletes understand that excessive oxida-tion or free radicals are not good and are a source of inflammation and cellular and DNA damage. Endurance athletes may realize they are promoting more oxidative damage and desire to counter it with *antioxidant nutrients* such as vitamins C and E, beta-carotene, lutein, or coenzyme Q. Interestingly, two studies of endurance athletes have suggested that athletes who consume antioxi-dants in dietary supplements actually have higher markers of oxidative damage after long-endurance feats than competitors who do not use the antioxi-dant supplements [65, 66]. This supports the theory that our body responds to reactive oxygen species with native antioxidant systems and that taking antioxidant supplements may dampen the native response [67]. There is great nutritional value to consuming a wide variety of vegetables and fruits instead of trying to consume them in pills.

There are a number of *ergogenic substances* that *may* improve endurance performance. Caffeine, nitrates, and beta alanine are examples of commonly used supplements in the current endurance culture. Some athletes would choose to consume foods containing these supplements, while others would choose to use an intentional dietary supplement. The quality of dietary sup-plements is poorly regulated, and it is wise for athletes to choose third-party verified products to ensure purity and potency [68].

Caffeine has been proven ergogenic in both cycling and running [69]. The American College of Sports Medicine (ACSM) provides a consumer-friendly "Current Comment" which addresses the dose of caffeine that is considered safe, legal, and efficacious for endurance exercise at 3–9 mg/kg [70]. While it is suggested that caffeine spares glycogen early in exercise, the exact mechanism is still under debate. Most athletes will choose to consume 5–6 mg/kg one hour before the performance activity to avoid gastrointestinal side effects yet target improved performance.

Nitrates have become a popular supplement for endurance athletes and are often consumed as beetroot juice. Current studies support an increase in skeletal muscle efficiency by decreasing the oxygen need at a given submaximal intensity for some athletes [71]. An interesting step in metabolism for this supplement is that it relies on the nitrate cycling through the system to the mouth where bacteria in the oral cavity will reduce the nitrate (NO_3^-) to nitrite (NO_2^-) as a mandatory conversion step; thus chewing gum and antibacterial mouthwashes are avoided for maximal conversion. Most reviews agree that more research is needed to identify the exercise intensity, duration, mode, and environments where nitrates are most ergogenic. There are still many research questions to be answered around this ergogenic, but high-level sport organizations are embracing the research [30].

Beta alanine is a precursor to muscle carnosine and may help buffer the acidity associated with high-intensity intervals or sprint performance in some endurance athletes [72]. The International Society for Sports Nutrition (ISSN) has published a position statement to outline the current dosing guidelines and applications [73]. This particular supplement appears to be safe, but does include an unusual side effect of paresthesias or tingling in the extremities for some individuals. The use of this supplement in combination with others (such as caffeine and/or creatine) appears to be the current trend [74–76].

Summary

There are numerous acceptable training diets to help endurance athletes achieve their desired performance and physique goals. The traditional training diet includes a high-carbohydrate routine to fuel the muscle with plenty of glycogen. The keto-adapted diet is not commonplace, but does seem to offer a reasonable fueling alternative for some endurance athletes. Some athletes choose to rely on dietary supplements for at-risk nutrients as well as a few ergogenic supplements. The bottom line is that endurance athletes need to approach the training diet with their personal needs and goals in mind.

References

1. Jacobs K, Sherman W. The efficacy of carbohydrate supplementation and chronic high carbohydrate diets for improving endurance performance. Int J Sport Nutr. 1999;9:92–115.
2. Sherman W, Brodowicz G, Wright D, Allen W, Simonsen J, Dernbach A. Effects of 4 hour pre-exercise carbohydrate feedings on cycling performance. Med Sci Sports Exerc. 1989;12:598–604.
3. Sherman W, Peden M, Wright D. Carbohydrate feedings 1 hour before exercise improves cycling performance. Am J Clin Nutr. 1991;54:866–70.
4. Jentjens RLPG, Underwood K, Achten J, Currell K, Mann CH, Jeukendrup AE. Exogenous carbohydrate oxidation rates are elevated after combined ingestion of glucose and fructose during exercise in the heat. J Appl Physiol. 2006;100(3):807–16.
5. Nieman DC. Immunonutrition support for athletes. Nutr Rev. 2008;66(6):310–20.
6. Bolster DR, Pikosky MA, Gaine PC, et al. Dietary protein intake impacts human skeletal muscle protein fractional synthetic rates after endurance exercise. Am J Physiol Endocrinol Metab. 2005;289(4): E678–83.
7. Maughan RJ. Nutritional status, metabolic responses to exercise and implications for performance. Biochem Soc Trans. 2003;31(Pt 6):1267–9.
8. Borsheim E, Tipton KD, Wolf SE, Wolfe RR. Essential amino acids and muscle protein recovery from resistance exercise. Am J Physiol Endocrinol Metab. 2002;283(4):E648–57.
9. Dougherty KA, Baker LB, Chow M, Kenney WL. Two percent dehydration impairs and six percent carbohydrate drink improves boys basketball skills. Med Sci Sports Exerc. 2006;38(9):1650–8.
10. Baker LB, Dougherty KA, Chow M, Kenney WL. Progressive dehydration causes a progressive decline in basketball skill performance. Med Sci Sports Exerc. 2007;39(7):1114–23.
11. Winnick JJ, Davis JM, Welsh RS, Carmichael MD, Murphy EA, Blackmon JA. Carbohydrate feedings during team sport exercise preserve physical and CNS function. Med Sci Sports Exerc. 2005; 37(2):306–15.
12. Romijn JA, Coyle EF, Sidossis LS, et al. Regulation of endogenous fat and carbohydrate metabolism in

relation to exercise intensity and duration. Am J Physiol. 1993;265(3):E380–91.

13. Brooks GA, Mercier J. Balance of carbohydrate and lipid utilization during exercise: the "crossover" concept. J Appl Physiol. 1994;76(6):2253–61.

14. Lim CL, Byrne C, Chew SA, Mackinnon LT. Leukocyte subset responses during exercise under heat stress with carbohydrate or water intake. Aviat Space Environ Med. 2005;76(8):726–32.

15. Morris JG, Nevill ME, Thompson D, Collie J, Williams C. The influence of a 6.5% carbohydrate-electrolyte solution on performance of prolonged intermittent high-intensity running at 30 degrees C. J Sports Sci. 2003;21(5):371–81.

16. Schröder S, Fischer A, Vock C, et al. Nutrition concepts for elite distance runners based on macronutrient and energy expenditure. J Athl Train. 2008;43(5):489–504.

17. De Souza MJ, Miller BE, Loucks AB, et al. High frequency of luteal phase deficiency and anovulation in recreational women runners: blunted elevation in follicle-stimulating hormone observed during luteal-follicular transition. J Clin Endocrinol Metab. 1998;83(12):4220–32.

18. Loucks AB, Kiens B, Wright HH. Energy availability in athletes. J Sports Sci. 2011;29 Suppl 1:S7–15.

19. Mountjoy M, Sundgot-Borgen J, Burke L, et al. The IOC consensus statement: beyond the female athlete triad-relative energy deficiency in sport (RED-S). Br J Sports Med. 2014;48(7):491–7.

20. Nattiv A, Loucks AB, Manore MM, et al. American College of Sports Medicine position stand. The female athlete triad. Med Sci Sports Exerc. 2007; 39(10):1867–82.

21. Hind K, Truscott JG, Evans JA. Low lumbar spine bone mineral density in both male and female endurance runners. Bone. 2006;39(4):880–5.

22. Hackney AC. Effects of endurance exercise on the reproductive system of men: the "exercise-hypogonadal male condition". J Endocrinol Invest. 2008;31(10):932–8.

23. Hetland ML, Haarbo J, Christiansen C. Low bone mass and high bone turnover in male long distance runners. J Clin Endocrinol Metab. 1993;77(3):770–5.

24. Stewart AD, Hannan J. Total and regional bone density in male runners, cyclists, and controls. Med Sci Sports Exerc. 2000;32(8):1373–7.

25. Loucks AB. Energy availability, not body fatness, regulates reproductive function in women. Exerc Sport Sci Rev. 2003;31(3):144.

26. Loucks AB, DiPietro L, Stachenfeld NS. The female athlete triad: do female athletes need to take special care to avoid low energy availability? Med Sci Sports Exerc. 2006;38(10):1694–700.

27. Holloway GP, Spriet LL. The metabolic systems: interaction of lipid and carbohydrate metabolism. In: Farrell P, Joyner M, Caiozzo V, editors. Advanced exercise physiology. 2nd ed. Philadelphia: Lippincott, Williams and Wilkins; 2012. p. 408–22.

28. Tipton KD. Protein requirements and recommendations for athletes: relevance of ivory tower arguments for practical recommendations. Clin Sports Med. 2007;26(1):17–36.

29. Rodriguez NR, Di Marco NM, Langley S. American College of Sports Medicine position stand. Nutrition and athletic performance. Med Sci Sports Exerc. 2009;41(3):709–31.

30. Proceedings of the IOC Consensus Conference on Nutrition in Sport, 25-27 October 2010, Lausanne, Switzerland. J Sports Sci. 2011;29:S:1–36.

31. Hawley JA, Burke LM, Phillips SM, Spriet LL. Nutritional modulation of training-induced skeletal muscle adaptations. J Appl Physiol. 2011;110(3): 834–45.

32. Cox GR, Clark SA, Cox AJ, et al. Daily training with high carbohydrate availability increases exogenous carbohydrate oxidation during endurance cycling. J Appl Physiol. 2010;109(1):126–34.

33. Spriet LL. New insights into the interaction of carbohydrate and fat metabolism during exercise. Sports Med. 2014;44 Suppl 1:S87–96.

34. Stellingwerff T, Spriet LL, Watt MJ, et al. Decreased PDH activation and glycogenolysis during exercise following fat adaptation with carbohydrate restoration. Am J Physiol Endocrinol Metab. 2006;290(2):380–8.

35. Timothy Allen Olson—mindful mountain ultra runner. http://www.timothyallenolson.com. Accessed Nov 20, 2015.

36. Zach bitter—ultra runner and coach. http://zachbitter.com/index.php. Accessed Nov 20, 2015.

37. Hawley JA, Gibala MJ, Bermon S. Innovations in athletic preparation: role of substrate availability to modify training adaptation and performance. J Sports Sci. 2007;25:S115–24.

38. Position of the American Dietetic Association. Dietitians of Canada, and the American College of Sports Medicine: nutrition and athletic performance. J Am Diet Assoc. 2009;109(3):509–27.

39. Berning J, Manore MM, Meyer NL. Nutrition and athletic performance before, during and after exercise: adapting the joint position statement into practical guidelines. Commissioned by Gatorade Sports Science Institute. 2010.

40. Currell K, Jeukendrup AE. Superior endurance performance with ingestion of multiple transportable carbohydrates. Med Sci Sports Exerc. 2008;40(2): 275–81.

41. Jeukendrup AE. Carbohydrate intake during exercise and performance. Nutrition. 2004;20(7–8):669–77.

42. de Oliveira EP, Burini RC, Jeukendrup A. Gastrointestinal complaints during exercise: prevalence, etiology, and nutritional recommendations. Sports Med. 2014;44 Suppl 1:79–85.

43. Leiper JB. Fate of ingested fluids: Factors affecting gastric emptying and intestinal absorption of beverages in humans. Nutr Rev. 2015;73 Suppl 2:57–72.

44. Jeukendrup A. The new carbohydrate intake recommendations. Nestle Nutr Inst Workshop Ser. 2013;75:63–71.

45. Adamo KB, Tarnopolsky MA, Graham TE. Dietary carbohydrate and postexercise synthesis of proglycogen and macroglycogen in human skeletal muscle. Am J Physiol. 1998;275(2 Pt 1):E229–34.

46. Nieman DC, Henson DA, Gojanovich G, et al. Influence of carbohydrate on immune function following 2 h cycling. Res Sports Med. 2006;14(3): 225–37.
47. Bryhn M. Prevention of sports injuries by marine omega-3 fatty acids. J Am Coll Nutr. 2015;34:60–1.
48. Jouris KB, McDaniel JL, Weiss EP. The effect of omega-3 fatty acid supplementation on the inflammatory response to eccentric strength exercise. J Sports Sci Med. 2011;10(3):432–8.
49. Mickleborough TD. Omega-3 polyunsaturated fatty acids in physical performance optimization. Int J Sport Nutr Exerc Metab. 2013;23(1):83–96.
50. Mori TA, Beilin LJ. Omega-3 fatty acids and inflammation. Curr Atheroscler Rep. 2004;6(6):461–7.
51. Tipton KD, Elliott TA, Cree MG, Aarsland AA, Sanford AP, Wolfe RR. Stimulation of net muscle protein synthesis by whey protein ingestion before and after exercise. Am J Physiol Endocrinol Metab. 2007;292(1):E71–6.
52. Nelson AR, Phillips SM, Faulkner JA, et al. Protein-leucine fed dose effects on muscle protein synthesis after endurance exercise. Med Sci Sports Exerc. 2015;47(3):547–55.
53. Sawka MN, Burke LM, Eichner ER, Maughan RJ, Montain SJ, Stachenfeld HS. Exercise and fluid replacement. Med Sci Sports Exerc. 2007;39(2): 377–390.
54. Hew-Butler T, Rosner MH, Fowkes-Godek S, et al. Statement of the 3rd international exercise-associated hyponatremia consensus development conference, Carlsbad, California, 2015. Br J Sports Med. 2015;49(22):1432–46.
55. Jeukendrup AE. Nutrition for endurance sports: marathon, triathlon, and road cycling. J Sports Sci. 2011;29:S91–9.
56. DellaValle DM, Haas JD. Iron status is associated with endurance performance and training in female rowers. Med Sci Sports Exerc. 2012;44(8):1552–9.
57. Clark SF. Iron deficiency anemia: diagnosis and management. Curr Opin Gastroenterol. 2009;25(2):122–8.
58. McClung JP, Gaffney-Stomberg E, Lee JJ. Female athletes: a population at risk of vitamin and mineral deficiencies affecting health and performance. J Trace Elem Med Biol. 2014;28(4):388–92.
59. Hinton PS, Sinclair LM. Iron supplementation maintains ventilatory threshold and improves energetic efficiency in iron-deficient nonanemic athletes. Eur J Clin Nutr. 2007;61(1):30–9.
60. Buratti P, Gammella E, Rybinska I, Cairo G, Recalcati S. Recent advances in iron metabolism: relevance for health, exercise, and performance. Med Sci Sports Exerc. 2015;47(8):1596–604.
61. Hinton PS, Sanford TC, Davidson MM, Yakushko OF, Beck NC, Hinton PS. Nutrient intakes and dietary behaviors of male and female collegiate athletes. Int J Sport Nutr Exerc Metab. 2004;14(4):389–405.
62. Hollis BW, Sorenson MB, Taft TN, Anderson JJB, Cannell JJ. Athletic performance and vitamin D. Med Sci Sports Exerc. 2009;41(5):1102–10.
63. Todd JJ, Pourshahidi LK, McSorley EM, Madigan SM, Magee PJ. Vitamin D: recent advances and implications for athletes. Sports Med. 2015;45(2): 213–29.
64. Calton EK, Keane KN, Newsholme P, Soares MJ. The impact of vitamin D levels on inflammatory status: a systematic review of immune cell studies. PLoS One. 2015;10(11), e0141770.
65. Knez, Wade L., Jenkins, David G., Coombes, Jeff S. Oxidative stress in half and full Ironman triathletes. Med Sci Sports Exerc. 2007;39(2):283–8.
66. Nieman DC, Henson, Dru A., Mcanulty, Steven R., Mcanulty, Lisa S., Morrow, Jason D., Ahmed, Alaa, Heward, Chris B. Vitamin E and immunity after the Kona Triathlon world championship. Med Sci Sports Exerc. 2004;36(8):1328–35.
67. Slattery K, Bentley D, Coutts AJ. The role of oxidative, inflammatory and neuroendocrinological systems during exercise stress in athletes: Implications of antioxidant supplementation on physiological adaptation during intensified physical training. Sports Med. 2015;45(4):453–71.
68. Buell JL, Franks R, Ransone J, Powers ME, Laquale KM, Carlson-Phillips A, National Athletic Trainers' Association. National Athletic Trainers' Association position statement: evaluation of dietary supplements for performance nutrition. J Athl Train. 2013;48(1): 124–36.
69. Spriet LL. Exercise and sport performance with low doses of caffeine. Sports Med. 2014;44(2):175–84.
70. Spriet LL, Graham TE. Caffeine and exercise performance. ACSM current comment http://www.acsm. org/docs/current-comments/caffeineandexercise.pdf. Accessed Nov 20, 2015.
71. Jones AM. Dietary nitrate supplementation and exercise performance. Sports Med. 2014;44:35–45.
72. Hobson RM, Saunders B, Ball G, Harris RC, Sale C. Effects of beta-alanine supplementation on exercise performance: a meta-analysis. Amino Acids. 2011; 43(1):25–37.
73. Trexler ET, Smith-Ryan A, Stout JR, et al. International society of sports nutrition position stand: beta-alanine. J Int Soc Sport Nutr. 2015;12:30.
74. Kendall KL, Moon JR, Fairman CM, et al. Ingesting a preworkout supplement containing caffeine, creatine, β-alanine, amino acids, and B vitamins for 28 days is both safe and efficacious in recreationally active men. Nutr Res. 2014;34(5):442–9.
75. McCormack WP, Stout JR, Emerson NS, et al. Oral nutritional supplement fortified with beta-alanine improves physical working capacity in older adults: a randomized, placebo-controlled study. Exp Gerontol. 2013;48(9):933–9.
76. Spradley BD, Crowley KR, Tai CY, et al. Ingesting a pre-workout supplement containing caffeine, B-vitamins, amino acids, creatine, and beta-alanine before exercise delays fatigue while improving reaction time and muscular endurance. Nutr Metab. 2012;9:28.

Darrin Bright and Ben Bring

Overview

Individual participation in mass sporting events, including full and half marathons, cycling races, and triathlons, is steadily gaining popularity in the United States. According to Running USA's annual Marathon Report, there were a record number of 541,000 finishers and more than 1100 marathon races across the country in 2013 [1]. The USA Triathlon set a record for annual membership in 2013 with an increase of 5.5 % from 2012 in both youth and adult categories [2]. Likewise, the USA Cycling has seen an increase in membership and license holder numbers over the past several years according to a membership analysis done in 2013 [3].

With the growth in size and number of competitions, well-organized medical coverage is essential. The major aspects of endurance medicine include professional medical staff, appropriate equipment and supplies, precise weather evaluation, effective communication systems, and a comprehensive security plan to ensure the health and safety of the participants, volunteers, and spectators. Each of these components can be organized by progressive phases: data collection and planning, event-day implementation, and follow-up and evaluation [4].

Anticipated Encounters

During the planning phase of a mass-participation event, gathering demographic data on all participants is imperative. Athletes should provide information regarding their medical history, as well as emergency contacts. This data can be obtained through a questionnaire on the back of participants' bibs or electronically prior to the event. The advantages and disadvantages to both formats must be assessed to determine the best method for a particular event. Some event planners may find it necessary for athletes to complete a Physical Activity Readiness Questionnaire (PAR-Q) to identify potential health risks that need to be evaluated by a physician prior to participation [5]. Knowledge of preexisting medical conditions of all participants can help prevent or treat an illness or injury as well as improve efficiency of care in medical tents. All patient's health information and medical encounters should be protected in compliance with HIPPA.

The medical staff should be prepared for a variety of medical issues at any mass-participation athletic event, including but not limited to exercise-associated collapse, musculoskeletal

D. Bright (✉)
Department of Family Medicine/Sports Medicine, OhioHealth, 3705 Olentangy River Road, Columbus, OH 43214, USA
e-mail: darrin.bright@ohiohealth.com

D. Bring (✉)
Department of Family Medicine, OhioHealth, 3705 Olentangy River Road, Columbus, OH 43214, USA

© Springer International Publishing Switzerland 2016
T.L. Miller (ed.), *Endurance Sports Medicine*, DOI 10.1007/978-3-319-32982-6_20

injuries, cardiac conditions, electrolyte abnormalities, dehydration, gastrointestinal complaints, dermal injuries, pulmonary conditions, and medication requests. All encounters should be promptly documented on a medical progress note that includes the vital signs (when appropriate), patient information, specific details about each injury, clinical evaluation, treatment, and final disposition. Medical progress notes serve as primary documentation to collect important data that can be used to identify common injuries and illnesses and time spent in the medical area. This information can improve efficiency of treatment at future races. The following image is an example of a medical encounter form (Fig. 20.1).

The Capital City Half Marathon is an annual race held in Columbus, Ohio, that includes a half marathon, quarter marathon, and 5-km run. A total of 68,038 runners participated over 11 years, and the medical usage rate at the Capital City Half Marathon was 97 encounters per 10,000 participants. The average number of participants per event over the past 3 years in the Capital City Half Marathon was about 10,500 runners, which supports the increasing popularity of mass endurance events. The most common injuries from the race were musculoskeletal injuries at 35.8%, exertional collapse at 17.4%, and skin and soft-tissue injuries at 11.5%. The figure below demonstrates the most common medical tent encounters at the Capital City Half Marathon events from 2005 to 2015 (Fig. 20.2).

In contrast to a similar mass event, a study done by Tan et al. reviewed injury data from the half marathon in Singapore. The data indicate a medical usage rate between 16.9 and 26.0 encounters per 10,000 participants over 3 years and include a total of 84,644 runners. Musculoskeletal and soft-tissue injuries were the most common injuries at 37.9%, followed by skin and soft-tissue injuries at 29.2%, physical exhaustion at 15.7%, and heat injury at 6.4%. Most of the musculoskeletal and soft-tissue injuries were evaluated at the race's end point. Runners were also most likely to become a medical encounter with longer event distances (21 km vs. 10 km) [5]. Other studies indicate a medical encounter rate between 2 and 10% depending on

number of participants, weather conditions, and length of the race [4]. Fortunately, the incidence of sudden cardiac death is rare at about 1:100,000 entrants, and the rate of sudden cardiac death was found to be significantly higher in full marathons compared to half marathons [6].

Triathlon events present a different set of conditions at medical tents. In contrast to marathons that involve running only, triathlons combine swimming, cycling, and running into one event. In addition to risk of injury in each phase of the competition, there are also risks during the two transition phases of the race. A study done by Gosling et al. evaluated 10,197 triathletes competing over a total of six races (combined group of sprint and Olympic distances) and found that 23% of all athletes were evaluated for medical assistance. The most common time of injury was during the run at 38.4% and cycling at 14.3%. This cohort had similar injury reporting in comparison to the marathon injuries referenced above. The most common injuries in triathletes were musculoskeletal, specifically lower limb injuries at 59.5%, and skin abrasions at 28.6%. The study also found that elite and Olympic-distance athletes ages 12–19 were at higher risk of injury during the running and cycling components of the race [7].

Medical Staff and Volunteer Management

Preparing and providing a well-organized medical staff is an essential component of any mass event to ensure the safety of all athletes. This is an important aspect of both the planning and implementation phases [4]. The medical team will be expected to collaborate with race organizers, city/state/federal government agencies, hospitals, and other medical personnel before, during, and after the event.

The most essential member of the medical team is the medical director, who coordinates care for injured athletes and provides direct communication with law enforcement and race officials. The responsibilities of the medical director include but are not limited to coordination with

Medical Progress Note
Quarter / Half / Full Marathon
(please circle)

Medical Tent: _____

Arrival Time (HH:MM)

Final Race Time (HH:MM)

Prev. Marathons _____

BIB # _____

Charity Runner? Y N

Age _____   Gender ☐ M ☐ F

Name

Address

Phone

Emergency Contact Name & Phone

Pre-Race Weight _____

Post-Race Weight _____

Past Med History

Current Medications / Allergies

CHIEF COMPLAINT:

☐ Collapse/Near Syncope   ☐ Hot   ☐ MSK

☐ Fatigue/Weakness   ☐ Cold   ☐ Chest Pain

☐ Dizziness   ☐ Cramping   ☐ SOB

☐ Nausea & Vomiting   ☐ Headache   ☐ Wheezing

Further History: _____
_____
_____

DIAGNOSIS:

☐ Dehydration   ☐ MSK _____

☐ Hyperthermia   ☐ Muscle Cramps

☐ Hypothermia   ☐ Hypoglycemia

☐ Hyponatremia   ☐ Ex Assoc Collapse

☐ Asthma/Respiratory   ☐ Other _____

☐ GI

☐ Laceration

DISPOSITION:

☐ Discharged Ambulatory

☐ Follow-up with PCP

☐ Refused Care

☐ Transferred to Hospital

Discharge Time (HH:MM)

Physician Signature (required)

VITAL SIGNS:

Time (HH:MM)   BP   P   RR   T
_____
_____
_____

EXAM:

Mental Status

☐ A&Ox3   ☐ Confused   ☐ Unresponsive

Cardiac

☐ Tachy   ☐ Murmur   ☐ Brady

Pulmonary

☐ Clear   ☐ Wheeze   ☐ Decreased

Abdomen   L / R (circle)

☐ Soft NT   ☐ Tender Location _____

MSK

☐ cramping (describe) _____

☐ other _____

Skin

☐ Blisters   ☐ Abrasions   ☐ Hot

☐ Dry   ☐ Sweaty   ☐ Cold

TREATMENT:

☐ ACE   ☐ Ice   ☐ Warming

☐ Oxygen   ☐ PO Fluids   ☐ IVF's

☐ Other: _____

Fig. 20.1 Medical progress note

event organizers, recruitment and leadership of the medical team, evaluation of weather conditions, and helping to ensure the safety of participants, volunteers, and spectators.

In addition to the medical director, it is crucial to have experienced professionals in sports medicine and/or emergency medicine for effective coverage. The core medical team consists of

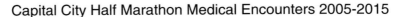

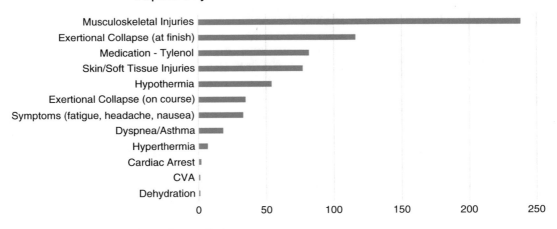

Fig. 20.2 Capital City Half Marathon medical encounters

physicians, acute care nurses, certified athletic trainers, emergency medical technicians (EMT), and persons trained in first aid [8]. Other members of the medical team can include podiatrists, physical therapists, massage therapists, and chiropractors. Medical staff at mass-participation events should follow predetermined protocols in all medical evaluations and effectively triage all athletes [9]. Members of the medical team should meet in advance of the race as part of the preplanning phase to review standard protocols for common injuries and conditions expected to be seen on race day [4]. Expectations and responsibilities for medical team members should be clearly communicated prior to the event. Medical team members are responsible for checking and documenting vital signs, recording all medical encounters including injuries and illnesses, and mobilizing athletes from the racecourse to the main medical tent or to local hospitals as needed. Documentation of all triaged athletes will aid in the post-race phase to determine quantity of supplies used, number and types of injuries/illnesses, as well as other pertinent demographic information.

Basic infrastructure of the medical team consists of course medical tents (located throughout the course), finish line medical tents (usually located near the finish line), an emergency communication/command center (arranged with

the race director), ambulance services, general transportation vehicles, and sag vehicles. Coordination with local police and fire departments prior to the event can also make operations more efficient; especially with vehicle transportation throughout the course [4]. A thorough knowledge of the event course as well as strategic planning to access all areas of the course will be helpful in transporting injured or ill participants during the race.

Designation and placement of both medical and nonmedical volunteers should be at the discretion of the medical director and other leadership. Ideally, at least one physician should be stationed at each of the medical tents throughout the course in addition to athletic trainers, nurses, or other medical professionals. Most events will require a large presence of medical volunteers at and around the finish line. Exercise associated collapse (EAC) is very common at the finish line of endurance events. The unexpected collapse of an exhausted participant at the finish line can lead to serious medical complications. Having a portion of the medical volunteers serving as "catchers" can minimize this risk. Frequently EAC can be prevented by supporting the athlete and encouraging them to continue moving through the finish chute. If they remain unstable or collapse having wheelchairs nearby will assist with transport to the finish line medical area.

Follow-up and evaluation meetings should be held between the medical director, medical staff, emergency medical services, police, command team, and event organizers to evaluate areas of weakness and identify opportunities to improve upon operational issues. These meetings should be conducted shortly after the conclusion of the race and are part of the post-race phase [4].

Equipment, Supplies, and Logistics

Medical tents should be strategically positioned throughout the course to provide medical attention during the event [5]. The number and location of these tents will be determined by the type of event, distance, individual course characteristics, anticipated needs, historical encounters, and available resources. The "main" medical tent should be in close proximity to the finish line and can be used to triage major injuries or illnesses as well as evaluate athletes that had been transported from the course. For larger venues, an additional tent is recommended in the athlete recovery area to provide basic first aid and serve as an extra location to provide medical care following the race.

Evaluation and distribution of medical supplies are an important component of the planning phase. Medical supplies can be distributed in pre-made "medical kits" and should be distributed to the medical tents along the course and at the main medical tent in the finish area. If multiple medical tents are stationed throughout the course, portable medical kits should be provided. Medical kits should include an AED, stethoscope, blood pressure cuff, and general wound care items such as Vaseline, Band-Aids, gauze, and Kerlix wrap. Large plastic containers or bins are ideal for packing portable medical kits for transportation. For cost purposes and to improve efficiency of treatment, items such as IV fluids, ACLS medications, and oxygen should be located only at the main medical tent. If athletes require invasive treatment measures, it is likely they will need more intensive monitoring and should be transported to the main medical tent or local hospital.

In cases where the course covers a smaller geographic footprint, it is possible to have one large medical tent at the finish area to triage illnesses and injuries. For larger events, the main medical tent should include an adequate number of cots to provide an appropriate area for the evaluation and recovery of athletes requiring medical care. The American College of Sports Medicine (ACSM) has developed a supply list in the team physician consensus statement [9]. The Columbus Marathon is an annual event with 19,000 registered participants (12,000 half and 7000 full). The following is a list of supplies utilized at the Columbus Marathon finish line medical tent:

1. Sterile gauze 2×2 in. pads
2. Sterile gauze 4×4 in. pads
3. Telfa pads
4. Flexible fabric bandages (variety)
5. Steri-Strips (1/4 in.)
6. Steri-Strips (1/2 in.)
7. Benzoin of tincture swabs
8. Elastic bandage (ace)
9. Paper, cloth, and clear tape
10. Alcohol prep swab pads
11. Antibiotic ointment
12. Betadine
13. Hydrogen peroxide
14. Sterile saline
15. Albuterol inhaler
16. Diphenhydramine
17. Dextrose 50 %
18. EpiPen
19. Lidocaine 1 %
20. Acetaminophen
21. Aspirin
22. Petroleum jelly
23. Tongue blades
24. Disinfectant spray
25. Antiseptic hand gel
26. Latex gloves (small, medium, and large)
27. Chucks
28. Ice coolers
29. Ice scoops
30. Ice bags
31. Pallet wrap
32. Trauma scissors
33. Blood pressure meter
34. Stethoscope
35. Pen lights

36. Rectal thermometer
37. Thermometer probe covers
38. Glucometer
39. Sterile lancets
40. Test strips
41. AED
42. Oxygen masks
43. Oxygen
44. Airway devices
45. Pulse oximeter
46. i-STAT
47. i-STAT cartridges
48. IV fluids
49. IV poles
50. IV syringes and catheters
51. IV starter kits
52. Scalpels
53. Syringes (5 and 10 cc)
54. Laceration kits
55. Suture material
56. Paper towels
57. Tissues
58. Tampons
59. Garbage container
60. Biohazard container and bag
61. Blankets
62. Folding chairs
63. Tables
64. Cots (50)
65. Wheelchairs (30)
66. Ice bath/immersion tubs (2)
67. Progress notes
68. Encounter logs
69. Clipboards
70. Pens
71. Name tags
72. Phone tree
73. Course map
74. Local map

Many of the supplies listed above can be very expensive and have a limited shelf life once they are opened. It is important to inspect all medical supplies and equipment prior to the event to ensure proper function and valid expiration dates. Positioning one or more EMS units at the finish line medical tent may reduce the need for some of the supplies listed above as they will have their own emergency medical equipment and supplies. Quantifying the total amount of supplies can be difficult and depends mostly on the number of athletes participating, the course distance, and weather conditions. Previous studies have evaluated average injury incidence for mass-participation events [5] and can be used to calculate needed supplies for a specific population or race. Estimating the number of medical encounters can be calculated by multiplying the number of participants by the average casualty incidence. This estimate can be used to calculate the appropriate number of medical volunteers, supplies, and equipment [8]. In order to calculate an accurate injury incidence, it is essential for the medical staff to document all medical encounters throughout the duration of the event. Data analysis of these encounters can assist in planning for future events. Mass events should also provide hydration stations that are easily accessible throughout the course for all participants. About 6–12 oz of fluid is recommended for every 15–20 min of continuous activity, and foods high in carbohydrates should be available to athletes at the finish of the event [9].

Weather Monitoring and Alerts

Monitoring extreme temperatures or severe weather conditions before and during the event is essential for the safety of all participants. The Wet-Bulb Globe Temperature (WBGT) is a measure of heat stress and should be used at mass-participation events. WBGT is more accurate than ambient temperature alone in predicting the effect that heat will have on a participant. The WBGT evaluates several variables, including temperature, humidity, wind speed, sun angle, and cloud cover (solar radiation) [10]. A digital or sling psychrometer can be purchased for a few hundred dollars and can aid in the decision-making process of weather safety prior to and during the event. The digital handheld devices can effectively and rapidly determine the WBGT. In 2007, American College of Sports Medicine (ACSM) issued a position statement on exertional heat illness during training and competition using WBGT to predict safe participation in practice and competition [11]. Individuals can be classified into non-acclimatized ("high risk") or acclimatized ("low risk") depending on baseline fitness level. WBGT levels can be used to modify or cancel competitions depending on WBGT measurements and level or duration of competition [11].

Predicting anticipated weather conditions provides important information when scheduling mass events. The use of a color-coded flag system is an effective means of communicating risks of participation to athletes and is based on the WBGT. The color-coded Event Alert System (EAS) developed by Chicago Event Management, Inc, producers of the Bank of America Chicago Marathon, allows the race organizer to effectively communicate to runners, spectators and volunteers prior to the race so they can prepare for varying weather conditions and on race day in the event that conditions changed for anything from weather, to a course reroute or cancellation. The EAS model is currently in place at all major American road races and is employed at many Chicago area events [4]. EAS uses the series of color-coded flags to indicate an "alert level" of low (green), moderate (yellow), high (red), or extreme (black) depending on event conditions.

With each alert level, there is a "recommended action," as noted in Fig. 20.3.

It is recommended that event organizers distribute alert level information via email, website communications, text messages, or with flyers/signs prior to the start of the event, so that athletes and volunteers are familiar with EAS. Color-coded flags should be placed throughout the course and at the finish line to keep the community and participants updated on current alert levels [12].

Figure 20.4 includes ACSM recommendations and guidelines on how a mass event should react to various weather conditions through the use of the Event Alert System. The Wet-Bulb Globe Temperature is used to determine the alert level [13].

A study conducted by Roberts calculated a "do not start" temperature of 20.5 °C for the Twin Cities Marathon in Minnesota. This statistic was calculated by plotting the number of unsuccessful starters per 1000 finishers against start WBGT. The article recommends calculating a "do not start" WBGT temperature for every race [14]. This calculation can be used in conjunction with the ACSM guidelines as noted above.

ALERT LEVEL	EVENT CONDITIONS	RECOMMENDED ACTIONS
EXTREME	EVENT CANCELLED/EXTREME AND DANGEROUS CONDITIONS	PARTICIPATION STOPPED/FOLLOW EVENT OFFICIAL INSTRUCTIONS
HIGH	POTENTIALLY DANGEROUS CONDITIONS	SLOW DOWN/OBSERVE COURSE CHANGES/FOLLOW OFFICIAL INSTRUCTIONS/CONSIDER STOPPING
MODERATE	LESS THAN IDEAL CONDITIONS	SLOW DOWN/BE PREPARED FOR WORSENING CONDITIONS
LOW	GOOD CONDITIONS	ENJOY THE EVENT/BE ALERT

Fig. 20.3 Event Alert System

WBGT	Flag Color	Level of Risk	Comments
<65°F (<18°C)	Green	Low	Risk low but still exists on the basis of risk factors
65°-73°F (18°-23°C)	Yellow	Moderate	Risk level increases as event progresses through the day
73°-82°F (23°-28°C)	Red	High	Everyone should be aware of injury potential; individuals at risk should not compete
>82°F (>28°C)	Black	Extreme or hazardous	Consider rescheduling or delaying the event until safer conditions prevail; if the event must take place, be on high alert. Take steps to reduce risk factors (e.g., more and longer rest breaks, reduced practice time, reduced exercise intensity, access to shade, minimal clothing and equipment, cold tubs at practice site, etc.).

Fig. 20.4 Wet-Bulb Globe Temperature risk chart

Historical weather conditions should be reviewed and are helpful in establishing the event date and start time. Earlier start times have been proven to have a decreased number of casualties due to lower temperatures at the beginning of the race [14]. Races held in fall months in the Northern Hemisphere (October/November) are ideal because runners can train in warmer weather during the summer and then run the event on a day with likely cooler temperatures [15]. Avoiding extremes in warm temperatures will provide a lower risk of heat-related illness and allows for large groups of athletes to participate safely.

Event-Day Communication

The largest marathons and mass events in the United States host up to 50,000 athletes. With this number of participants, communication among event personnel is essential for rapid response to incidents during the race [16]. Communication begins with dissemination of information to a large number of participants before, during, and after the race.

It is important to have direct communication between medical staff members throughout the event. All event course volunteers, including course marshals, medical tent personnel, and fluid station volunteers, should be informed on protocols for identifying injured athletes, so that the appropriate medical personnel can be notified when a participant needs medical attention [15].

Course spectators can also be urged to notify emergency personnel of athletes that are injured along the course. Emergency contact information can be distributed and posted to inform spectators how to report an incident. Additionally, many large events have partnered with the American Red Cross to provide demonstrations on bystander CPR during the event expo.

It is essential for the medical director to communicate with emergency services about the exact start time so that 911 calls related to the mass event can be triaged appropriately. Emergency operators should ask for the participant's name, location, and bib number in order to assist emergency medical personnel in identifying and responding to the appropriate athlete requiring aid. Communication methods should not rely on any single technology and should incorporate voice, data, video, PA systems, and digital message boards in case any system fails during an emergency situation. Any and all communication methods should be tested to ensure that the selected method is fully functional prior to the start of the event. Megaphones can also be used to give instructions to athletes or for crowd control [17].

The use of two-way radios is a simple and cost-effective way of direct communication between the medical director and other medical staff members. It is helpful to have these radios placed with the medical team captains stationed throughout the course and finish area. Medical team captains are designated prior to the start of the race and serve to communicate directly with the medical director about injuries at various points along the course.

Two-way radios are an important alternative to cell phones due to decreased cellular coverage and increased demand with a large number of individuals on a network. Two-way radios also allow for an individual to communicate simultaneously to everyone on a particular channel allowing for more rapid dissemination of information in an emergency situation. Cell phones should be used in addition to two-way radios, and all pertinent phone numbers should be collected, printed on small cards, and distributed to all medical staff prior to the start of the race. For patient privacy, medical personnel should be advised to refer to athletes requiring medical attention by bib number as opposed to their name.

An Emergency Command Center (ECC) can serve as the central hub for all emergency communications relative to an event. It is advised to have the ECC in close proximity to the finish line to allow for direct access to this area by the medical director, race director, and other important race personnel. Depending on the distance, size, and geographic footprint of the course, it may be necessary to have representatives from the EMS, fire and police departments, American Red Cross, and race operations. Having all emergency services around the same table ensures a more effective and collaborative response to participants requiring medical attention.

Larger events should utilize police officers and other law enforcement personnel positioned throughout the course to provide additional monitoring and direct communication with the police dispatcher and command center [15]. Social media such as Twitter or Facebook can provide fast communication to emergency services or hospitals in a disaster scenario. The use of social media can also serve as an effective means of communicating updates and status reports to athletes and spectators. If desired, the race director or medical director can create a social media account specific to the mass-participation event. Information about how to use social media to report events should be distributed prior to the start of the race.

Event Security

Mass events including marathons, triathlons, or cycling events often host up to tens of thousands of participants and should be designated as a potential "mass casualty event." In case of extreme weather, natural disasters, terrorist attack, or other mass casualty situation, emergency services and hospitals may be overwhelmed by a high volume of patients in a catastrophe situation. In order to minimize risk of a mass casualty event, race directors, law enforcement, and other essential personnel should work together during the planning process.

Implementation of organized security measures at mass events is of utmost importance because of the high volume of potential casualties. Recent mass event tragedies, such as the 2013 Boston Marathon bombing, highlight the importance of well-organized security measures when planning a large race. The use of a unified command approach has proven to be an effective means of organizing a mass-participation event with assistance from both local police and fire departments [4]. Event organizers are encouraged to be familiar with and receive training in emergency operations management developed by the Federal Emergency Management Agency (FEMA) including but not limited to National Incident Management System (NIMS), Incident Command Systems (ICS), and Unified Command (UC). In the event of a disaster scenario, it is imperative that the medical director has experience with ICS to ensure efficient operations and avoid duplication of tasks and misinformation. The unified command approach allows all of the various agencies (police, fire department, Red Cross) to work together to direct an emergency action plan (EAP) [4]. Every mass event should have a prepared EAP with designated incident commander in case of an emergency or mass casualty incident [17]. The medical director should have close communication with the race director and the central command center in order to disseminate information to medical volunteers as needed in the event of an emergency.

In order to mitigate potential disaster risks, the University of Southern Mississippi created the

"National Marathon Safety and Security Best Practices Guide" (NMSSBP) in July 2015. The guide was developed with representatives from the public safety agencies, USA Track and Field, Running USA, Ironman World Championships, and individuals with experience in marathon and endurance event planning. Race directors and medical directors can use this document as a standardized approach for best practices in safety and security for any mass event. One of the challenges of providing security for running and cycling events in urban environments is that racecourses may involve many miles of roadway and streets through densely populated areas that can be difficult to secure. Creating a culture of hyper-vigilance and increased awareness among race spectators, participating athletes, and EMS/law enforcement/fire departments is a key component of implementing a secure course [17]. Topics addressed in the NMSSBP guide include event and race-day planning, crowd management, emergency action planning, risk and threat assessment, staff development and training, creating a culture of safety and awareness, and the use of technology.

Security planning should occur throughout the entire year to consistently improve existing protocols and evaluate new security risks. A "risk assessment team" including local/state/federal law enforcement, fire departments, EMS, and medical staff is essential for any mass event. The medical director should have direct communication with the risk assessment team prior to the race. Roles and responsibilities of all above parties should be defined prior to the event in order to avoid confusion and wasted time during a disaster scenario. Meetings to outline the roles and responsibilities of each team member should occur well in advance to the race and follow existing protocols for emergency response. Medical staff should be briefed prior to the start of the event to review protocols for evacuation during a potential disaster event. All staff and volunteers should be trained to be observant and report suspicious activity to law enforcement and be organized in a "command matrix" system. The command matrix provides a tiered system that organizes personnel so that each member knows which management

system to report to in the event of an emergency [17]. All medical staff should report directly to the medical director who can then report to the other management systems as needed.

In addition to the organization of personnel as outlined above, there are several other recommendations to mitigate security risks for mass events. The NMSSBP recommends that law enforcement should conduct a full crime analysis prior to the race to evaluate the types of crime that occur in the event area independent of race-day activities. This may require coordination and cooperation among different jurisdictions and is important to anticipate potential events before they may happen. Mobile barriers should be placed along the racecourse and around the start and finish line areas to create a "buffer zone" between the racecourse and the general public [17]. Barricades should be utilized around areas that may be vulnerable to forced vehicle entry and includes large trucks or buses, concrete walls, or anti-ram fences. Uniformed law enforcement and race security staff should be present, when feasible, at the starting line, finish area, and perimeter entry/control points. Areas of the course can be divided into the inner, middle, and outer areas as described by the NMSSBP.

All volunteers should be provided with appropriate credentialing to avoid confusion in areas where workers are allowed to be present during a race. Credentials and race assignments can be provided at a single "check in" location prior to the start of the race and should be displayed at all times for identification purposes. It is helpful to designate specific areas of the course with a number so that assigned credentials can identify where volunteers are able to access the course.

In addition to personnel credentials, all vehicles requiring access into the inner area of the race should be designated prior to race day and should be provided with a separate set of credentials. A "no reentry policy" should be established at the end of the race in order to maintain control of the inner access areas, as well as a designated "secure exit" point that prevents spectators from entering the secured course. Once athletes go past this exit point, they should not be allowed to return to the race area. The NMSSBP best practices document contains additional information regarding security measures. The medical director should discuss all security measures with law enforcement and the race director depending on the location of the race and should follow protocols related to specific city jurisdictions.

Conclusion

As participation in mass endurance events continues to grow, it is essential to develop a well-organized medical plan. An appropriate medical plan should include professional medical staff, appropriate equipment and supplies, precise weather evaluation, proper placement of equipment and personnel, an effective communication system, and a comprehensive security plan to ensure the health and safety of the participants, volunteers, and spectators. An effective medical plan can mean the difference between life and death.

References

1. Harshbarger R, Jacobson J. Running USA's Annual Marathon Report. Running USA. 2014. http://www.runningusa.org/marathon-report-2014?returnTo=annual%20-reports. Accessed 3 Dec 2015
2. United States Olympic Committee. USA Triathlon Membership Report. USA Triathlon. 2014. https://www.teamusa.org/usa-triathlon/about/multisport/demographics. Accessed 3 Dec 2015
3. Larson D. Membership Survey and Analysis. USA Cycling, INC. 2013. https://s3.amazonaws.com/USACWeb/forms/encyc/2013-USAC-Membership-Survey-Report.pdf. Accessed 3 Dec 2015
4. Chiampas G, Jaworski CA. Preparing for the surge. Curr Sports Med Rep. 2009;8(3):131–5.
5. Tan CM, Tan I, Kok W, Lee MC, Lee VJ. Medical planning for mass-participation running events: a 3-year review of a half-marathon in Singapore. BMC Public Health. 2014;14(1):1109.
6. Kim JH, Malhotra R, Chiampas G, et al. Cardiac arrest during long-distance running races. Race Associated Cardiac Arrest Event Registry (RACER) study group. N Engl J Med. 2012;366(2):130–40.
7. Gosling CM, Forbes AB, Mcgivern J, Gabbe BJ. A profile of injuries in athletes seeking treatment during a triathlon race series. Am J Sports Med. 2010;38(5):1007–14.
8. Roberts WO. Event coverage. In: Safran MR, McKeag DB, Van Camp SP, editors. Manual of sports medicine. Philadelphia, PA: Lippincott-Raven Publishers; 1998. p. 54–69.
9. Herring Stanley A, Bergfeld John A, Boyajian-O'Neill Lori A, Indelicato Peter, Jaffe Rebecca, Kibler W Ben, O'Connor Francis G, Pallay Robert, Roberts William O, Stockard Alan, Taft Timothy N, Williams James, Young Craig C. Mass participation event management for the team physician: a consensus statement. MSSE. 2004;36:2004–2008
10. National Weather Service. WetBulb Globe Temperature. National Weather Service Forecast Office. 2015. http://www.srh.noaa.gov/tsa/?n=wbgt. Accessed 3 Dec 2015
11. Armstrong LE, Casa DJ, Millard-Stafford M, Moran DS, Pyne SW, Roberts WO. Exertional heat illness during training and competition. Med Sci Sports Exerc. 2007;39(3):556–72.
12. Bank of America Chicago Marathon. Public Safety—Event Alert System. Chicago Marathon. 2015. https://www.chicagomarathon.com/participant-information/public-safety/. Accessed 3 Dec 2015
13. Armstrong LE, Epstein Y, Greenleaf JE, et al. American College of Sports Medicine position stand: heat and cold illnesses during distance running. Med Sci Sports Exerc. 1996;28:i–x.
14. Roberts WO. Determining a "do not start" temperature for a marathon on the basis of adverse outcomes. Med Sci Sports Exerc. 2010;42(2):226–32.
15. Ewert GD. Marathon race medical administration. Sports Med. 2007;37:428–30.
16. Harshbarger R, Jacobsen J. National Runner' Survey. http://www.runningusa.org/2015-nationalrunner. Accessed 3 Dec 2015
17. University of Southern Mississippi. National Center for Spectator Sports Safety and Security (NCS4). Marathon Safety and Security Best Practices Guide. 2015. https://www.ncs4.com/about/best-practices. Accessed 3 Dec 2015

Return to Sport Decision-Making for Endurance Athletes

21

Brett Toresdahl, Polly deMille, Julia Kim,
Jason Machowsky, Mike Silverman,
and Scott Rodeo

Identification and Correction of Predisposing Factors

Although an athlete can recover from an isolated injury without understanding the exact cause, the athlete's ability to return to competition quickly and avoid recurrent injury is dependent on identifying the cause. In the case of an acute injury, the culprit is often apparent [1]. However, a chronic overuse injury may have a more subtle cause that is amplified through hours of training. A thorough history and examination can often reveal the most likely cause of an injury and involves evaluation of biomechanics, equipment, training pattern, and nutrition. In all athletes and especially in multisport endurance athletes, there may be more than one contributing factor so care must be taken to identify and address each one.

Biomechanics and Equipment

Running

Poor and inefficient running mechanics are often associated with—if not the direct cause of—lower extremity injuries in athletes. Runners with anterior knee pain attributed to patellofemoral syndrome should be observed running to look for excessive hip adduction and hip internal rotation, which result in greater stress on the patellofemoral joint [2–4]. A runners' ability to control hip adduction may appear sufficient in the biomechanics lab. However, with prolonged running and fatiguing of the hip abductors, a runner can develop increased hip adduction and internal rotation, resulting in patellofemoral pain [4, 5]. Stride length and cadence has also been shown to directly affect ground reaction forces with a shorter stride and higher cadence being associated with a decrease in ground reaction force, peak hip adduction, hip flexion, and knee flexion angles at impact [6].

Lower extremity injuries in runners should prompt not only a reevaluation of running biomechanics but also shoe selection. While often

B. Toresdahl (✉)
Primary Care Sports Medicine Service, Department of Medicine, Hospital for Special Surgery, 535 East 70th Street, New York, NY 10021, USA
e-mail: toresdahlb@hss.edu

P. deMille • J. Machowsky
Sports Rehabilitation and Performance, Hospital for Special Surgery, 525 East 71st Street, New York, NY 10021, USA

J. Kim
Medicine, Hospital for Special Surgery, 535 East 70th Street, New York, NY 10021, USA

M. Silverman
Sports Rehab, Hospital for Special Surgery, 108 East 96th Street, Apt 10-E, New York, NY 10128, USA

S. Rodeo
Sports Medicine and Shoulder Service, Department of Orthopedic Surgery, Hospital for Special Surgery, 535 East 70th Street, New York, NY, USA

© Springer International Publishing Switzerland 2016
T.L. Miller (ed.), *Endurance Sports Medicine*, DOI 10.1007/978-3-319-32982-6_21

considered when addressing a foot or ankle complaint, a shoe that does not fit the runner's natural stride can contribute to injuries in the knee, hip, and lumbar spine. Running shoes can be classified as cushioning, stability, motion control, and minimalist. Cushioned shoes are best suited for runners with pes cavus alignment and those who are observed to have excessive supination. Stability shoes, which balance cushioning and pronation control, can be used by runners who have a neutral foot and normal running mechanics. Motion control shoes are designed for runners with flat feet and who need to accommodate for both rear and mid-foot pronation. Minimalist shoes are meant to simulate barefoot conditions while running, allowing a runner to land with a flatter foot. This flatter foot, which creates more of a forefoot strike pattern, decreased stride length and the vertical force at initial contact [7–9]. Additionally, orthotics are commonly used to further alter lower extremity mechanics in runners, particularly in those with abnormal foot types and dysfunction. The potential benefit of orthotics has been shown in studies of lower extremity stress injuries among military recruits [10].

Biking

A proper bike fit has the ability to prevent injury as well as improve performance, increase comfort, and maximize aerobic efficiency [11]. However, some adjustments that can increase efficiency and aerodynamics come at the cost of comfort and risk of injury [12]. Although the typical cyclist will deal with major injuries such as fractures, dislocations, ligament ruptures, as well as concussions, the most common types are overuse injuries, especially involving the knee. If a cyclist presents with anterior knee pain, consider that the saddle may be too low or too far forward, causing excessive patellofemoral loading throughout the pedal cycle. Iliotibial band friction syndrome can also be seen with improper cleat position, which can lead to excessive internal tibial rotation [13].

Swimming

In swimming, athletes strive to achieve ideal stroke mechanics and technique to maximize performance and efficiency [14]. If an athlete has a limitation in strength, coordination, or range of motion anywhere along the kinetic chain, performance is affected [15]. Among endurance athletes, the freestyle stroke is one of the most commonly performed. The continuous repetition of this stroke puts strain on the shoulder and can lead to problems, particularly shoulder impingement. A common error is dropping the elbow during the pull through and recovery phase of swimming, which externally rotates and horizontally adducts the shoulder. Additionally, an elbow that enters the water before the hand can lead to superior translation of the humeral head. These alterations in normal stroke mechanics can result in shoulder impingement [16–20].

Rowing

The repetitive motion of the rowing stroke can result in overuse injuries of the spine and extremities [21–23]. Compared to open water training or competition, injuries and specifically back pain occur at a higher frequency when training on an ergometer [24, 25]. This should be considered when caring for athletes who primarily train indoors during the winter months. Knee pain can be the result of improper position of the foot stretcher, causing an increased knee flexion angle at the catch. By elevating the foot stretcher, this angle can be decreased, which in turn decreases stress on the patellofemoral joint. Other adjustments that can alleviate undue stress on the knee include altering the toe-in versus toe-out position in the setting of functional knee varus or valgus alignment and the use of stops on the front or back to limit the arc of knee flexion or extension [23].

Training

The most critical factor in the success of an endurance athlete, both in improving performance and voiding, is the training program. Overuse injuries are by definition an error of training—too much, too hard, too often. Studies of risk factors for injuries in endurance athletes have identified correlations between injury and training volume, training frequency, and training intensity [7, 26–30]. When evaluating an athlete's training program, consider whether it follows basic principles of any effective training program: progressive overload, specificity, periodization, and individualization [31–33].

The principle of progressive overload states that a system must be exposed to a stress greater than that to which it is accustomed in order for positive adaptations to occur. Training load is progressively increased so that after the adaptations gained in the recovery periods, fitness has improved and a proportionately greater training stimulus must be applied. Specificity in the context of training refers to the concept that in order for a system to adapt to a specific requirement, it must be stressed in a manner similar to that requirement. Training adaptations are specific to the type, volume, and intensity of the training. Periodization is a system of progressively cycling various aspects of a training program to achieve peak fitness for competition while avoiding injury and overtraining. Finally, individualization is the concept that individuals respond differently to identical training regimens. Genetic characteristics play a major role in the response to a training stimulus. Training programs should take into account the individual athlete's current level of fitness, training history in the sport, competitive level in the sport, injury history, medical history, and other life stresses (work and travel demands, family obligations, etc). Training is a form of stress, and the cumulative effect of training load in addition to major life stress should be considered.

When evaluating the injured athletes, consider training errors that could have contributed to the occurrence of the injury. Many common training mistakes listed below can be identified without examining every detail of an athlete's training log.

- Is the athlete following a training plan? If so, how was the training plan created and individualized?
- Is the athlete working with a coach?
- Is the training plan periodized?
- Do they follow their training plan even if they feel fatigued from the previous workout?
- How many hours per week are spent training?
- Do the workouts vary from day to day?

- Does the athlete have any rest days during the week?
- Does the athlete limit sleep hours to fit in training?
- How many hours per night is the athlete sleeping?
- Does the training plan include cross-training?
- How frequently does the athlete compete and are there varying levels of competition among the events?

A qualified exercise physiologist is a valuable resource when evaluating the contribution of an athlete's training plan to the development of an injury and how to minimize risk of recurrence. The same focused determination to achieve a goal that often leads to success in endurance sports can have a downside when an athlete inappropriately adheres to a poorly suited training program. Failure to identify and correct training errors risks recurrent injury and further time lost from competition.

Nutrition

While endurance athletes tend to have lower body mass indexes (BMI) and body fat percentages to maximize competitiveness at their sport, clinicians must understand the nutritional tightrope that these athletes walk [34, 35]. The signs of compromised nutritional state must be recognized, including chronic fatigue, immune system suppression, anemia, electrolyte abnormalities, and recurrent overuse injuries [36–39].

Most athletes require an energy availability (EA = energy intake − energy expenditure) of greater than 30–45 kcal/kg fat to maintain normal physiological function [40]. Fueling based on hunger and satiety alone may still result in an EA deficit, especially when performing rigorous training over weeks to months [41]. Moreover, athletes with disordered eating—most notably as part of the female athlete triad—represent some of the most challenging cases of under-fueling, as the psychological component may be the primary driver of eating behavior [42].

Alternatively, an athlete may have sufficient caloric intake, but a nutrient poor diet. Particular nutrients of interest for endurance athletes include those related to bone health (calcium, vitamin D), recovery/immune system (vitamin C, vitamin E, beta-carotene, zinc, and selenium), muscular function (magnesium), metabolism (B vitamins, particularly B6 and folate), and oxygen transport (iron). While adequate intake of a range of vegetables, fruits, lean proteins, healthy fats, and whole grains to meet daily energy requirements should provide enough of these nutrients, restricted intakes or nutrient poor diets may require a multivitamin with mineral until eating habits are improved [43]. Identification of any clinical nutrient deficiencies may require specific supplementation as well.

Additional factors that can add further stress to an athlete's nutritional demands that could exacerbate illness or injury include travel, changes in training environment (e.g., altitude, heat), increased training volume, and medical conditions leading to GI distress and/or malabsorption of nutrients [43, 44].

Restoration of Function

Following the appropriate diagnostic workup to determine the etiology and pathophysiology an athlete's injury, the rehabilitation process can begin. Initial treatments are focused on reducing pain and inflammation using a combination of rest, ice, anti-inflammatory medication, compression, bracing, gentle stretching, and electrotherapeutic modalities. Depending on the injury, concurrent cross-training can be done to maintain aerobic fitness, such as with a stationary bike for a swimmer or rower with a shoulder injury. Once the pain has subsided, the rehabilitation process can proceed, first with a focus on regaining range of motion, followed by strength, neuromuscular training, and sport-specific training until finally returning to competition. As an athlete progresses through the rehabilitation process, any recurrence of symptoms should prompt the athlete to step back until the symptoms subside before continuing on. Frequent communication between the medical team and the coaching staff helps assure a smooth transition back to competition.

Range of Motion

If limitations in range of motion were identified in the initial post-injury evaluation, this should be addressed in the initial phase of rehabilitation as optimal muscle and joint function require satisfactory flexibility. Frequency and intensity of stretching is dependent on the athlete's pain, and care should be given to not exacerbate the symptoms by overstretching. Additionally, the flexibility of the muscle tendon unit and adjacent tissue should be addressed and optimized. Restoration of appropriate muscle flexibility is an important part of the overall rehabilitation program.

Strength

As pain subsides and flexibility is addressed, the focus can begin to transition to strengthening. The clinician needs to assess baseline strength and symmetry of all muscle groups relevant for the specific activity. For example, swimmers need adequate strength of the rotator cuff and scapular-stabilizing muscles, while runners will need to focus more on the lower extremity. Core strengthening can be easily overlooked but is critical for any of these athletes and should be evaluated as well. In addition to measuring strength of isolated muscle groups, another important consideration is the balance between different major muscle groups. Various agonist and antagonist groups need to work in concert. In swimmers, there is often an imbalance at the shoulder with internal rotators being relatively stronger than the external rotators, due to the activity of internal rotators during the swimming stroke [45].

Muscle endurance is especially important for the endurance athlete. Assessment of endurance and muscle fatigability by testing with lower resistance and higher repetitions is often necessary, especially when an endurance athlete has normal biomechanics when observed outside of competition but has symptoms with extended training sessions or competition. Generally, athletes are recommended to regain at least 90 % of strength in the affected muscle group compared to the contralateral side prior to proceeding through the rehabilitation program.

Neuromuscular Training

Compared to the relatively straightforward areas of flexibility, strength, and endurance, the assessment of neuromuscular function, coordination, and proprioception are often more difficult to quantify objectively. Various functional tests can be used to provide information about muscle coordination and proprioception. Examples include jump landing, triple hop tests, and more challenging tasks. An athlete must first be evaluated to ensure readiness for completing these more challenging functional tasks. As neuromuscular deficits that affect coordination and proprioception are starting to be recognized more frequently as the underlying primary factors that led to injury, an experienced physical therapist is a valuable member of the treatment team. The physical therapist can both perform an advanced neuromuscular assessment and create a comprehensive rehabilitation program to address the deficits identified.

Sport-Specific Training

After determining that the athlete has developed an adequate baseline level of muscle strength, endurance, flexibility, and neuromuscular function, more sport-specific activities can be introduced into the rehabilitation and training regimen. Training activities that mimic and simulate the specific movements of the sport are well-established as being the optimal way to prepare an athlete for return to sport. These activities should be introduced gradually, taking care to monitor the athlete's symptoms as they increase their training. At this stage of the rehabilitation program, the physician and physical therapist should also coordinate with other members of the athlete's support team, which may include a coach athletic trainer, and strength and conditioning specialist. This will help the medical team to better understand the specific requirements of the sport and allow a rehabilitation plan that accounts for the specific physical demands of the sport.

Returning to Competition

A careful and detailed plan for return to competition should be devised in conjunction with the medical team and the other members of the athlete's support team. When an athlete is cleared to begin competing again, this does not necessarily mean the athlete can compete without limitations. The frequency, intensity, and volume of competition activities should be carefully planned so as to avoid competing too much too soon and risking reinjury. All of these factors may be gradually increased over time to ensure a safe and effective return to competition.

A number of variables need to be considered in planning the return to competition schedule. Such factors include consideration of the competition schedule, what phase of the season the athlete or team is currently in, where the athlete is in their career, and the athlete's goals. There is no "one-size-fits-all" approach to returning an athlete to competition. A highly individualized plan needs to be devised for that athlete based on a number of these considerations. For example, the plan may be different for a young scholastic athlete versus a mature collegiate athlete who is entering their final year of competition. Upcoming major events on the competitive calendar, such as Olympic trials, will affect the decision to have the athlete compete in earlier events.

Managing Challenges During Rehabilitation

Given the inevitability of injury in endurance sports, great athletes are often those who are able to quickly and fully recover from injury. A comprehensive approach to injury management provides the best opportunity to ensure an optimal return to competition. Without consideration for all aspects of the athlete's rehabilitation, an injury may be fully healed, but the athlete may be far from being ready for competition because of the fitness, nutritional, or psychological effects of the injury. The rehabilitation from an injury affects each athlete differently, so there is not a one-size-fits-all treatment. The medical team must frequently monitor the various aspects of the athlete's health and well-being and intervene accordingly.

Maintaining Fitness Level

An endurance athlete who sustains an injury is faced not only with the challenge of rehabilitation but also with the loss of hard-earned fitness as a result of cessation or significant interruption of training. Significant changes can occur fairly rapidly in cardiorespiratory, metabolic, and muscular fitness when training is interrupted [1, 31, 46–48]. The magnitude of loss of fitness is dependent on the initial fitness level and the amount of time without a sufficient training stimulus. Even short-term (<4 weeks) cessation of training can result in a wide range of physiological changes that negatively impact endurance performance (Table 21.1).

The loss of fitness in the context of injury can often be attenuated. Training volume can be reduced by as much as 70 % from previous weekly volume and training frequency by up to 30 % as long as training intensity is maintained [1, 47, 49, 50]. Exercise intensity seems to be the critical component needed to maintain training-induced adaptations. The optimal intensity needed to maintain fitness is unknown. Continuous work performed at an intensity of 70–85 % of VO2max and intervals performed at 90–100 % of VO2max have been shown to maintain training adaptations during short periods of reduced training volume and frequency [31, 48, 50–53].

If the injury precludes training in the primary sport, then the athlete should train in as similar of a mode as possible [54]. For example, a runner with a stress fracture could perform deep-water running as an alternative during rehabilitation. Using a dissimilar training mode may sometimes be necessary; for example, swimming with a pull-buoy may be possible when use of the lower

Table 21.1 Physiologic changes that occur in context of short-term cessation of training

Cardiorespiratory parameter
↓ Maximal oxygen uptake
↓ Blood volume
↑ Maximal and submaximal heart rate
↓ Cardiac output
↓ Exercise stroke volume
↓ Ventricular mass
↓ Maximum ventilatory volume
Metabolic parameters
↑ Maximal and submaximal respiratory exchange ratio
↓ Muscle GLUT-4 protein content
↓ Muscle lipoprotein lipase activity
↓ Insulin-mediated glucose activity
↑ Submaximal blood lactate
↓ Lactate threshold
↓ Muscle glycogen
Muscular parameters
↓ Capillary density
↓ Oxidative enzyme activities
↓ Glycogen synthase activity
↓ Mitochondrial ATP production

Adapted from Mujika and Padilla [46, 47, 72]

extremities is contraindicated in a cyclist or runner. Although not ideal, training in dissimilar modes may help delay the loss of training adaptations [54]. Given the extensive literature documenting the negative effects of detraining that occur with complete cessation of training, the medicine team should make every attempt to provide an alternative training plan to support the athlete's fitness during rehabilitation. Collaboration between the physical therapist, exercise physiologist, and coach can provide an individualized plan for maintaining training adaptations during recovery from injury.

Dietary Changes

In the initial phase of rehabilitation, nutritional guidance should promote weight maintenance since significant weight loss or weight gain can impair healing [55, 56]. Although total calorie requirements will decrease in relation to training volume, a very low-calorie diet is not recommended.

Significant injury, e.g., fracture or surgery, may increase basal metabolic rate by 20 %, and crutching can burn 2–3 times more calories than walking [57, 58]. Lean mass can be maintained through adequate intake of lean protein spaced even throughout the day, but higher amounts of protein may be warranted for bone healing or promoting satiety in athletes who are susceptible to weight gain during inactivity [55]. Other nutrients involved in wound healing and anti-inflammatory processes, such as omega 3 fatty acids, vitamin A (beta-carotene), vitamin C, vitamin E, zinc, and selenium, may be worth extra attention [59]. Increased amounts of calcium and vitamin D may be needed in the presence of fractures or bone-related surgeries [60]. While adequate intake would ideally be achieved through food-based sources, a comprehensive multivitamin with minerals may be useful. Large doses of any single nutrient are not recommended unless indicated for the treatment of a clinical deficiency. Adequate fluids should be consumed, and excessive alcohol should be avoided as it is a low nutrient source of calories and has been shown to impair muscle protein synthesis, which likely affects recovery [61]. Supplement recommendations to preserve muscle mass (leucine, beta-hydroxy-beta-methylbutyrate, creatine, etc.) or decrease inflammation (fish oil, curcumin, ginger, etc.) should be individualized, and their effectiveness is still equivocal in many cases [55, 62–65]. Limited mobility can make food preparation or consumption difficult, and accommodations should be made when possible.

To avoid setbacks or delayed healing, the athlete must continue to consume enough food and nutrients to absorb the increased demands of increasing training. Protein requirements will likely stay constant in the presence of adequate calories. Fluid needs will increase with return to activities that significantly increase sweat rate. Changes in body composition, strength, and desired athletic adaptations should be tracked throughout this period to guide nutrition recommendations. An athlete should develop a fueling plan before returning to full training and competition to ensure they are able to adapt their eating habits to the season-specific demands of their sport. The requirements of daily physiological function, training, and recovery need to be considered. Greater detail can be found in Chap. 18, Optimizing Nutrition for Endurance Sports Training. The athlete is ideally returning to competition with well-established proper eating habits, a fueling plan for in-season and off-season, any nutrition-related symptoms controlled, nutritional deficiencies corrected, a healthy body composition, and a positive outlook on returning to their sport.

Psychological Challenges

Endurance athletes are self-motivated and have the persistence to endure physical and mental obstacles. The mental strength required to succeed can also be an obstacle when mental enthusiasm does not match an athlete's physical capabilities due to injury. A successful return to competition requires mental, emotional, and physical readiness to be in-line. An injury can cause an athlete to lose a sense of identity and community, daily structure, self-esteem due to lack of consistent positive reinforcement from training and competition, confidence in the strength and resilience of their body, and a constructive form of stress release [66]. Athletes can experience stages of emotion following an injury that are similar to the Kubler-Ross' stages of coping with loss: denial, anger, bargaining, depression, and acceptance [67]. How one approaches these losses can influence one's expectations, goals, and therefore readiness to return to sport.

The biggest challenge an endurance athlete has is to temporarily change expectations in order to safely return to sport. The key is to view the injury as another challenge to overcome and apply the same mental and physical resilience in recovery as in training and competition. Adjusting and maintaining a strong mind helps an athlete take control of the situation and maintain self-esteem (Table 21.2).

Psychological skills that have been shown to improve performance for endurance athletes include goal-setting, self-talk, and imagery [68].

Table 21.2 Managing psychological challenges following injury

Grief	Feeling sad and disappointed allows an athlete to mourn the loss and express feelings in a healthy manner. This prevents internalized anger from turning into more debilitating depression and externalized anger from detracting from responsibility
Acceptance	Allowing one to mourn loss can help one come to terms with the situation and not stay stuck in the past. By accepting the situation, an athlete can set realistic goals to prepare for recovery and successful return to sport
Commitment	Committing to rehabilitation can help an athlete to use existing strengths, such as drive, dedication, and perseverance, to adhere to a rehabilitation plan
Responsibility	Athletes must take an active role in their recovery and identify what areas of their recovery are within their control
Listen to body with patience	Endurance athletes are trained to push through the pain of extreme exertion. When injured, training in a similar way by ignoring pain will lead to delay in recovery and potentially further injury. Athletes need to listen to their bodies and adjust accordingly
Support and guidance	Support from family, friends, and coaches can help boost morale and alleviate depression and isolation. Support from coaches, medical team, and psychologists can help guide recovery for a successful return to sport

When injured, these skills must be reapplied to the new challenges and goals of rehabilitation.

- Goal setting: In order to achieve the long-term goal of returning to sport, the long-term goal will need to be broken down into short-term goals, whether on a daily or weekly basis. Short-term and achievable goals allow an athlete to monitor and to experience success during recovery.
- Positive self-talk: An injured athlete often engages in negative and self-defeating talk, particularly when the injury has not been fully processed and accepted. Positive self-talk can

help athletes focus on healthy goals and stay motivated during a difficult recovery period. It allows athletes to control aspects of rehabilitation, particularly when so many factors seem out of their control.

- Imagery: During rehabilitation imagery can help mentally practice process goals, such as activities used for pain management, motor coordination, and timing. Additionally, research has shown that mental imagery can evoke physiological responses (i.e., increased heart rate, respiratory rate, and oxygen consumption) as if the movement or exercise was being performed [69, 70].
- Relaxation: Various relaxation techniques can help an athlete cope with the stressors associated with injury aiding in the acceptance of injury and rehabilitation. Systematic relaxation techniques can help with pain perception, breathing patterns, and muscle tension. This provides the athlete with greater awareness of his or her body and the ability to adapt to physical needs [71].

Integrating the Treatment Team

Each athlete and each injury is unique in what is needed to achieve an optimal rehabilitation and return to racing. Minor injuries may not require more than a brief adjustment in training coordinated by the athlete or in conjunction with a coach. Conversely, significant injuries that result in prolonged time away from training and competition are best managed by a team of experts in rehabilitation, exercise physiology, coaching, nutrition, psychology, and medicine related to endurance sports. Assembling the appropriate team to support an injured athlete requires experience to know when and who to involve. Local knowledge of the experts and services available in the athlete's area is invaluable. Detailed descriptions of the most common members of an endurance athlete's care team are listed below. Additional providers not listed but who are also often included in the care team include certified athletic trainers, massage therapists, acupuncturists, podiatrists, orthotists, and chiropractors.

Physical Therapy

Finding the right physical therapist for the right athlete can be a challenging. Not all physical therapists have the same training and experience, and many have specialties within specialties. Within large sports medicine centers and physical therapy clinics, there are often physical therapists that specialize in each of the major endurance sports. Given the frequency of physical therapy visits required for an injured athlete, often the location of the physical therapy practice influences the selection of the right physical therapist. Knowledge of the various physical therapist specialists and services within a community is necessary for being able to make an appropriate referral for an injured athlete. One indication that a physical therapist is specialized in an endurance sport is by having become a certified coach through various organizations, such as United States Track and Field Association, Road Runners Clubs of America, United States Triathlon Association, USA Cycling, Iron Man Coaching, United States Swimming, or US Rowing.

Exercise Physiology

Referral to a clinical exercise physiologist can facilitate a safe return to endurance training. Time lost from training as a result of the injury may have resulted in significant detraining leading to changes in maximal and submaximal heart rate, lactate threshold, and metabolic efficiency [46–48, 72]. If the athlete had been using individualized training zones, these zones will no longer be valid after an injury and detraining. An exercise physiologist can also review the athlete's goals and training plan to ensure that it is appropriate considering the time lost to injury and the athlete's abilities. The periodization of the training schedule will need to be adjusted as well as the intensity of training and the schedule of races will be affected. Alternative approaches for future training can be discussed when athletes have been injured potentially due in part to a faulty training program. A resource for finding a

local clinical exercise physiologist is American College of Sports Medicine (ACSM) Certified Pro Finder website.

Coaching Staff

Communication with the athlete's coaching staff can help guide the training adjustments during rehabilitation and ensure a safe return to training once rehabilitation has been completed. Specific recommendations regarding mode, frequency, and duration of exercise that are appropriate during the athlete's rehabilitation can provide the coach with guidelines for developing a program aimed at maintaining, or minimizing the loss of, fitness without exacerbating the injury. Similarly, specific recommendations regarding a timeline to return to a full training load after discharge from physical therapy can be extremely valuable in assisting the coach in developing the initial phase of training after injury. In addition, if the sports medicine team has concerns that the training program was inappropriate to the athlete's abilities and led to the injury, then these concerns should be shared with the coaching staff to ensure that adjustments are made going forward. The physician, physical therapist, and the exercise physiologist are all appropriate members of the healthcare team to create open lines of communication with the coaching staff.

The hand off from the sports medicine team back to a qualified coach or coaching staff is a critical step in ensuring the athlete's success in returning to their sport. In some cases, goals may need to be adjusted. If the physician feels that the athlete's immediate goal is too aggressive and will likely lead to reinjury, a discussion with the coach may be helpful. Having all members of the athlete's team on the same page will lead to a unified, cohesive plan consistent with the athlete's strengths and limitations.

In some cases, endurance athletes may not have a coach at all. Post collegiate endurance athletes may be self-coached, using a generic training plan, or part of a local club without organized coaching. In these cases, referral to a qualified coach is warranted particularly in the case when a poorly designed training plan has contributed to an overuse injury. The governing agencies of the sports have lists of local certified coaches.

Nutrition

Injury can provide an opportunity for the dietitian to work with an athlete to educate them on how to properly fuel in order to recover better, train harder, and ultimately reach higher levels of performance. Nutrition professionals can work with the athlete to identify areas for improvement, determine readiness to change, and create actionable plans that the athlete is ready and willing to work on. Regular follow-up with the athlete for at least a few months is ideal to track progress, problem solve challenges, and modify the nutrition action plan based on the athlete's feedback and experiences. Having an expert available for motivation, guidance, and accountability will ideally maximize the athlete's chances of achieving sustainable results.

Coaches and athletic training staff can further support an athlete in complying with a fueling plan due to their frequent contact and high level of influence on the athletes. In ideal circumstances, the treating dietitian can provide the coach with a copy of the athlete's nutrition plan and relay pertinent details through a brief conversation. The coach can help keep the athlete motivated and accountable. Unfortunately, the pursuit of performance can sometimes lead coaches or training staff to recommend nutritional changes that may lead to inadequate intake or nutrient deficiencies, and the coach's high level of influence can prevail over evidence-based advice.

Communication with the athlete's healthcare team is essential for providing the best care possible. Reasons for communication with other healthcare practitioners include obtaining additional information that may impact the dietitian's recommendations or providing nutrition, eating habit, or body composition feedback that can impact the athlete's course of care.

Sport Psychology

Sports psychologists have unique training in the developmental and social issues related to sports participation, organizational and systemic aspects of sports consulting, biobehavioral basis of sport and exercise, and have specific knowledge of training science and technical requirements of sport and competition. They have an understanding of issues related to specific sports and utilize sport-specific psychological assessment and mental skills training to enhance performance and an athlete's satisfaction. The inclusion of a sports psychologist to the treatment team can help an athlete understand the mental and emotional barriers to adjusting to a modified training protocol, which includes processing and accepting the injury itself. How an individual responds to an injury is unique and is based on preexisting coping and personality styles. A psychologist can help an athlete understand his/her personal reaction to injury and develop a personalized plan to successfully return to sport. As part of an integrated treatment team, communication is essential. A sports psychologist who is aware of the recommendations of other team members can help facilitate communication, education, and adherence to a rehabilitation program by personalizing information in ways best processed by the athlete.

Sports Medicine Physicians and Surgeons

An athlete often seeks the guidance of a sports medicine physician or surgeon at the onset of the injury or after having persistent symptoms after a period of conservative care. Diagnostic evaluation and initial treatment recommendations are provided, which involves determining which additional team members are needed to ideally support the athlete during the rehabilitation process. As previously discussed, communication with the other members of the treatment team is crucial for providing the best opportunity for the athlete to quickly and safely return to competition. Since the athlete has less contact with the physician or surgeon compared to a physical therapist or coach, communicating the care plan in detail to the other individuals involved in the athlete's recovery can improve compliance and as a result improve outcome. If the treating provider is a non-surgeon, involving an orthopedic surgeon is valuable not only when consideration of surgical intervention is indicated but also when a subspecialist evaluation is required for determining the etiology of the injury. Collaboration among sports medicine specialists of various disciplines and areas of expertise can produce a more accurate diagnostic evaluation and more effective treatment plan.

References

1. Neufer PD. The effect of detraining and reduced training on the physiological adaptations to aerobic exercise training. Sports Med. 1989;8(5):302–20.
2. Noehren B, Sanchez Z, Cunningham T, McKeon PO. The effect of pain on hip and knee kinematics during running in females with chronic patellofemoral pain. Gait Posture. 2012;36(3):596–9.
3. Souza RB, Powers CM. Differences in hip kinematics, muscle strength, and muscle activation between subjects with and without patellofemoral pain. J Orthop Sports Phys Ther. 2009;39(1):12–9.
4. Dierks TA, Manal KT, Hamill J, Davis I. Lower extremity kinematics in runners with patellofemoral pain during a prolonged run. Med Sci Sports Exerc. 2011;43(4):693–700.
5. Dierks TA, Manal KT, Hamill J, Davis IS. Proximal and distal influences on hip and knee kinematics in runners with patellofemoral pain during a prolonged run. J Orthop Sports Phys Ther. 2008;38(8):448–56.
6. Heiderscheit BC, Chumanov ES, Michalski MP, Wille CM, Ryan MB. Effects of step rate manipulation on joint mechanics during running. Med Sci Sports Exerc. 2011;43(2):296–302.
7. van Gent RN, Siem D, van Middelkoop M, van Os AG, Bierma-Zeinstra SM, Koes BW. Incidence and determinants of lower extremity running injuries in long distance runners: a systematic review. Br J Sports Med. 2007;41(8):469–80. discussion 80.
8. Hall JP, Barton C, Jones PR, Morrissey D. The biomechanical differences between barefoot and shod distance running: a systematic review and preliminary meta-analysis. Sports Med. 2013;43(12):1335–53.
9. Davis IS. The re-emergence of the minimal running shoe. J Orthop Sports Phys Ther. 2014;44(10): 775–84.
10. Milgrom C, Giladi M, Kashtan H, Simkin A, Chisin R, Margulies J, et al. A prospective study of the effect of a shock-absorbing orthotic device on the incidence of stress fractures in military recruits. Foot Ankle. 1985;6(2):101–4.
11. Silberman MR, Webner D, Collina S, Shiple BJ. Road bicycle fit. Clin J Sport Med. 2005;15(4):271–6.
12. Dahlquist M, Leisz MC, Finkelstein M. The club-level road cyclist: injury, pain, and performance. Clin J Sport Med. 2015;25(2):88–94.
13. Asplund C, St Pierre P. Knee pain and bicycling: fitting concepts for clinicians. Phys Sportsmed. 2004;32(4):23–30.
14. Evershed J, Burkett B, Mellifont R. Musculoskeletal screening to detect asymmetry in swimming. Phys Ther Sport. 2014;15(1):33–8.
15. Roy JS, Moffet H, McFadyen BJ. Upper limb motor strategies in persons with and without shoulder impingement syndrome across different speeds of movement. Clin Biomech (Bristol, Avon). 2008; 23(10):1227–36.
16. Richardson AB, Jobe FW, Collins HR. The shoulder in competitive swimming. Am J Sports Med. 1980; 8(3):159–63.
17. Scovazzo ML, Browne A, Pink M, Jobe FW, Kerrigan J. The painful shoulder during freestyle swimming. An electromyographic cinematographic analysis of twelve muscles. Am J Sports Med. 1991;19(6): 577–82.
18. Stocker D, Pink M, Jobe FW. Comparison of shoulder injury in collegiate- and master's-level swimmers. Clin J Sport Med. 1995;5(1):4–8.
19. Yanai T, Hay JG, Miller GF. Shoulder impingement in front-crawl swimming: I. A method to identify impingement. Med Sci Sports Exerc. 2000; 32(1):21–9.
20. Virag B, Hibberd EE, Oyama S, Padua DA, Myers JB. Prevalence of freestyle biomechanical errors in elite competitive swimmers. Sports Health. 2014;6(3):218–24.
21. Morris FL, Smith RM, Payne WR, Galloway MA, Wark JD. Compressive and shear force generated in the lumbar spine of female rowers. Int J Sports Med. 2000;21(7):518–23.
22. Smoljanovic T, Bojanic I, Hannafin JA, Hren D, Delimar D, Pecina M. Traumatic and overuse injuries among international elite junior rowers. Am J Sports Med. 2009;37(6):1193–9.
23. Hosea TM, Hannafin JA. Rowing injuries. Sports Health. 2012;4(3):236–45.
24. Wilson F, Gissane C, Gormley J, Simms C. A 12-month prospective cohort study of injury in international rowers. Br J Sports Med. 2010;44(3): 207–14.

25. Wilson F, Gissane C, McGregor A. Ergometer training volume and previous injury predict back pain in rowing; strategies for injury prevention and rehabilitation. Br J Sports Med. 2014;48(21):1534–7.

26. Jacobs SJ, Berson BL. Injuries to runners: a study of entrants to a 10,000 meter race. Am J Sports Med. 1986;14(2):151–5.

27. Korpelainen R, Orava S, Karpakka J, Siira P, Hulkko A. Risk factors for recurrent stress fractures in athletes. Am J Sports Med. 2001;29(3):304–10.

28. Egermann M, Brocai D, Lill CA, Schmitt H. Analysis of injuries in long-distance triathletes. Int J Sports Med. 2003;24(4):271–6.

29. Nielsen RO, Buist I, Sorensen H, Lind M, Rasmussen S. Training errors and running related injuries: a systematic review. Int J Sports Phys Ther. 2012;7(1):58–75.

30. Ristolainen L, Kettunen JA, Waller B, Heinonen A, Kujala UM. Training-related risk factors in the etiology of overuse injuries in endurance sports. J Sports Med Phys Fitness. 2014;54(1):78–87.

31. Wilmore J, Costill DL. Physiology of Sport and Exercise. 3rd ed. Champaign, IL: Human Kinetics; 2004.

32. Zaryski C, Smith DJ. Training principles and issues for ultra-endurance athletes. Curr Sports Med Rep. 2005;4(3):165–70.

33. McGregor SJ. Periodization. In: Freil J, Vance J, editor. Champaign, Triathlon Science, IL: Human Kinetics; 2013. p. 311–25.

34. Fleck SJ. Body composition of elite American athletes. Am J Sports Med. 1983;11(6):398–403.

35. Legaz Arrese A, Gonzalez Badillo JJ, Serrano OE. Differences in skinfold thicknesses and fat distribution among top-class runners. J Sports Med Phys Fitness. 2005;45(4):512–7.

36. Halson SL, Jeukendrup AE. Does overtraining exist? An analysis of overreaching and overtraining research. Sports Med. 2004;34(14):967–81.

37. Ivkovic A, Franic M, Bojanic I, Pecina M. Overuse injuries in female athletes. Croat Med J. 2007;48(6):767–78.

38. Cosca DD, Navazio F. Common problems in endurance athletes. Am Fam Physician. 2007;76(2):237–44.

39. Hinton PS. Iron and the endurance athlete. Appl Physiol Nutr Metab. 2014;39(9):1012–8.

40. Loucks AB, Kiens B, Wright HH. Energy availability in athletes. J Sports Sci. 2011;29 Suppl 1:S7–15.

41. Loucks AB. Low energy availability in the marathon and other endurance sports. Sports Med. 2007;37(4-5):348–52.

42. De Souza MJ, Nattiv A, Joy E, Misra M, Williams NI, Mallinson RJ, et al. 2014 Female Athlete Triad Coalition Consensus Statement on Treatment and Return to Play of the Female Athlete Triad: 1st International Conference held in San Francisco, California, May 2012 and 2nd International Conference held in Indianapolis, Indiana, May 2013. Br J Sports Med. 2014;48(4):289.

43. American Dietetic A. Dietitians of C, American College of Sports M, Rodriguez NR, Di Marco NM, Langley S. American College of Sports Medicine position stand. Nutrition and athletic performance. Med Sci Sports Exerc. 2009;41(3):709–31.

44. Reilly T, Waterhouse J, Edwards B. Jet lag and air travel: implications for performance. Clin Sports Med. 2005;24(2):367–80. xii.

45. Pink MM, Tibone JE. The painful shoulder in the swimming athlete. Orthop Clin North Am. 2000;31(2):247–61.

46. Mujika I, Padilla S. Detraining: loss of training-induced physiological and performance adaptations. Part I: Short term insufficient training stimulus. Sports Med. 2000;30(2):79–87.

47. Mujika I, Padilla S. Detraining: loss of training-induced physiological and performance adaptations. Part II: Long term insufficient training stimulus. Sports Med. 2000;30(3):145–54.

48. Marles A, Legrand R, Blondel N, Mucci P, Betbeder D, Prieur F. Effect of high-intensity interval training and detraining on extra VO2 and on the VO2 slow component. Eur J Appl Physiol. 2007;99(6):633–40.

49. Hickson RC, Kanakis Jr C, Davis JR, Moore AM, Rich S. Reduced training duration effects on aerobic power, endurance, and cardiac growth. J Appl Physiol Respir Environ Exerc Physiol. 1982;53(1):225–9.

50. Hickson RC, Foster C, Pollock ML, Galassi TM, Rich S. Reduced training intensities and loss of aerobic power, endurance, and cardiac growth. J Appl Physiol. 1985;58(2):492–9.

51. Neary JP, Bhambhani YN, McKenzie DC. Effects of different stepwise reduction taper protocols on cycling performance. Can J Appl Physiol. 2003;28(4):576–87.

52. Houmard JA, Kirwan JP, Flynn MG, Mitchell JB. Effects of reduced training on submaximal and maximal running responses. Int J Sports Med. 1989;10(1):30–3.

53. Houmard JA, Scott BK, Justice CL, Chenier TC. The effects of taper on performance in distance runners. Med Sci Sports Exerc. 1994;26(5):624–31.

54. Loy SF, Hoffmann JJ, Holland GJ. Benefits and practical use of cross-training in sports. Sports Med. 1995;19(1):1–8.

55. Tipton KD. Nutrition for acute exercise-induced injuries. Ann Nutr Metab. 2010;57 Suppl 2:43–53.

56. Biolo G, Agostini F, Simunic B, Sturma M, Torelli L, Preiser JC, et al. Positive energy balance is associated with accelerated muscle atrophy and increased erythrocyte glutathione turnover during 5 wk of bed rest. Am J Clin Nutr. 2008;88(4):950–8.

57. Frankenfield D. Energy expenditure and protein requirements after traumatic injury. Nutr Clin Pract. 2006;21(5):430–7.

58. Waters RL, Campbell J, Perry J. Energy cost of three-point crutch ambulation in fracture patients. J Orthop Trauma. 1987;1(2):170–3.

59. Chow O, Barbul A. Immunonutrition: role in wound healing and tissue regeneration. Adv Wound Care (New Rochelle). 2014;3(1):46–53.

60. Borrelli Jr J, Pape C, Hak D, Hsu J, Lin S, Giannoudis P, et al. Physiological challenges of bone repair. J Orthop Trauma. 2012;26(12):708–11.
61. Vargas R, Lang CH. Alcohol accelerates loss of muscle and impairs recovery of muscle mass resulting from disuse atrophy. Alcohol Clin Exp Res. 2008;32(1):128–37.
62. Molfino A, Gioia G, Rossi Fanelli F, Muscaritoli M. Beta-hydroxy-beta-methylbutyrate supplementation in health and disease: a systematic review of randomized trials. Amino Acids. 2013;45(6):1273–92.
63. Sharma RA, Gescher AJ, Steward WP. Curcumin: the story so far. Eur J Cancer. 2005;41(13):1955–68.
64. Baptista IL, Leal ML, Artioli GG, Aoki MS, Fiamoncini J, Turri AO, et al. Leucine attenuates skeletal muscle wasting via inhibition of ubiquitin ligases. Muscle Nerve. 2010;41(6):800–8.
65. Hespel P, Op't Eijnde B, Van Leemputte M, Urso B, Greenhaff PL, Labarque V, et al. Oral creatine supplementation facilitates the rehabilitation of disuse atrophy and alters the expression of muscle myogenic factors in humans. J Physiol. 2001;536(Pt 2):625–33.

66. Winsberg M. The psychology of the injured athlete: endurance corner. 2015. http://www.endurancecorner.com/Mimi_Winsberg/psychology_injuries.
67. Kübler-Ross EB. On death and dying. New York: Scrobmer; 2014.
68. McCormick A, Meijen C, Marcora S. Psychological determinants of whole-body endurance performance. Sports Med. 2015;45(7):997–1015.
69. Wang Y, Morgan WP. The effect of imagery perspectives on the psychophysiological responses to imagined exercise. Behav Brain Res. 1992;52(2):167–74.
70. Papadelis C, Kourtidou-Papadeli C, Bamidis P, Albani M. Effects of imagery training on cognitive performance and use of physiological measures as an assessment tool of mental effort. Brain Cogn. 2007;64(1):74–85.
71. Taylor J. A conceptual model for integrating athletes' needs and sport demands in the development of competitive mental preparation strategies. Sport Psychol. 1995;9(3):339–57.
72. Mujika I, Padilla S. Cardiorespiratory and metabolic characteristics of detraining in humans. Med Sci Sports Exerc. 2001;33(3):413–21.

Index

Printed in the United States
By Bookmasters